江苏大学英文教材基金资助出版

U0890756

CLINICAL NEUROLOGY

临床神经病学

名誉主编　徐　运
主　　审　刘春风　王小姗
主　　编　于　明　李敬伟　蒋　萍
副 主 编　夏海平　杨　溢　徐宇浩
编　　委　卜　浪　蔡志荣　陈思远　陈晓鹏
韩　薇　何　悦　蒋　萍　李敬伟
刘春风　马　瑞　佟学志　王小姗
武文琦　夏海平　徐建慧　徐宇浩
徐　运　杨　溢　于　明　张　雷
张婷婷　郑秋月　朱文利　朱　颖
邹　容
参编单位　江苏大学
南京大学
南京医科大学
首都医科大学
苏州大学

江苏大学出版社
JIANGSU UNIVERSITY PRESS
镇　江

图书在版编目(CIP)数据

临床神经病学 = Clinical Neurology：英文／于明，李敬伟，蒋萍主编. -- 镇江：江苏大学出版社，2021.12
ISBN 978-7-5684-1776-1

Ⅰ.①临… Ⅱ.①于… ②李… ③蒋… Ⅲ.①神经病学－英文 Ⅳ.①R741

中国版本图书馆 CIP 数据核字(2022)第 003028 号

临床神经病学
Clinical Neurology

主　　编/于　明　李敬伟　蒋　萍
责任编辑/仲　蕙
出版发行/江苏大学出版社
地　　址/江苏省镇江市梦溪园巷 30 号(邮编：212003)
电　　话/0511-84446464(传真)
网　　址/http://press.ujs.edu.cn
排　　版/镇江文苑制版印刷有限责任公司
印　　刷/江苏凤凰数码印务有限公司
开　　本/787 mm×1 092 mm　1/16
印　　张/20
字　　数/716 千字
版　　次/2021 年 12 月第 1 版
印　　次/2021 年 12 月第 1 次印刷
书　　号/ISBN 978-7-5684-1776-1
定　　价/68.00 元

如有印装质量问题请与本社营销部联系(电话：0511-84440882)

Foreword

As the Ministry of Education reported, the number of international medical students in China ranks first among majors of academic education. When medical students and residents are asked about their expectations for text book, their responses are in agreed: they want to learn how to conduct effective neurologic examinations and how to evaluate and manage common neurologic conditions. However, there are very few neurological textbooks in English for MBBS (Bachelor of Medicine and Bachelor of Surgery) in China, and their contents are too outdated to reflect the scientific developments. It is imperative and highly beneficial to tailor an English text book of neurology for an undergraduate program designed for those students. After practicing neurology for more than 30 years in an academic setting, I prefer my colleagues to share their valuable erudition with medical students here.

Clinical Neurology is a general teaching material for clinical majors written in a suitable format for MBBS students in China. It covers a broad spectrum of clinical and basic neuroscience. As is well known, modern imaging techniques, the new molecular biological development, as well as recent innovations in the treatment of disorders, have brought about substantial progress in our knowledge in the field of neuroscience. This textbook consists of 3 sections, comprising of 18 chapters, introducing the basic knowledge of nervous system and the common clinical diseases first and covering the recent advances in neurointervention, treatment of neurologic complications of general medical disorders. In clinical theories, we tried to systematize the theoretical knowledge and emphasize training in medical thinking by some practical cases. We have accumulated a lot of practical resource matching with contents, enabling students to understand the details of neurological diseases better. Updated concept is another feature that has been introduced in this book, such as important updates on seizure and NMOSD (neuromyelitis optica spectrum disorder). Virtually each chapter is coauthored by at least one expert with dual backgrounds in academic medicine and practice in the respective area.

This book represents efforts by a talented group of authors. I am grateful that we have received full support from experts in Jiangsu University, Nanjing Medical University and other institutions in close cooperation. Our goal is to facilitate clinical practice ability of neurology trainees. Last, we look forward to receiving comments in any form that readers choose.

Xu Yun
May, 2022

Contents

SECTION I Neurological Foundation

SECTION II Common Clinical Diseases

SECTION III Disciplines Linked to Neurology

Appendixes

SECTION I

Neurological Foundation

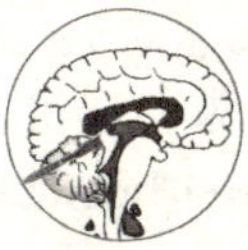

Chapter 1
Introduction of Neurology

Neurology, a part of neuroscience, is based on neuroanatomy, neurophysiology, neurobiochemistry, neuroimmunology, neuropharmacology, neurogenetics, neuropathology, neuroepidemiology, neuropsychology, neurobiology and experimental neurology, etc. Meanwhile, neurology is a branch of clinical medicine, which is closely linked to many other clinical disciplines, and it is also a highly logical and theoretical clinical discipline. This chapter will briefly introduce the concept, history and basic knowledge of neurology.

1.1 Concept and Category

Neurology is a clinical discipline, which studies the etiology, pathogenesis, clinical manifestations, diagnosis and differential diagnosis, prevention, treatment and rehabilitation of neurological and muscle diseases. According to anatomic structures, the nervous system is divided into two parts: the central nervous system (brain and spinal cord) and the peripheral nervous system (cranial and spinal nerves). The former is responsible for analyzing and reacting to information from internal and external environment, while the latter is responsible for conducting nerve impulses. According to function, it is divided into somatic nervous system and autonomic nervous system, the former is responsible for adjusting the body to adapt the external environment, while the latter is responsible for stabilizing the internal environment. Muscles contain striated muscle, smooth muscle, and myocardium. Striated muscle is also called voluntary muscle or skeletal muscle. The muscle diseases in this textbook mainly refer to skeletal muscle diseases.

Neurology is a clinical branch of neuroscience, which permeates and promotes other branches of neuroscience. Advances in neuro-anatomy, neuro-pathology, neuro-biochemistry, neuro-imaging, neuro-genetics and neuro-molecular biology have brought about rapid development of neurology, making neurology become a hot topic in the field of medical science.

1.2 Brief History

The development of modern neurology began in the 16th century. Vesalius (1514—1564) detailed the anatomy of the brain and other parts. Thomas Willis (1621—1675) published the *Anatomy of the Brain* in 1664 and the *Pathology of the Brain* in 1676. Willis Circle was named after Thomas Willis for description of it, which lasted for now. His vague ideas about reflexes and localization are the first foundation to understand the function of the brain, besides he also described neurological signs such as epilepsy, stroke and hemiplegia. The term "neurology" was first used in his literature.

The application of microscopy led to further advances in the study of neurology in the 19th century. Purkinje (1787—1869) firstly described the morphology of neurons in 1837, after that, Golgi and Cajal discovered branches and synapses of nerve cells. Luigi Galvani (1737—1798) found that electrical stimulation of nerves caused muscle contractions. Charles Bell (1774—1842) and Francois Magendie (1783—1855) found that the anterior horn of the spinal cord was associated with movement and the posterior horn was associated with sensation. Hereafter, the functional orientation of the nervous system has been fully understood with the efforts of many neurologists. With the development of physiology, pathology, microbiology and immunology and the progress of experimental technology, the diagnosis and treatment level have been improved, and neurology has been improved to a new phase of development.

The 20th century was a period of rapid development in neurology. Neurology has achieved great progress based on previous achievements in neuroanatomy, neurophysiology and neuropathology. Computed tomography (CT) and successive magnetic resonance imaging (MRI) have greatly improved the diagnostic level of neurological diseases, accelerated the development of clinical neurology, and benefited countless patients with neurological diseases. In addition, the human genome project started in 1990 completed the complete sequencing of human genes, revealing the mystery of genes, which will provide new methods and ideas for the genetic diagnosis and treatment of hundreds of various neurogenetic diseases and degenerative diseases.

The 21st century is a century of vigorous development in neurology. After the US Congress approved the American Academy of Neurology to propose the "Decade of the Brain" (1991—2000), the US government proposed that the 21st century is the "Century of the Brain", and neuroscience research has become the most active research field. Progresses in neuropathology, neuroimmunity, neuroviruses, genes and proteomics enable people to understand the etiology and pathology of neurological diseases at multiple levels. The development of neuroimaging and interventional technology provide new methods of diagnosis and treatment for many diseases. Researches at gene and protein molecular level promote development of neuropharmacology and make great progress in drug research and development. Stem cell technology offer new hope for treatment of neurological diseases. The researches on neural network and functional reconstruction help stroke patients get better neurological rehabilitation.

1.3 Composition of Nervous System

The central nervous system (CNS) comprises the brain and spinal cord. The brain is divided into cerebrum, diencephalon, brainstem, cerebellum and other parts. The spinal cord is composed of gray matter containing nerve cells and white matter containing upper and lower conduction tracts.

1.3.1 Cerebral Hemisphere

The surface of the cerebral hemispheres is covered by the cerebral cortex, forming sulcus and gyri on the surface, the inside contains white matter, basal ganglia and lateral ventricles.

The sides of cerebral hemispheres are connected by the corpus callosum. Each side of cerebral hemisphere is divided into frontal lobe, parietal lobe, temporal lobe and occipital lobe by the central sulcus, the lateral fissure and its extension, the connection between the parietal occipital sulcus and the anterior occipital notch. In addition, the brain also includes the insula located in the deep part of the lateral fissure of the brain and the limbic system, which is composed of limbic lobes, amygdala, anterior thalamus and hypothalamus and located in the medial sides of hemisphere. The function of the two cerebral hemispheres is not completely symmetrical, which is divided into the dominant hemisphere and the non-dominant hemisphere according to the function. The dominant hemisphere is dominant in language, logical thinking, analytical synthesis, and computational functions, most of which are located on the left side. Only few right-handed people and about half of left-handed people may be on the right side. The non-dominant hemisphere is mostly the right one, which is dominant in music, art, general ability, spatial, geometric and facial recognition and visual memory functions. Damages on different parts lead to different clinical symptoms.

1.3.2 Interal Capsule

Interal capsule is a broad layer of white matter composed of longitudinal fiber bundles that radiate upwards to the cortex, which locates in the caudate nucleus, the pellucid nucleus, and the thalamus. On the horizontal section, the internal capsule forms an obtuse angle with the tip turning inward and is divided into the forelimb, hind limb and knee. The fore limb of the inner capsule is located between the caudate nucleus and the pellucid nucleus. The ascending fibers are the fibers from the medial thalamic nucleus to the frontal cortex, and the descending fibers are the pons of the frontal lobe. The knee of the inner capsule is located in the anterior and posterior limbs, where the cortical medulla bundle passes through. The posterior limb of the internal capsule is located between the thalamus and the pellucid nucleus, and is divided into corticospinal tract, thalamocortical tract from the thalamus to the posterior central gyrus, followed by auditory radiation, temporal pontine tract, posterior thalamic radiation, visual radiation. (Fig. 1.1)

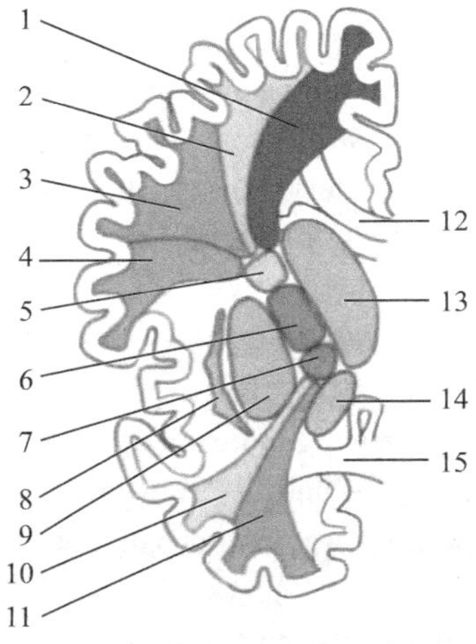

1—Optic radiation;
2—Posterior thalamic radiation;
3—Temporopontine tract;
4—Auditory radiation;
5—Central thalamic radiation;
6—Corticospinal tract;
7—Corticobulbar tract;
8—Claustrum;
9—Lenticula;
10—Anterior thalamic radiation;
11—Frontopontine tract;
12—Splenium of the corpus callosum;
13—Thalamus;
14—Head of caudate nucleus;
15—Genu of the corpus callosum.

Fig. 1.1 Fiber bundles through interal capsule

1.3.3 Basal Ganglia

Basal ganglia, also called basal nucleus, is located in the deep parts of cerebral white matter, and consists of caudate nucleus, lenticular nucleus, claustrum and amygdala. The red nucleus, substantia nigra, and subtha-lamic nucleus are also involved in the basal ganglia system. Caudate nucleus and piliform nucleus are together called striatum, and piliform nucleus is divided into putamen and globus pallidus. The species lines of caudate nucleus and putamen occur later, which is called neostriatum. Globus pallidus appears earlier, known as the old striatum. The amygdala is the oldest part of the basal ganglia, known as the palaeostriatum. The basal ganglia is the relay station of the extrapyramidal system, and there are close fibrous connections between the nucleus, which upload information to the cerebral cortex through the thalamus and transmit the impulse to the globus pallidus through the thalamus, and then affect the motor neurons under the spinal cord through the red nucleus, substantia nigra and reticular structure. The basal ganglia, in coordination with the cerebral cortex and cerebellum, regulates voluntary movements, muscle tone and postural reflexes, and also participates in the regulation of complex behaviors. (Fig. 1.2)

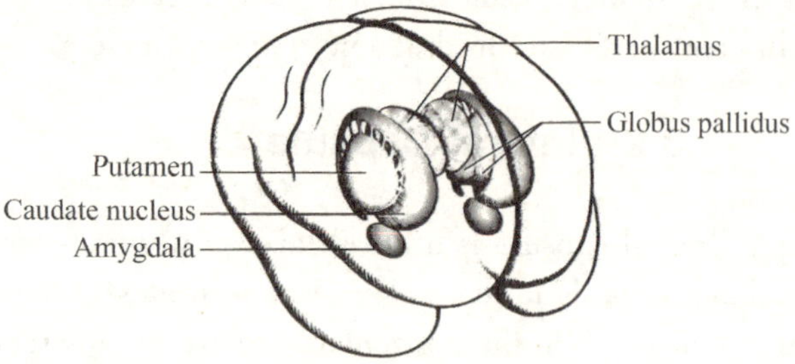

Fig. 1.2 Basal ganglia

1.3.4 Diencephalon

Diencephalon located between the two hemispheres of the brain, is a relay station between the brainstem and the hemispheres of the brain, containing four parts: thalamus, hypothalamus, epithalamus and subthalamus.

Thalamus, the largest ovoid mass of gray matter in the diencephalon, is symmetrically distributed on both sides of the third ventricle. The thalamus is separated by a thin layer of Y-shaped white matter fibers (internal medullary plate) into several nuclear groups, mainly the anterior, medial and lateral nuclear groups. The thalamus is a subcortical center and relay station for the conduction of various senses (except olfactory sense). It plays a significant role in the activity of the motor system, sensory system, limbic system, ascending reticular system and cerebral cortex.

Hypothalamus is located under the subthalamic sulci, composed of gray matter around the third ventricle. It has close connection with the brainstem, basal ganglia, thalamus, limbic system and cerebral cortex. Hypothalamus is subcortical center that regulates visceral and endocrine activities. Certain cells in the hypothalamus are both neurons and endocrine cells. The hypothalamus regulates body temperature, food intake, water and salt balance and endocrine activities, and involves in emotional activities.

Epithalamus is located in the interior of thalamus and around the top of the third ventricle. The main structures contain a. pineal gland: locates between two epithalamuses and its base is attached to the habenular commissure; b. habenular commissure: locates between two epithalamuses, in front of the pineal gland and is composed of transverse fibrous bundles; c. posterior conjunctions: locates below the pineal gland and also is composed of transverse fiber bundles.

Subthalamus is located in the external of internal capsules and in anterior medial area of the hypothalamus. It is the transitional area between the tegmental area of midbrain tegmentum and the dorsal thalamus. The upper end of the red nucleus and substantia nigra also extend into this area. The main structure is the subthalamic nucleus, which is a part of the extrapyramidal system that receives fibers from the globus pallidus and the premotor region of the frontal lobe, emits fibers to the globus pallidus, substantia nigra, the red nucleus and the midbrain tegmentum.

1.3.5 Brain Stem

Brain stem is connected to diencephalon forwardly and the spinal cord downwardly, including the midbrain, pons and medulla oblongata. The main internal structures are neural nucleus, upstream and downstream conduction bundles and reticular structures. Except the cerebral nucleus, there are also relay nucleus (thin-fasciculus nucleus and wedge-fasciculus nucleus), red nuclei and substantia nigra, which are related to the extrapyramidal system. Brainstem conduction tracts are white matter in brain stem, including light and depth sensory conduction tracts, pyramidal tracts, extrapyramidal pathways, medial longitudinal tracts and so on. (Fig. 1.3)

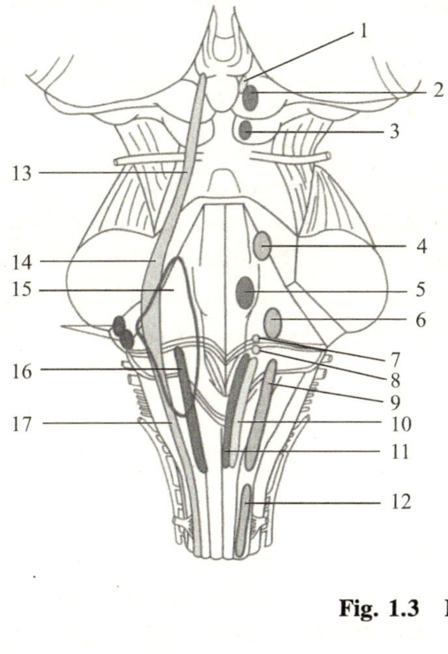

1—(Ⅲ) Accessory oculomotor nucleus;
2—(Ⅲ) Oculomotor nucleus;
3—(Ⅳ) Trochlear nucleus;
4—(Ⅴ) Trigeminal motor nucleus;
5—(Ⅵ) Abducent nucleus;
6—(Ⅶ) Facial nucleus;
7—(Ⅶ) Superior aslivatory nucleus;
8—(Ⅸ) Inferior salivatory nucleus;
9—(Ⅸ, Ⅹ, Ⅺ) Ambiguous nucleus;
10—(Ⅹ) Vagal dorsal motor nucleus;
11—(Ⅻ) Hypoglossal nucleus;
12—(Ⅺ) Accessory nucleus;
13—(Ⅴ) Mesencephalic nucleus of trigeminal nerve;
14—(Ⅴ) Pontine nucleus of trigeminal nerve;
15—(Ⅷ) Nucleus vestibularis;
16—(Ⅶ, Ⅸ, Ⅹ) Solitary nucleus;
17—(Ⅴ) Trigeminal spinal nucleus.

Fig. 1.3 Brainstem nuclei

1.3.6 Cerebellum

Cerebellum locates in the posterior fossa, which is below the tentorium and on the back of the pons and medulla oblongata. Cerebellum is connected with the medulla oblongata, pons and midbrain by the lower foot of cerebellum (rope body), middle foot (pontine arm) and upper foot (combined arm) respectively. It does not send out motor impulses, but connects with spinal cord, vestibule, brain stem, basal nucleus and cerebral cortex through afferent fibers, so as to regulate motor neurons. The cerebellum maintains body balance, controls posture and gait, regulates muscle tension and coordinates the accuracy of voluntary movements. The efferent fibers of cerebellum cross twice in the conduction pathway, playing the role of ipsilateral coordination of body activities, and have representative regions of various body parts. For example, cerebellum hemisphere is the representative region of limbs, its upper part represents the upper limb, the lower part represents the lower limb and the vermis represents the trunk. There are two main symptoms after cerebellar injury: ataxia and imbalance disorder.

1.3.7 Extrapyramidal System

Extrapyramidal system in a broad sense refers to the nervous system structure of all body movements in the pyramidal system, including striatum system and vestibulocochlear system. At present, the anatomy and physiology of extrapyramidal system is not completely clear, and its structure is complex and its fiber connections are extensive, involving many structures in the brain, including cerebral cortex, striatum, thalamus, subthalamic nucleus, midbrain parietal gland, corpora rubrum, substantia nigra, pontine, vestibular nucleus, cerebellum, some reticular nuclei of brain stem and their connecting fibers, etc. These structures together constitute many complex neural circuits: a. cortex-neostriatum-pallium-thalamus-cortex circuits; b. cortex-pontine-cerebellum-cortex loop; c. cortex-pontine-cerebellum-thalamus-cortex loop; d. new striatum-substantia nigra-new striatum loop; e. cerebellar dentate nucleus-thalamus-cortex-pontine-cerebellar dentate nucleus loop. The main functions of extrapyramidal system are: regulating muscle tension and coordinating muscle movement; maintaining and adjusting posture; responsible for semi-automatic rigid movements and reflective movements, such as walking with two arms swinging, expression movements, defensive reactions and eating movements. There are mainly two kinds of symptoms for extrapyramidal system injury: muscle tension change and involuntary movement. Globus pallidus and substantia nigra lesions are mostly hypokinesia and high muscle tension syndrome, such as Parkinson's disease. The lesions of caudate nucleus and psoas nucleus are mostly manifested as increased exercise and decreased muscle tone syndrome, such as chorea. Unilateral throwing may occur in subthalamic nucleus lesions.

1.3.8 Spinal Cord

The spinal cord consists of gray matter containing nerve cells and white matter containing upper and lower conduction tracts. Normal spinal cord activity is performed under the control of brain. The function of the spinal cord is mainly revealed in two aspects: one is the relay station of the upward and downward conduction pathways, and the other is the reflex center. Sensory conduction bundles in spinal cord mainly include spinal thalamus bundles (lateral spinal thalamus bundles and anterior spinal thalamus bundles), thin bundles and wedge bundles, spinal cerebellum bundles, etc. The arrangement of sensory conduction bundles in medulla is different. The lateral bundles of spinal thalamus are lined with fibers from neck, chest, waist and gingiva from inside to outside. Thin bundle and wedge bundle are located in the posterior cord, inside the thin bundle and outside the wedge bundle, and are arranged by fibers from the mandible, waist, chest and neck from inside to outside. This hierarchical arrangement of intramedullary sensory conduction bundles is of great value for the diagnosis of intramedullary and extramedullary lesions of spinal cord. For example, intramedullary tumors in the cervical segment, superficial sensory disturbance develops from top to bottom in the order of neck, chest, waist and sacrum. However, in the case of cervical extramedullary tumor, the development order of sensory disturbance is opposite. (Fig. 1.4)

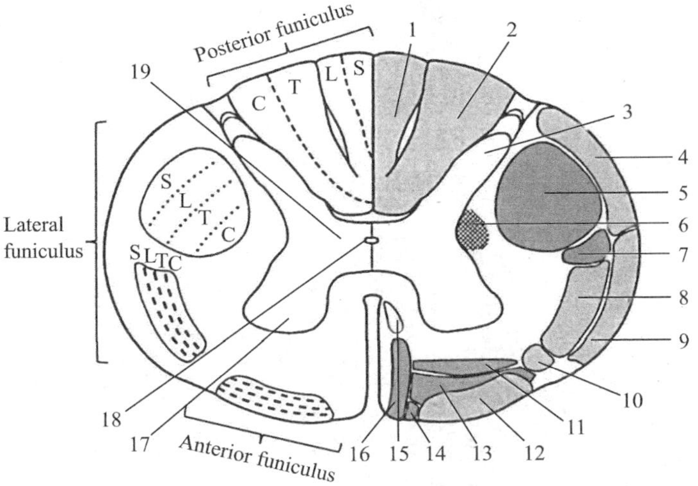

1—Fasciculus gracilis;
2—Fasciculus cuneatus;
3—Posterior horn;
4—Posterior spinocerebellar tract;
5—Corticospinal tract;
6—Reticular formation;
7—Rubrospinaol tract;
8—Lateral spinothalamic tract;
9—Anterior spinocecebellar tract;
10—Spinotectal tract;
11—Reticulospinal tract;
12—Anterior spinothalamic tract;
13—Vestibulospinal tract;
14—Tectospinal tract;
15—Medial longitudinal fasciculus;
16—Anterior corticospinal tract;
17—Anterior horn;
18—Central canal;
19—Gary commissure;
C—Cervical segments;
T—Thoracic segments;
L—Lumbar segments;
S—Sacral segments.

Fig. 1.4 Anatomy of the spinal (cross-section)

The spinal cord sends 31 pairs of spinal nerves to the extremities and trunk. The upper limit of the spinal injury should be 1 ~ 2 segments higher than the sensory disturbance plane of physical examination. This segmental sensation distribution is most obvious in the thoracic segment, such as T4 in the nipple plane, T10 in the umbilical plane, T12 and L1 in the groin. The segmental sensory distribution of upper limbs and lower limbs is complex, but there are still some rules of segmental dominance, such as C5 ~ C7 on the radial side of upper limbs, C8 and T1 on the ulnar side of forearm and hand, T2 on the inner side of upper arms, L1 ~ L3 in front of thigh, L4 ~ L5 in front of calf, S1 ~ S2 in the back of calf and thigh, S4 ~ S5 in the saddle area around anus. This segmental sensory innervation of spinal cord is of great significance for clinical diagnosis. (Fig. 1.5)

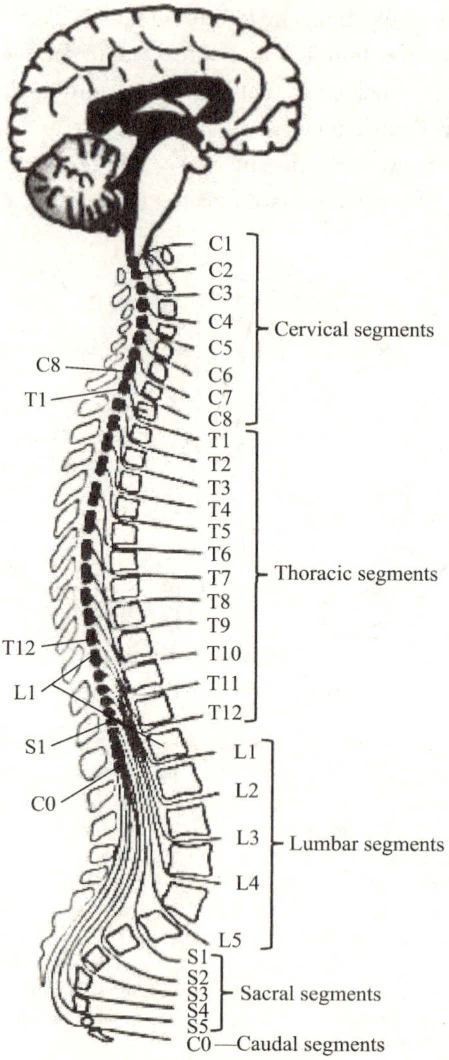

Fig. 1.5 Spinal cord and vertebral body

In addition, the unique feature of the spinal cord or spinal reflex is divided into body reflection and internal reflection, the former refers to skeletal muscle reflex activity, such as stretch reflexes, buckling reflection and light reflection; the latter refers to some body-internal reflection, reflection of viscera internal reflection and internal organs-body, such as pilomotor reflex, bladder reflex and rectum defecation reflex.

1.3.9 Peripheral Nerve

Peripheral nerves indicate all the nerve structures outside of the spinal cord and pia matter of brain stem, namely, all cranial nerves and spinal nerves except the olfactory and optic nerves. Most peripheral nerves are mixed nerve, containing sense fiber, movement fiber, sympathetic fiber, parasympathetic fiber, and also packaged with connective tissue membrane, blood vessel, lymphatic and so on. Cranial, spinal and visceral nerves all contain sensory and motor components respectively. The sensory afferent nerves are composed of the posterior root of the spinal nerves, the posterior root ganglion and the ganglion of the cerebral nerves, and transmit the impulses from the skin, joints, tendons and visceral nerves to the central nervous system through sensory receptor; motor efferent nerves are composed of the anterior roots of spinal nerves deriving from the anterior and lateral horns of the spinal cord and the cranial nerves deriving from the motor nuclei of the brain stem, and transmit nerve impulses from the central nervous system to the surrounding effectors. The efferent part of visceral nerves is also known as autonomic nerve, because it specially innervates the movement of smooth muscle, heart muscle, and glands that are not directly controlled by the human mind. Autonomic nerve is divided into sympathetic nerve and parasympathetic nerve according to their morphologies and functions.

(1) Cranial nerves

Cranial nerves contain 12 pairs of peripheral nerves connected to the brain. The order of their arrangement is determined by the order of their parts in and out of the brain. The Ⅰ and Ⅱ pairs of cranial nerves belong to the components of the brain and diencephalon. The Ⅱ and Ⅲ pairs of cranial nerves are the fiber bundles of their neurons in the brain. The brain stem has the nerve nucleus corresponding to each brain nerve, the general motor nucleus is close to the midline, the sensory nucleus is in its lateral. The nucleus Ⅲ and Ⅳ are located in the midbrain, the nucleus Ⅴ, Ⅵ, Ⅶ and Ⅷ are located in the pons, and the nucleus Ⅸ, Ⅹ, Ⅺ and Ⅻ are located in the medulla oblongata. Only a portion of the accessory nerve arises from the anterior horn of the upper 4 segments of the cervical spinal cord. According to function, cranial nerves can be divided into a. motor nerves (Ⅲ, Ⅳ, Ⅵ, Ⅺ and Ⅻ pairs); b. sensory nerves (Ⅰ, Ⅱ and Ⅷ pairs); c. mixed nerves (Ⅴ, Ⅶ, Ⅸ and Ⅹ pairs) (Tab. 1.1). Certain cranial nerves (Ⅲ, Ⅶ, Ⅸ and Ⅹ pairs) also contain parasympathetic nerve fibers. Except for the lower part of the facial nucleus and the sublingual nucleus which are only innervated by the contralateral cortical brainstem tract, other motor nucleus of cerebral nerves are innervated bilaterally.

Tab. 1.1 Physiological functions of cranial nerves

No.	Cranial nerves	Nature	Function
Ⅰ	Olfactory	Sensory	Conduct smell
Ⅱ	Optic	Sensory	Conduct vision
Ⅲ	Oculomotor	Motor	Manage palpebrae superioris, superior rectus, inferior rectus, internal rectus, inferior oblique, pupil sphincter and ciliary muscle
Ⅳ	Trochlear	Motor	Manage oblique
Ⅴ	Trigeminal	Mixed	Conduct facial, nasal and oral mucosa sensation and manage masticatory muscles
Ⅵ	Abducent	Motor	Manage external rectus muscle
Ⅶ	Facial	Mixed	Manage facial expression muscles, lacrist glands and salivary glands, and transmits the anterior 2/3 taste and external auditory canal sensation
Ⅷ	Vestibulocochlear	Sensory	Conduct hearing and balance

Continued

No.	Cranial nerves	Nature	Function
Ⅸ	Glossopharyngeal	Mixed	Conduct taste in the posterior 1/3 of tongue and pharyngeal feeling and manage pharyngeal muscle and parotid gland
Ⅹ	Vagus	Mixed	Manage the activities of the pharynx, laryngeal muscles and visceral movements of the chest and abdomen
Ⅺ	Accessory	Motor	The sternocleidomastoid and trapezius muscles
Ⅻ	Hypoglossal	Motor	Manage tongue muscle

(2) Spinal nerve

The peripheral nerves connected to the spinal cord are called spinal nerves, and each pair of spinal nerve is connected to a segment of the spinal cord by anterior (movement fiber) and posterior (sense fiber) roots. The 31 pairs of spinal nerves can be divided into 5 parts: 8 pairs of cervical nerves, 12 pairs of thoracic nerves, 5 pairs of lumbar nerves, 5 pairs of sacral nerves and 1 pair of caudal nerves. Immediately after exiting the foramen, each spinal nerve trunk is divided into anterior branch, posterior branch, meningeal branch and communicating branch. The anterior branches interlace into a plexus, that is, the cervical plexus, the brachial plexus, the lumbar plexus and the sacral plexus, from which branches are distributed to the muscles and skin of the anterolateral trunk and the limbs, which are used for muscle movement and skin sensation.

(3) Autonomic nerve

Autonomic nerve including sympathetic nerve and parasympathetic nerve, regulates the physiological activities of organs through hypothalamus, brainstem and spinal cord under the antagonistical and harmonious regulation of cerebral cortex. All the regulation activities are performed without the control of will. The function of autonomic nerve is completed by neurotransmitters released from nerve endings, which can be divided into cholinergic nerve and adrenergic nerve. The former contains sympathetic and parasympathetic preganglionic fibers, parasympathetic postganglionic fibers, and sympathetic postganglionic fibers that innervate blood vessels, sweat glands and uterus. The latter contains the sympathetic postganglionic fibers that innervate the heart, gut and vasoconstriction. Internal organs are innervated by both sympathetic nerve and parasympathetic nerve, which are antagonistic and coordinating, and can maintain the balance of body function, integrity, make the body adapt to the change of internal and external environment.

1.3.10 Muscle

Skeletal muscle is an effector unit executing motor function and an important organ of energy metabolism. It is innervated by motor nerves. A motor neuron sends out an axon, which divides into many nerve endings before reaching muscle fiber. Each end reaches a muscle fiber to form a neuromuscular junction (synapse). A motor neuron innervates many muscle fibers simultaneously. Electrical impulses from the motor nerve induce the contraction of skeletal muscles through chemical transmission of the neuromuscular junctions, thus to perform various voluntary movements.

1.3.11 Reflex

The anatomical basis of reflex is reflex arc. The reflex arc consists of receptors, afferent neurons (sensory neurons), intermediate neurons, efferent neurons (spinal cord anterior horn cells or brainstem motor neurons), peripheral nerves (motor fibers) and effector organs (muscles, secretory glands and so on). The reflex activity depends on the complete reflex arc, and any interruption in the reflex arc can cause the reflection to weaken and disappear. At the same time, reflex arc is also inhibited and facilitated by higher-level nerve center, so when the higher-level central disease occurs, the originally inhibited reflex (deep reflex) can be strengthened, and the facilitated reflex (shallow reflex) can be weakened. Each reflex arc has its fixed spinal cord segment and peripheral nerve, so the location of lesion can be determined by the change of reflex in clinic.

Physiological reflex is the reflex that normal people should have which includes deep reflex and superficial reflex.

(1) Deep reflex

Deep reflex is the rapid contraction of muscles caused by the proprioceptors stimulating tendons and periosteum, also known as tendon reflex or muscle stretch reflex, and its reflex arc is a synaptic reflex arc composed of sensory neurons and motor neurons directly connected. Usually, tapping tendon causes deep reflex, and muscle contraction reaction is most obvious in the stretched muscle. Clinical tendon reflexes are biceps brachii reflex (C5 ~ C6), triceps brachii reflex (C6 ~ C7), radial membrane reflex (C5 ~ C8), knee tendon reflex (L2 ~ L4), achilles tendon reflex (S1 ~ S2) and so on.

(2) Superficial reflex

Superficial reflex is the rapid contraction of muscles caused by stimulation of skin, mucous membrane and cornea. The reflex arc of shallow reflex is complex, besides segmental reflex arc of spinal cord, there are impulses reaching cerebral cortex (central front and back), and then descending to the anterior horn cells of spinal cord with pyramidal tract. Therefore, both central nervous system lesions and peripheral nervous system lesions can show the weakening or disappearance of shallow reflex. Commonly used reflex clinically are abdominal wall reflex (T7 ~ T12), cremaster reflex (L1 ~ L2), plantar reflex (S1 ~ S2), anal reflex (S4 ~ S5), corneal reflex and pharyngeal reflex, etc.

References

[1] LOUIS E D, MAYER S A, NOBLE J M. Merritt's neurology [M]. New York: Lippincott Williams and Wilkins, 2021.

[2] ROPPER A H, SAMUELS M A, KLEIN J, et al. Adams and Victor's principles of neurology [M]. New York: McGraw-Hill Education/Medical, 2019.

[3] STEPHEN G M. Clinical neuroanatomy [M]. New York: McGraw-Hill Education, 2013.

(Ma Rui, Chen Siyuan)

Chapter 2
Common Neurological Symptoms

Neurological symptoms are usually the only things given by the patients. Physicians use examinations and history according to the symptoms to make diagnosis and therapy. Common symptoms in nervous diseases include impaired consciousness, cognitions defection, vision disturbance and vertigo, sense loss, paralysis ataxia and sleep disorder. In order to understand these signs and symptoms, it is necessary to review the normal anatomy in Chapter 1 as it pertain to disease. Each symptom begins with a consideration of basic facts, followed by the manner in which they are affected by disease states and give rise to observable changes.

2.1 Impaired Consciousness

2.1.1 Consciousness Disorders According to Degrees of Awareness

(1) Somnolence

Somnolence is the early show of impaired awareness. It is a state of sleeping for unusually long periods, which can be awakened, after awakeness patients can grudgingly matching the examination and answer simple questions, in the absence of these stimuli, and quickly fall back into the original state, which could be caused by circadian rhythm disorders and physical ill-health.

(2) Coma

Coma is a state of unconsciousness from which the individual cannot be aroused. The levels of coma according to severity are shown in Tab. 2.1. The most common cause is poisoning, followed by lack of oxygen and trauma.

Tab. 2.1 Levels of coma

Levels of coma	Responses to stimuli	Voluntary movements	Responses to reflexes	Vital signs
Light coma	Show pain expressions and evading	Still a few	Still normal	Normal
Middle coma	No responses to normal stimuli	Few	Decrease	Change
Deep coma	No responses to any stimuli	No	No	Obvious change, irregular respiratories

2.1.2 Consciousness Disorders According to Conscious Contents

(1) Confusion

Confusion state includes disorientation, bewilderment, emotional disturbance and difficulty in following commands, which could be caused by drug poisoning, acute stress reaction, alcoholism.

(2) Delirium

Delirium is a syndrome containing disturbances in attention, consciousness, and cognition, which contains agitation, confusion, drowsiness, hallucinations, delusions and memory problems.

2.1.3 Special Consciousness Disorders

(1) Decorticated syndrome

The arms are bent in toward the body and the wrists and fingers are bent and held on the chest. This type of posturing is a sign of severe damage in the brain. Decorticate posturing can occur in structural or metabolic disorders and indicates hemispheric damage with preservation of motor centers in the upper portion of the brain stem (e.g., rubrospinal tract).

(2) Decerebrate rigidity

Decerebrate rigidity indicates that the upper brain stem motor centers, which facilitate flexion, have been structurally damaged and that only the lower brain stem centers (e.g., vestibulospinal tract, reticulospinal tract), which facilitate extension, are responding to sensory stimuli. The differences between decorticate syndrome and decerebrate rigidity are shown in Fig. 2.1.

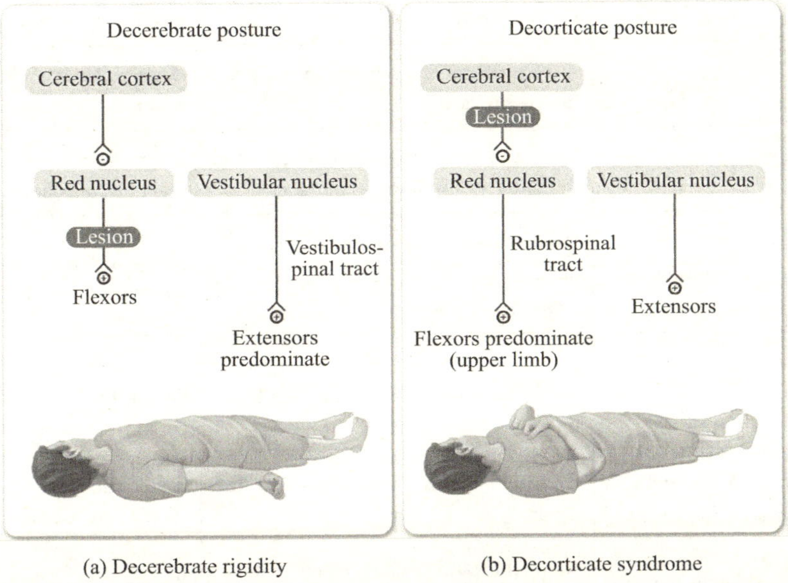

Fig. 2.1 Differences between decerebrate rigidity and decorticate syndrome

(3) Akinetic mutism

Akinetic mutism is a silent and inert state without voluntary motor activity despite preserved sensorimotor pathways and vigilance.

(4) Vegetative state

A vegetative state is absence of responsiveness and awareness due to overwhelming dysfunction of the cerebral hemispheres, with sufficient sparing of the diencephalon and brain stem to preserve autonomic and motor reflexes and sleep-wake cycles.

2.1.4 Differential Diagnosis of Consciousness Disorders

(1) Locked-in syndrome

Locked-in syndrome is complete paralysis of voluntary muscles in all parts of the body except for those that control eye movement. It may result from traumatic brain injury, diseases of the circulatory system, diseases that destroy the myelin sheath surrounding nerve cells, or medication overdose.

(2) Abulia

Abulia is a loss of drive, expression, behavior and speech output, with slowing and prolonged speech latency, and reduction of spontaneous thought content and initiative.

(3) Stupor

Stupor can be a serious mental state where people cannot respond to normal conversation. Instead, they respond only to physical stimulation. It is marked by absence of spontaneous movement and usually impaired consciousness.

The classification of impaired consciousness is concluded in Tab. 2.2.

Tab. 2.2 Classification of impaired consciousness

Classification	Symptom	Definition	Cause
Degrees of awareness	Somnolence	A state of long sleeping, which can be awakened	Circadian rhythm disorders, physical ill-health
	Coma	A state of unconsciousness which can not be aroused	Drug poisoning, lack of oxygen, trauma
Conscious contents	Confusion	Disorientation, bewilderment, and difficulty in following commands	Drug poisoning, acute stress reaction, alcoholism
	Delirium	Disorientation, agitation, confusion, drowsiness, hallucinations, delusions, memory problems	Toxic/metabolic conditions or structural brain lesions
Special consciousness disorders	Decorticate posturing	Arms close to one's sides and bend in at the elbows, extension of lower limbs	Severe damage in the brain
	Decerebrate rigidity	Extension of all four limbs and the trunk	Structurally damaged upper brain stem motor centers
	Akinetic mutism	A silent and inert state without voluntary motor activity	Bilateral frontal lobes lesions
	Vegetative state	Functioning brain stem but no consciousness or cognitive function	Severe brain damage

Continued

Classification	Symptom	Definition	Cause
Differential diagnosis of consciousness disorders	Locked-in syndrome	Complete paralysis of voluntary muscles in all parts of the body except for those that control eye movement	Infarction, hemorrhage, infection, tumor, multiple sclerosis
	Abulia	A state of diminished motivation with slowing and prolonged speech latency, and reduction of spontaneous thought content and initiative	Bilateral frontal lobes lesions
	Stupor	A serious mental state where people don't respond to normal conversation	Schizophrenia, severe depression

2.2 Aphasia, Apraxia and Agnosia

2.2.1 Aphasia

(1) Paralateral sulcus aphasia

1) Broca aphasia

The lesion of Broca aphasia is commonly located in the left frontal or frontoparietal area (including the Broca area), which is usually caused by infarction hemorrhage trauma or tumor. This aphasia shows anomia in oral and written language, nonfluent speech (with slow, effortful production, short phrase length, impaired prosody, and reduced use of prepositions and conjunctions), good comprehension, impaired repetition, impaired writing (nonfluent agraphia).

2) Wernicke aphasia

The lesion of Wernicke aphasia is in the left temporoparietal area, including the Wernicke area, which shows anomia in oral and written language, fluent speech (with paraphasias, a variety of grammatical forms, but often conveying little meaning), poor auditory and written comprehension, impaired repetition, errors in reading (alexia), fluent agraphia. The locations of Broca area and Wernicke area are shown in Fig. 2.2.

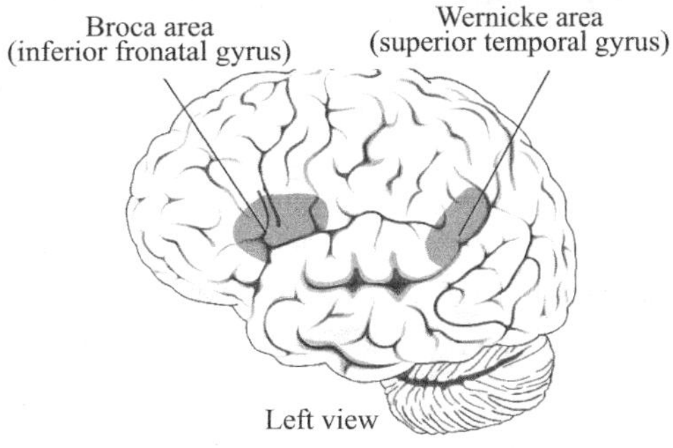

Fig. 2.2 Locations of Broca area and Wernicke area

3) Conduction aphasia

Conduction aphasia is characterised by intact auditory comprehension, coherent (yet paraphasic) speech production, but poor speech repetition. It is caused by damage to the parietal lobe of the brain. The arcuate fasciculus, which connects Broca's area and Wernicke's area, is affected.

(2) **Transcortical aphasia**

1) Transcortical motor

The lesion is in temporoparietal area, excluding Broca and Wernicke areas, which is caused by infarction, encephalitis, hemorrhage, trauma or tumor.

2) Transcortical sensory aphasia

The lesion is in left temporoparietal area, the Wernicke area, excluding the Broca and Wernicke areas, which is caused by infarction, encephalitis hemorrhage, trauma, or tumor. This aphasia is similar to Wernicke aphasia, except with normal repetition.

3) Global aphasia

The lesion is in the left frontotemporal area, which is caused by infarction hemorrhage, trauma or tumor. It shows severe anomia in oral and written language, nonfluent speech (often with sparse output), poor comprehension, impaired repetition, alexia and agraphia.

4) Anomic aphasia

The lesion of anomic can be anywhere of the left hemisphere language areas, which may be caused by infarction, hemorrhage, trauma or tumor. It shows anomia in oral and written language, fluent speech, good auditory and reading comprehension and normal repetition.

5) Subcortical aphasia

The lesion of subcortical aphasia under the superior temporal gyrus or the inferior parietal lobe in the left hemisphere, which is caused by infarction, hemorrhage or tumor.

2.2.2 Apraxia and Agnosia

Apraxia is the inability to perform certain purposeful voluntary movements but with normal consciousness, motor and language functions. The classification includes ideational apraxia, ideomotor apraxia, melokinetic apraxia and constructional apraxia. Patients may behave weirdly, e.g., putting their shoes on before socks, or being unable to copy a simple geometric shape despite the fact that see and recognize it, hold and use a pen, and understand the task.

Agnosia is the inability to comprehend the meaning or recognize the importance of various forms of stimulation that cannot be attributed to impairment of a primary sensory modality. Diagnosis is clinical, often including neuropsychologic testing, with brain imaging to identify the cause. Prognosis depends on the nature and extent of damage and patient age. Visual agnosia located in occipital lobe is the most common classification of apraxia, which includes prosopagnosia (inability to recognize human faces), simultanagnosia (inability to recognize and sort out objects when they appear together and achromatopsia (inability to distinguish different colors). Auditory agnosia, located in the superior temporal gyri, means inability to distinguish environmental and non-verbal auditory cues. Tactile agnosia is an inability to recognize or identify objects by touch alone located in bilateral angular and supramarginal gyri. Other special agnosia include finger agnosia (disability to distinguish or name the fingers) and anosognosia (lack of awareness that a deficit exists or lack of insight into an existing deficit) often accompanies with damage of the non-dominant parietal lobe.

2.3 Disturbance of Vision and Nystagmus

Disturbance of vision is caused by any lesion from visual organ to occipital cortex center which contains visual impairment and visual field impairment. In addition, nystagmus is an important sign in neurology.

2.3.1 Visual Impairment

(1) Monocular visual impairment

1) Acute monocular impairment

This impairment includes a. ophthalmic artery occlusion, central retinal artery occlusion; b. amaurosis fugax (transient vision loss). Symptoms include the sudden loss of vision in one or both eyes. It usually lasts for 1~5 minutes followed by recovering. After 10~20 minutes, vision returns to normal, which is caused by transient ischemic attack to carotid system.

2) Progressive monocular visual impairment

This impairment develops in several minutes to several hours, include a. optic neuritis; b. giant cell (temporal) arteritis; c. optic nerve compression.

(2) Binocular visual impairment

1) Transient binocular impairment

This impairment develops quickly and recovers after several minutes to several hours, which is caused by transient ischemic attack to the occipital cortex. Cortical blindness is the total or partial loss of vision in a normal-appearing eye caused by damage to the bilateral occipital cortex.

2) Progressive visual impairment

This impairment develops slowly and increasingly to blind, optic atrophy or optic papilla edema.

2.3.2 Visual Field Impairment

a. Bitemporal hemianopia is a loss of vision in the temporal half of visual field in both eyes. The condition manifests when there is compression in the optic chiasm which is usually caused by tumor in pituitary gland.

b. Contralateral homonymous hemianopia is a loss of vision in the same half of visual field in both eyes. This type of visual field loss is indicative of a lesion involving the visual pathway posterior to the chiasm.

c. Contralateral homonymous superior quadrantanopia is a loss of vision in the same upper quadrant of visual field in both eyes, which is usually caused by the lesion in posterior part of temporal lobe. Lesion could be tumors or vascular diseases.

d. Contralateral homonymous inferior quadrantanopia is a loss of vision in the same lower quadrant of visual field in both eyes, which is usually caused by lesion in parietal lobe. Lesion could be tumors or vascular diseases. The visual field impairments are shown in Fig. 2.3.

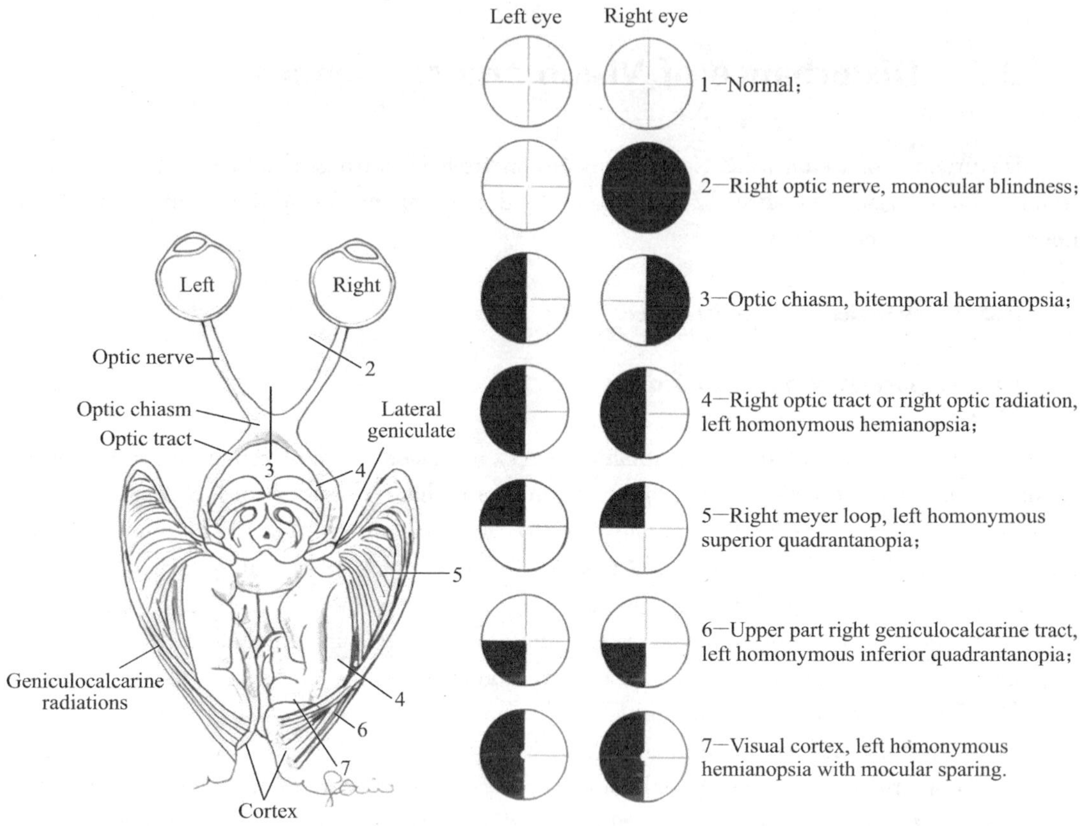

Fig. 2.3 Visual field impairments

2.3.3 Nystagmus

Nystagmus is involuntary rhythmic, oscillating motions of eyes when gazing at a point. It may be noticed in a person being evaluated for dizziness, vertigo and other balance problems. Nystagmus contain horizontal, vertical, rotatory, or mixed types according to directions. These eye movements typically appear as one of two types according to rhythm: pendular nystagmus or jerk nystagmus. In pendular nystagmus, the oscillations of eyes have an equal rate, amplitude, direction, and type of movement. Pendular nystagmus usually occurs as a result of poor central vision (ocular nystagmus) as in bilateral chorioretinitis, total colour blindness, albinism, congenital cataract, corneal scarring, amblyopia or in coal miners after many years of working in the dark. Depending on associated symptoms, tests (brain MRI or blood work) can help to rule out potentially dangerous causes such as stroke or demyelination. Jerk nystagmus is one in which there is a slow and fast phase, the nystagmus being conventionally defined by the direction of the fast phase. It is usually associated with a motor defect that may be induced by brainstem or cerebellar lesions (central nystagmus); drug intoxication, a lesion of the vestibular nerve or nuclei (vestibular nystagmus); disease or injury to the labyrinth; multiple sclerosis.

2.4 Vertigo

Vertigo is a sensation of movement of the self or the environment when there is no actual movement. Usually the perceived movement is rotary, a spinning or wheeling sensation, but some patients simply feel pulled to one side. Vertigo is not a diagnosis—it is a description of a sensation. Vertigo is classified into either peripheral or central, depending on the location of the dysfunction of the vestibular pathway. The differences between peripheral and central vertigo are shown in Tab. 2.3.

Tab. 2.3 Differences between peripheral and central vertigo

Clinical feature	Peripheral vertigo	Central vertigo
Lesion	Labyrinth and peripheral part of vestibular nerve	Cerebellum, cerebrum, brainstem
Cause	Benign paroxysmal positional vertigo (BPPV), Ménière disease, vestibular neuronitis, labyrinthitis	Vertebrobasilar insufficiency (VBI), brainstem stroke, demyelinating disorder, tumors in temporal lobe or fourth ventricles
Onset, duration, intensity	Sudden, short, severe	Slow, long, light
Nystagmus	Torsional/horizontal	Vertical
Nausea	Frequent	Infrequent
CNS sign	Absent	Usually present
Tinnitus/hearing loss	Can be present	Absent
ANS symptom	Frequent	Infrequent

Note: ANS, autonomic nerve system.

2.5 Syncope

Syncope is a sudden loss of consciousness and postural tone from a lack of blood flow to the brain. Causes of syncope are shown in Tab. 2.4.

Tab. 2.4 Causes of syncope

Classification of syncope	Disease
Reflex syncope (neurally mediated syncope, vasodepressor syncope, common faint)	Vasovagal syncope (orthostatic hypotension defecating/swallowing/coughing/urinating), carotid sinus syncope
Cardiac syncope (serious cardiovascular conditions)	Arrhythmia and abnormal heart rhythm: cardiomyopathy, mitochoencephalopathy, aortic dissection, aortic valve stenosis, aortic arch syndrome
Cerebral syncope	Cerebrovascular occlusion, hypertensive encephalopathy
Others	Hyperventilation syndrome, hypoglycemia

2.6 Seizure

Seizure is a transient brain dysfunction caused by abnormal discharge of cortical neurons. According to the location of cerebral focus and seizure time, seizure can have the following clinical manifestations. a. Disturbance of consciousness: a sudden loss of consciousness, and after the seizure, there may be a short-term confusion of consciousness and disorientation, etc.; b. Abnormal movement: convulsions and clonus of limbs; c. Paresthesia; d. Mental disorders; e. Autonomic nerve dysfunction. Common causes of seizure can be seen in Tab. 2.5.

Tab. 2.5 Common causes of seizure

Classification	Causes of seizure
Neural diseases	Epilepsy
	Lack of sleep
	Head trauma
	Stroke
	Meningitis
	Brain tumor
	Abnormalities of the blood vessels in the brain
Somatic diseases	Hyponatremia
	Hypoglycemia
	Hypocalcemia
	Uremia
	Hepatic encephalopathy
	Hypertensive encephalopathy
	Hypertension encephalopathy
	High fever
	COVID-19

2.7 Somatic Sensation Impairment

Somatic sensation refers to the perception formed in the human brain of acting of various stimuli on somatic receptors. Sensory consists of two categories: special senses (sight, hearing, taste and smell) and general senses (superficial sense, deep sense and compound sense). Sensory impairments can be divided into inhibitory symptoms and irritant symptoms. The distribution and characteristics of sensory disturbance in different parts of sensory conduction pathway are different, which provides an important clue for localized diagnosis.

2.7.1 Classifications According to the Damaged Parts

(1) Nerve trunk type of sensory disorder

Nerve trunk type of sensory disorder is characterized by the decline or disappearance of various senses in a damaged nerve trunk distribution area, such as radial nerve paralysis, ulnar nerve paralysis, common peroneal nerve injury and lateral femoral cutaneous neuritis.

(2) Terminal sensory disorder

Terminal sensory disorder is characterized by various sensory disorders (temperature, pain, touch and deep feeling) at the symmetrical ends of limbs, which is distributed like gloves and socks, and the distal end is heavier than the proximal end, often accompanied by autonomic nerve dysfunction, which is common in polyneuropathy and so on.

(3) Posterior root sensory disorder

Posterior root sensory disorder is unilateral segmental sensory disorder, and the scope of sensory disorder is consistent with the distribution of nerve roots. It is often accompanied by severe radiation pain (neuralgia), such as lumbar intervertebral disc detachment and extramedullary tumors.

(4) Intramedullary sensory disorder

1) Posterior horn type

Posterior horn damage is characterized by segmental dissociated sensory disturbance on the injured side, with pain and dysesthesia on the diseased side, while the sense of touch and deep feeling is preserved. This is because pain and warm sensation fibers enter the posterior horn, while some tactile and deep sensation fibers directly enter the posterior cord without passing through the posterior horn. It can be seen in syringomyelia, spinal cord tumors, etc.

2) Posterior cable type

If the thin bundle and wedge bundle of posterior cable are damaged, deep sensory disturbance and fine tactile disturbance below the damaged plane will result in sensory ataxia. It can be seen in diabetes, spinal cord rot or subacute combined degeneration.

3) Lateral cord type

As the lateral bundle of spinal cord and thalamus are affected, it shows pain below the contralateral plane of the lesion, loss of temperature sensation and preservation of touch and deep sensation (dissociative sensory disorder).

4) Anterior commissure type

Anterior commissure is the cross fiber concentration of both sides of the spinal thalamus. When an injury occurs, symmetrical separation dysesthesia with bilateral segmental distribution will appear, showing that pain and warm sensation disappear and deep sensation and touch exist. It can be seen in syringomyelia and early stage of intramedullary tumors.

5) Semi-severed spinal cord type

Brown-sequard syndrome presents with deep sensory disturbance and upper motor neuron paralysis below the injury plane on the diseased side, pain and lack of temperature sensation below the injury plane on the opposite side. It can be seen in extramedullary space occupying lesions, spinal cord trauma, etc.

6) Transversal spinal cord injury

It means all sensations (temperature, pain, touch and depth) below the lesion plane are lost or weakened, and there may be allergic zone in the upper part of the lesion plane. For example, the cervical and thoracic segment may be accompanied by signs of pyramidal tract injury, which is characterized by paraplegia or quadriplegia and dysfunction of size. It is common in myelitis and spinal cord tumor.

7) Cone-shaped horsetail

It presents mainly saddle-shaped sensory loss around anus and perineum, and root-type sensory disturbance present severe pain after horsetail disease, which can be seen in tumor and inflammation, etc.

(5) Brainstem sensory disorder

Brainstem sensory disorder is contralateral sensory disturbance. The lesions on the lateral medulla oblongata, the inferior pontine damage the lateral spinal thalamic bundle and the spinal bundle and nucleus of the trigeminal nerve, and there are dissociative sensory disorders on the ipsilateral side and the opposite side (pain, lack of warm sensation and tactile sensation), such as Wallenberg syndrome. The lesions in the medulla oblongata damage the medial colliculus system, causing deep sensory loss on the opposite side, while the spinal thalamus bundle located outside the medulla oblongata is not damaged, so the pain and warm sensation is unobstructed, that is, the deep and superficial sensory separation disorder appears. However, the medial colliculus system, trigeminal colliculus system and spinal thalamus bundle of the upper pontine and midbrain merge together, and all kinds of sensations on the side and half body are obstructed when the injury occurs, but most of them are accompanied by ipsilateral cranial nerve paralysis, which can be seen in inflammation, cerebrovascular disease, tumor and so on.

(6) Thalamic sensory disorder

Thalamus is the starting point of the third-level neurons of deep and superficial sensation, and when it is damaged, the complete sensory loss or decrease of contralateral deviation (including face) occurs. It is characterized by deep sensory and tactile disorders, which are more important than pain, warm sensation and the distal end is more important than the proximal end, often accompanied by spontaneous pain (thalamic pain) of the affected limb. It is more common in cerebrovascular diseases.

(7) Internal capsule sensory disorder

The inner capsule sensory disorder is hemiparesis, that is, the loss or decline of the feeling of hemiparesis (including face), often accompanied by hemiplegia and hemianopia, which is called trisection syndrome. It is found in cerebrovascular diseases.

(8) Cortical sensory disorder

Cortical sensory centers are located in the posterior central gyrus of cerebral cortex and the posterior part of the lateral central lobule. When damaged, there are two characteristics: a. Complex sensory (fine sensory) obstacles can appear on the opposite side of the lesion. Obstacles of entity perception, figure perception, two-point discrimination perception, and orientation perception are more common, while pain and temperature perception obstacles are light; b. The cortical sensory area has a wide range. If some areas are damaged, there may be sensory loss or decrease in the distribution of one upper limb or one lower limb on the opposite side, which is called sensory loss or loss of one limb. If it is an irritant lesion, there will be localized sensory epilepsy (paroxysmal sensory abnormality).

2.7.2 Categories According to the Impaired Sensory Conduction Pathway

(1) Inhibitory symptoms

Various sensory deficits in one region are called complete sensory deficits. Separation disorder refers to sensory disorder in a certain part and the preserver of other senses. Patients with normal depth perception, but without visual participation, who can not distinguish the stimulation position, object shape and weight, are called cortical sensory loss. When there is spontaneous pain in the nerve distribution area, and there is hypoesthesia at the same time, it is called painful hypoesthesia.

(2) Irritating symptoms

When the sensory pathway is stimulated or the excitability is increased, there are irritating symptoms, which can be divided into the following types.

1) Sensory hypersensitivity

Sensory hypersensitivity refers to the micro-sensation that will not cause discomfort or only slight sensation in normal people, but will cause very strong or even unbearable sensation in patients. It is common in shallow sensory disorders.

2) Hyper pathia

Hyper pathia generally occurs on the basis of sensory impairment, which has the following characteristics: a. long latency; b. the sensitivity decreased and the excitation threshold increased; c. an unpleasant feeling; d. expanding; e. delay.

3) Sensory inversion

Sensory inversion refers to the wrong feeling to the stimulation, such as cold stimulation produces hot feeling, touch and other stimulation are mistaken for pain. It is common in parietal lobe lesions or hysteria.

4) Paresthesia

Paresthesia refers to that the patient feels a sense of acupuncture, cold and hot, swelling in some parts without any external stimulation. It is common in peripheral nerve or autonomic neuropathy.

5) Pain

Pain is the body feeling when sensory fibers are stimulated, and it is the body's defense mechanism. Common clinical pain can be as follows. a. Local pain: It is localized pain of local lesions; b. Radiation pain: When the central nerve, nerve root or trunk are stimulated, the pain not only occurs locally, but also disperses to the innervated area of the affected nerve, such as swelling and pain of the nerve root or pressure of the intervertebral disc; c. Diffuse pain: It is the pain caused by stimulating the dispersion of one nerve branch to another nerve branch. For example, when one has toothache, the pain spreads to the branch areas of other trigeminal nerves; d. Referred pain: Pain is in the corresponding body surface area when visceral lesions occur. e. Phantom limb pain: After amputation, patients feel the severed limb still exists and there is pain. This phenomenon is called phantom limb pain, which is related to the loss of descending inhibitory system; f. Burning neuralgia: Severe burning-like pain is often seen after median nerve or sciatic nerve injury.

2.8 Paralysis

Paralysis is the temporary or permanent loss of movement in one or more parts of the body. According to the location of motor pathway, paralyses can be divided into upper motor neuron paralysis and lower motor neuron paralysis.

(1) Upper motor neurons (pyramidal system)

The upper motor neurons include the pyramidal cells (Betz cells) in the motor area of the frontal central gyrus and the cortical spinal cord bundle (fiber bundle from cerebral cortex to anterior horn of spinal cord) and cortical brainstem bundle (fiber bundle from cerebral cortex to motor nucleus of brain nerve). The function of the upper motor neurons is to send and transmit voluntary movement impulse to the lower motor meridian elements and control and dominate their activities. The upper motor neurons can produce central (spasticity) paralysis after injury. Its clinical manifestations are as follows.

a. Strength weakening: Paralysis caused by muscle strength weakening and motor neuron damage on one side can be a paralysis of one upper or lower limb, which is called monoplegia; it can also be a paralysis of upper and lower limbs, which is called hemiplegia. When the meridians of bilateral upper motor species are damaged, the performance is paralysis of both lower limbs, which is called diplegia. It can also be a quadriplegia (Fig. 2.4).

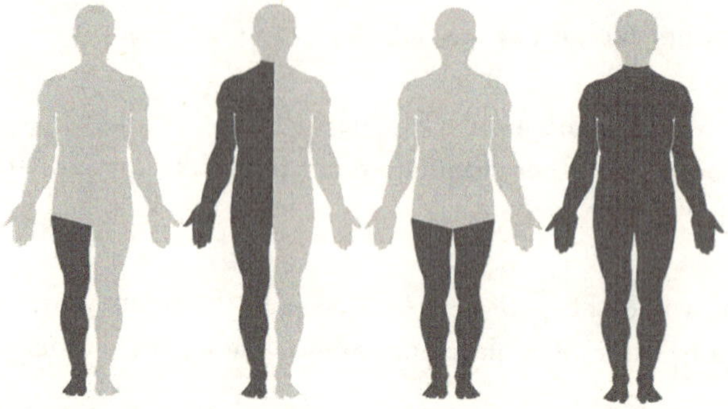

Fig. 2.4 Classification of paralyses according to the distribution

b. Increased muscle tension: When the mechanical tension increases, the muscle tension of the affected limb increases, which can present a special hemiplegic posture. Due to the increase of muscle tension, when the affected limb is pulled and extended by external force, resistance appears at the beginning. When the traction continues to a certain extent, the resistance suddenly disappears and the affected limb is pulled and extended rapidly. It is called "clasp knife phenomenon".

c. Active or hyperactive tendon reflex: There can also be reflex diffusion. For example, knocking on the radial periosteum can not only lead to the contraction of the radial muscle of the limb, but also lead to the reflex of the biceps or flexor digitorum of the limb. In addition, there may be clonus when the tendon reflex is excessively hyperactive.

d. Decrease or disappearance of superficial reflex: When the upper motor neuron is paralyzed, the injury can lead to the decrease and disappearance of superficial reflex, including abdominal wall reflex, testicular reflex and plantar reflex.

e. Pathological reflex: When the upper motor neuron is paralyzed, the pyramid tract is damaged. Pathological reflex will be released.

f. No obvious atrophy of muscle.

The characteristics of paralysis in each part of the upper motor neuron are as follows.

a. Cortical type: Because the cortical motor area is a long belt, a central paralysis of the upper limb, lower limb or face may appear in the local lesion, which is called monoplegia. It is called tumor compression, arterial cortical branch infarction, etc.

b. Internal capsule type: The internal capsule is the focus of sensory and motor conduction bundles, and the "three deviation" syndrome occurs when injured, namely hemiplegia, hemiparesis and hemianopia. It is more common in acute cerebrovascular diseases.

c. Brainstem type: Cross paralysis, that is, cranial nerve paralysis on the diseased side and central paralysis on the opposite limb. It is more common in brain stem tumors and/or cerebral vascular occlusion.

d. Spinal cord type: When the spinal cord is damaged transversely, paralysis of bilateral limbs, such as paraplegia or quadriplegia, occurs due to damage of bilateral pyramidal tracts. It is more common in spinal cord compression caused by myelitis, trauma or tumor. Fig. 2.4 demonstrates the classification of paralyses according to the distribution.

(2) Lower motor neurons

The lower motor neurons include the anterior horn cells of spinal cord, the motor nucleus of cranial nerve and its axon C. Its function is to combine these impulses from pyramidal system, extrapyramidal system or cerebellar system, and transmit them to the motor endplate through peripheral nerves, causing muscle contraction. The cranial nerves composed of axons from the motor nucleus of the cranial nerves directly reach the muscles they dominate. Axons from motor neurons in the anterior horn of spinal cord pass through the anterior root and nerve plexus (cervical plexus: C1 ~ C4; brachial plexus: C5 ~ T1; lumbar plexus: L1 ~ L4; gingival plexus: S5 ~ C0), the peripheral nerve reaches the muscle innervated by them. Peripheral (flaccid) paralysis can occur after injury of lower motor neurons.

Lower motor neuron paralysis is characterized by a. decreased muscle strength innervated by damaged inferior motor neurons; b. decreased or disappeared muscle tension, relaxed muscle, and there is no resistance when pulled by external force; c. weakened or disappeared wall reflection; d. obvious muscle atrophy. The comparison of upper motor neuron and lower motor neuron paralysis can been shown in Tab. 2.6.

The characteristics of paralysis in various parts of lower motor neuron are as follows.

a. Anterior horn cells of spinal cord: segmental and flaccid paralysis without sensory disturbance. For example, C5 anterior horn damage causes deltoid paralysis and atrophy, C8 ~ T1 damage causes hand small muscle atrophy, L3 damage causes quadriceps atrophy and weakness, L5 damage causes ankle joint and toe dorsiflexion, and acute onset is more common in poliomyelitis. Muscle bundle tremor can also occur in slowly progressive diseases, which can be seen in motor neuron diseases.

b. Anterior root: The injured segment shows flaccid paralysis and no sensory disturbance. It often damages the posterior root at the same time, resulting in root pain and segmental sensory disturbance. It can be seen in the compression of extramedullary tumors, inflammation of spinal membranes or vertebral lesions.

Tab. 2.6 **Comparison of upper motor neuron and lower motor neuron paralysis**

Feature/sign	Upper motor neuron paralysis	Lower motor neuron paralysis
Paralysis	Present-spastic paralysis	Present-flaccid paralysis
Muscles affected	Regional paralysis	Segmental paralysis
Muscle tone	Increased tone-spasticity. with "Clasp-Knife rigidity"	Leading to "hypotonia/flaccidity" muscle tone
Deep tendon reflex	++ Exaggerated – Hyperreflexia	Absent/reduced areflexia/hyporeflexia
Superficial reflexes	– Abdominal and cremasteric	Only if particular neuron supplying muscle is affected
Babinski sign	+ (Extensor plantar response. Indicates corticospinal tract involvement)	– (Plantar reflex flexor)
Clonus	+	–
Fasciculations	–	+
Wasting contractures	–	+

c. Nerve plexus: Nerve plexus contains motor fibers and sensory fibers. Lesions often involve most peripheral nerves of one limb, leading to flaccid paralysis, sensory disturbance and autonomic nerve dysfunction, which may be accompanied by pain.

d. Peripheral nerve: The muscles in innervated area appear flaccid paralysis, accompanied by sensory and autonomic nerve dysfunction or pain. Symmetrical distal limb muscle paralysis occurs in multiple peripheral neuropathy, accompanied by glove-sock-like sensory disturbance.

2.9 Ataxia

Ataxia refers to the clumsy and uncoordinated movement caused by the dysfunction of cerebellum, proprioception and vestibule. When the trunk, limbs and pharyngeal muscles are involved, it can cause the disorder of body balance, posture, gait and speech. Clinically, there are several types of ataxia.

(1) Cerebellar ataxia

Cerebellar ataxia is characterized by irregular strength, speed, amplitude and rhythm of voluntary movement, that is, coordinated movement disorder, which can be accompanied by decreased muscle tone, eye movement disorder and speech disorder.

a. Abnormal posture and gait: Cerebellar vermis lesions can cause ataxia of head and trunk, balance disorder and abnormal posture and gait. The patient stands unsteadily and staggers. When walking, his legs are separated to form an ataxia gait. When the upper vermis is diseased, the patient tilts forward, and when the lower vermis is diseased, the patient tilts backward.

b. Voluntary motor coordination disorder: Cerebellar hemispheric lesions can cause ataxia of ipsilateral limbs, manifested in that the movement is easy to exceed the target (poor distance discrimination), the tremor becomes more and more obvious when the movement is closer to the target (intentional tremor), and the coordination disorder of fine movement, such as the writing increasing sizes of letters.

c. Speech disorder: The patient is characterized by slow speech, unclear pronunciation and intermittent, faltering or violent voice, showing explosive or poetic language.

d. Eye movement disorder: Ataxia of extraocular muscles can lead to eye movement disorder. Most patients show large nystagmus in both eyes, and jumping nystagmus and rebound nystagmus are seen in a few patients.

e. Decreased muscle tension: Cerebellar lesions often have decreased muscle tension and weakened or disappeared tendon reflex. When the patient takes the sitting position, his legs sag naturally. After tapping the tendon, the lower leg swings like a pendulum (pendulum like tendon reflex).

(2) Cerebral ataxia

The frontal, temporal and occipital lobes and the cerebellar hemisphere form fiber connections through the frontopontine and the tempor occipitopontine bundle. Due to the fiber crossing between cerebral cortex and cerebellum, one side of brain lesion causes contralateral limb ataxia. Cerebral ataxia is smaller and its symptoms are mild.

a. Frontal ataxia: The patient's symptoms appear in the contralateral limb and are similar to cerebellar ataxia, such as postural balance disorder, unstable gait, backward or unilateral dumping, but the symptoms are milder. Romberg sign, poor distance discrimination and nystagmus are rare. Frontal ataxia is often accompanied by increased muscle tension, positive pathological reflex, mental symptoms, strong grip reflex and frontal lobe damage.

b. Temporal ataxia: The patient shows temporal ataxia of the contralateral limb with mild symptoms which are difficult to find in the early stage. It can be accompanied by other symptoms or signs of temporal lobe damage, such as tropism quadrant blindness and aphasia.

c. Parietal ataxia: Parietal ataxia shows different degrees of ataxia in the contralateral limb. The symptoms are obvious when the eyes are closed, and the deep sensory disturbance is not serious or transient. The posterior part of the lateral central lobule is damaged, which can lead to sensory ataxia of both lower limbs and dysuria.

d. Occipital ataxia: The patient is characterized by ataxia of the contralateral limb. The symptoms are mild, often accompanied by deep sensory impairment aggravated when the eyes are closed, and may be accompanied by other symptoms or signs of occipital lobe damage, such as visual impairment.

(3) Sensory ataxia

Deep sensory ataxia can occur in the damage of posterior root of spinal nerve, posterior cord of spinal cord, thalamus to parietal lobe of cerebral cortex. It is characterized by unstable standing, uncontrollable distance of walking, no depth of landing, and a sense of stepping on cotton. There is visual assistance when eyes are open. The symptoms are mild, and will be aggravated in the dark or when eyes are closed.

(4) Vestibular ataxia

Vestibular ataxia occurs due to the loss of body spatial orientation in vestibular damage. Standing unsteadily is the clinical manifestation and changing the head position can be an aggravation. Patients lean to the affected side when walking, accompanied by obvious dizziness, nausea, vomiting and nystagmus.

2.10 Sleep Disorders

Sleep-wake rhythm is regulated by three systemic factors: homeostasis system, circadian biological rhythm system and sub-circadian biological rhythm system. Sleep disorders can be divided into the following types.

a. Insomnia is a common sleep disorder, which refers to problems in the depth and length of sleep or awakening, manifested as difficulty in falling asleep, difficulty in maintaining sleep, early awakening and inability to recover spirit and physical strength after waking up.

b. Circadian rhythm sleep disorder refers to the disorder of patients' sleep work and rest rhythm, which is easy to fall asleep during the day, but difficult to fall asleep during the normal sleep period at night.

c. Sleep related breathing disorders are a group of respiratory disorders that occur only during sleep, including obstructive sleep apnea syndrome, central sleep apnea syndrome, upper airway resistance syndrome and obesity hypoventilation syndrome.

d. Parasomnias mainly occurs in the wake-up period of partial wake-up, complete wake-up or different stages of sleep, including night terrors and nightmares, sleeping sickness, enuresis and sleep behavior disorders in REM (rapid eye movements).

e. Sleep-related movement disorder refers to a group of diseases caused by relatively simple and rigid movement in sleep, resulting in sleep disorder and daytime dysfunction. These include restless legs syndrome, periodic limb dyskinesia, sleep related leg spasms, sleep related bruxism and sleep related rhythmic dyskinesia.

References

[1] KUKS J B M, SNOEK J W. Textbook of clinical neurology[M]. New York: Bohn Stafleu van Loghum, 2007:75-81.

[2] STANDRING S. Gray's anatomy: the anatomical basis of clinical practice[M]. 41st ed. Amstel dam: Elsevier Pte Ltd., 2016:216-222.

[3] MCGUINNESS B, BARRETT S L, MCLLVENNA J, et al. Predicting conversion to dementia in a memory clinic: a standard clinical approach compared with an empirically defined clustering method (latent profile analysis) for mild cognitive impairment subtyping [J]. Alzheimers & Dementia: Diagnosis Assessment & Disease Monitoring, 2015,1(4):447-454.

[4] WAHLSTER S, WIJDICKS E F M, PATEL P V, et al. Brain death declaration: practices and perceptions worldwide[J]. Neurology, 2015,84(18):1870-1879.

[5] TAUSCHER R G, SIMON S S, VOLPE N J. Retinal disease in the neurology clinic [J]. Current Opinion in Neurology, 2021,34(1):122-132.

[6] RIZZO J-R, BEHESHTI M, DAI W, et al. Eye movement recordings: practical applications in Neurology[J]. Seminars in Neurology, 2019,39 (6):775-784.

(Li Jingwei, Xia Haiping)

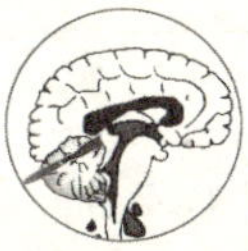

Chapter 3
Neurological Physical Examinations

The neurological examination is an assessment method to determine an examinee's neurologic function, which is central to the evaluation of patients with neurologic complaints. It relies heavily on the medical history and on directed, hypothesis-driven physical testing containing: mental status, cranial nerves, spinal nerves, motor system, muscle strength, gait, stance, coordination, sensation, reflexes and autonomic nervous system examination.

PE of CNS

3.1 Mental Status Examination

A mental status examination is an evaluation of a patient's level of cognitive ability, emotion, speech and thinking at the time of assessment. It can be helpful to distinguish the mental diseases from neurological diseases, to discern neurological mechanism for mental symptoms, to recognize focal cranial lesions from diffused lesions. Abnormal mental status may be caused by stroke, tumor, infection and metabolic disease and dementia disease. The specific cognitive functions of orientation, language, attention concentration, memory, computing ability, judgment and abstract reasoning are the most clinically relevant. Orientation is the ability to recognize one's place in time and space. Attention is the ability to focus based on internal or external priorities. Memory can be grouped into three kinds: immediate recall, short-term memory, and long-term storage. Judgement is the ability to make a decision according to information.

3.1.1 Consciousness

Consciousness impairment can be classified according to the degrees of awareness (drowsiness, somnolence and coma), according to conscious contents (confusion and delirium), special consciousness disorders (decorticate posturing, decerebrate rigidity, akinetic mutism and vegetative state), differential diagnosis of consciousness disorders (locked-in syndrome, abulia and stupor). Glasgow coma scale (GCS) is the used-widely tool now, including eye-pening response, verbal response and motor response (Tab. 3. 1).

Tab. 3.1 Glasgow coma scale (GCS)

Behavior	Score					
	1	2	3	4	5	6
Eye opening response	No response	Feel pain only (not applied to face)	Verbal stimuli, command, speech	Spontaneous open with blinking at baseline		
Verbal response	No response	Incomprehensible speech	Inappropriate words	Confusing conversation, but able to answer questions	Oriented	
Motor response	No response	Extension in response to pain	Flexion in response to pain	Withdraws in response to pain	Purposeful movement to stimulus	Obeys commands

Note: Severe head injury, GCS score≤8; moderate head injury, GCS score of 9~12; mild head injury, GCS score of 13~15.

The physical examination in conscious impairment contains: eye signs, autonomic dysfunction, motor dysfunction, brain stem reflex.

Specific PE of patient in coma

a. Eye signs: Dilated, pinpoint, or unequal pupils are all possible. Unilateral or bilateral pupils may be fixed in center. Eye movement may be dysconjugate or paresis or ocular bobbing, ocular dipping, opsoclonus. Homonymous hemianopia may be present. Other signs include absence of blinking in response to visual threat (almost touching the eye) and oculoreflex.

b. Autonomic dysfunction: Patients may have hypertension and bradycardia (cushing reflex) and abnormal breathing patterns (Cheyne-Stokes or Biot respirations). Abrupt respiratory and cardiac arrest may occur. However, hypotension may occur if impaired consciousness is caused by severe infection, severe dehydration, major blood loss, or cardiac arrest.

c. Motor dysfunction: Signs include flaccidity, hemiparesis, asterixis, multifocal myoclonus, decorticate posturing (elbow flexion and shoulder adduction with leg extension), and decerebrate posturing (limb extension and internal shoulder rotation). The limb drop test, flexing and lifting the patient's knees by hands with the heel on bed, can check the paralyzed part. When suddenly releases the hand, the paralyzed limb cannot straighten automatically and tilts outward. While normal limbs will drop in a bouncing manner and can maintain the vertical position of the foot.

d. Brain stem reflexes: The oculocephalic reflex is also called "doll's eye reflex" as doll's eyes move towards the contralateral side if the head is tilted to one side. In a conscious patient, such movement is inhibited. In a comatose patient, doll's eye reflex is present. And in a comatose patient with brainstem reflexes compromised, the oculocephalic reflex is absent. Other reflexes can be summarized in Tab. 3. 2.

e. Signs of meningeal irritation: Signs of meningeal irritation contain nuchal rigidity, brudzinski's sign and kernig's sign, which may be caused by infectious meningitis, subarachnoid hemorrhage, neoplasms of the brain and meninges.

f. Other signs of consciousness disorder: The perception ability, recognition ability of environment and self-care ability of patients with consciousness disorder may change, especially those in coma. As the patient's cough, swallowing and other reflexes weaken or disappear, the patient cannot control defecation, urination, indwelling catheterization and other factors.

Tab. 3.2 Brain stem reflexes

Reflex	Performance	Positive sign	Implication
Ciliospinal reflex	Stimulus to the neck causes mydriasis	Absent	Lower brainstem to upper thoracic and sympathetic are affected
Corneal reflex	Stimulus to the cornea causes blink	Absent	Nerves or midbrain are compromised
Oculocephalic reflex	Rotate the head to one direction	Eyes follow the rotation	Cortical influence on the brainstem has weakened
Oculovestibular reflex	Introduce iced water into the external ear canal	No response or ipsilateral dysconjugate deviation	Structural or metabolic dysfunction

3.1.2 Mental State and Advanced Cortical Function Examination

Mental state and advanced cortical function examination are used to judge whether the patient is suffering from neurological disease or mental disease, clarify the underlying neurological disease basis behind mental symptoms, and help determine whether it is focal brain damage or diffuse brain damage. In addition to primary mental diseases, in neurological diseases, mental state and higher cortical dysfunction can be caused by the following reasons: frontal and temporal lobe lesions caused by stroke or tumor, intracranial infection, metabolic encephalopathy, neurodegenerative diseases represented by Alzheimer's disease, etc. When checking the mental state of patients, attention should be paid to their appearance, behavior, conversation and thinking. Higher cortical function can be divided into cognitive function and non-cognitive function. Cognitive function examination mainly includes memory, computing power, orientation, aphasia, apraxia, agnosia, abstract thinking and judgment, visuospatial skills and so on; non-cognitive function tests include personality changes, behavioral abnormalities, mental symptoms (hallucinations, illusions and delusions) and emotional changes. This section mainly introduces the examination methods of cognitive impairment.

(1) Memory

Memory is the process of acquiring, storing and reproducing past experience, including three links: information recognition, retention and reproduction. Memory contains three subunits: immediate recall, short-term memory, and long-term storage. Short-term memory is the most clinically pertinent, and the most important to be tested. Short-term memory may be tested by having the patient learn 3 ~ 7 unrelated objects or concepts, a short sentence, or a five-component name and address, and then asking the patient to recall the information in 1 ~ 3 minutes after performing a second, unrelated mental task.

Orientation largely reflects recent memory function. Questions, such as "Where are you right now? What's the date today?" Immediate recall can be tested once again by repeating some words back to examiner. Long-term memory can be tested by the patient's ability to recall remote personal or historic events (e.g., where is your middle school?)

(2) Computational force

Computational power can be checked by asking the examinee a question about maths. It starts with the simplest calculation, such as: celery is 2 dollars per pound, then how many celeries can you buy with 10 dollars? At this time, we also need the participation and assistance of attention and concentration.

(3) Directional force

The examination can be divided into time orientation (day, month and season), place orientation (location of hospital or home) and character orientation (whether family members and familiar people can be recognized). This examination requires the patient to be in a state of concentration.

(4) Aphasia

Before examination, make sure that the patient is aware and cooperate with the examination. Clinical examination includes six aspects: oral expression, listening comprehension, retelling, naming, reading and writing ability. Comprehensive evaluation is helpful to the clinical diagnosis of aphasia.

1) Oral expression

During oral expression examination, pay attention to the patient's conversation volume, tone and pronunciation, whether it is laborious to speak, whether there are grammatical functions or sentence structure errors, whether there are substantive words or wrong words, word finding difficulty, rigid language, whether it can reach meaning, etc. It is divided into the following categories.

a. Speech fluency: Determine whether there is a change in speech fluency, which can be divided into fluent speech and non-fluent speech.

b. Speech disorder: Determine whether there is ambiguity in speech when there is no obstacle to pronunciation and vocal organs, and whether it affects tone and rhythm.

c. Word finding difficulty: Determine whether patients can think of appropriate words freely in speech, or the time of word finding is prolonged.

d. Wrong words, new words, meaningless clutter and stereotyped words: Determine whether the following words are used in expression: words with phonetic or semantic errors; meaningless newly created words; a string of sounds or words whose meaning is completely unknown; the stereotyped repetition of the same meaningless word, phrase or sentence.

e. Grammatical barriers: Determine whether it is difficult for patients to use a correct sentence pattern. Grammatical disorder is manifested in the misuse of auxiliary words or the position and order of words which do not conform to grammatical rules.

2) Hearing comprehension disorder

It means that the patient can hear the sound, but the semantic understanding is incomplete. The specific examination method: asking the patient to perform simple oral instructions (such as "open your mouth" "open your eyes" "close your eyes") and compound sentences with grammar (such as "touch your nose with your left hand" "touch your left ear with your right hand").

3) Retelling

Retell the words, phrases or sentences used by the examiner, including common words (such as pencil, apple, coat), uncommon words, abstract words, phrases, short sentences and long compound sentences. Pay attention to whether patients can retell the words correctly or without omission, whether there is difficulty in retelling, wrong language retelling, shortening, prolonging or completely unable to retell the original words and sentences, etc.

4) Naming

Ask the patient to say the name of the commonly used items referred to by the examiner, such as flashlight, cup, toothbrush, pen or body part, and describe the purpose of the items if the patient cannot name them.

5) Reading

Reading can be checked by asking the patient to read the text in books and newspapers and execute instructions written on paper, thus the patient's ability to read and understand the text can be determined.

6) Writing

Ask the patient to write their names, addresses, serial numbers, brief narrative, dictation or transcription, etc., to determine their writing ability.

(5) Apraxia

Apraxia is usually undetectable for patients themselves and often ignored by doctors. Oral and written orders can be given during the examination, and the ability of patients to execute orders, imitate actions and physical demonstration can be observed. Observe whether the patient's actions such as dressing, washing face, combing hair and dining are orderly and coordinated. Observe whether the patient can complete simple purposeful actions, such as tongue extension, eye closure, hand raising, writing and button fastening. Let the patient do simple actions (such as brushing teeth, dialing phone numbers, holding a pen, writing) first, and then move to complex actions (such as dressing, striking matches, lighting cigarettes).

(6) Agnosia

Agnosia refers to the abnormal sensory pathway and the patient can not distinguish familiar objects through a certain feeling. This disorder is caused by sensory, speech, intelligence and consciousness disorders, mainly including visual agnosia, auditory agnosia and tactile agnosia. Body image agnosia is also a kind of agnosia. Due to its own cognitive defects, it is not used as a routine physical examination. Visual agnosia is examined by showing patients some common objects, photos, landscape paintings and other objects, to see if they can recognize and express the items in language or writing. Auditory agnosia is examined by asking patients to recognise familiar sounds, such as bell, alarm clock, knocking tea cup and music, etc. Tactile agnosia refers to examination to make the patient close his eyes and let him touch the object in his hand for recognition.

(7) Visuospatial skills and executive functions

Visuospatial skills and executive functions can be checked by asking patients to draw a clock face, fill in numbers, and draw a watch needle at the specified time. To complete the task, the cooperation of spatial skills and executive function is required. If the clock face is missing or the pointer is incomplete, it indicates the dysfunction of both.

(8) Spatial orientation

Spatial orientation can be checked by drawing a triangle and asking patient to draw the same shape upside down.

(9) Abstract reasoning

Abstract reasoning can be checked by asking the examinee to identify a unifying theme of 3 or 4 objects (e.g., all the objects are fruit, vehicles of transportation or musical instruments).

For example, "Can you put the following items (an apple, a banana and an orange) into one group?" (Tab. 3.3)

Tab. 3.3 Methods and sample questions of mental status examination

Item	Method	Sample question
Direction force	Person	"What's your name?"
	Time	"What's the date today?"
	Place	"Where is your home?"
Attention concentration	Observe whether the examinee remain focused on all the interview	"Spell the word 'world.' Now spell the word 'world' backwards."
Immediate recall	Repeat some words back to examiner	"Could you recall the word I just said?"
Short-term memory	Ask the examinee to recall 3 ~ 7 objects after about 1 ~ 3 minutes	N/A
Long-term memory	Ask the examinee a question about the past	"Where is your middle school?"
Math	Ask the examinee a question about calculation	"How many dime coins can be changed for 1 dollar?"
Word finding	Ask the examinee to tell as many objects in a single category, such as articles of stationery and birds, as possible in certain time	"Can you say some names of birds?"
Naming objects	Present an article, and ask the examinee to name the object and a part of it	"How to call it?"
Writing	Ask the examinee to write a sentence. The sentence should contain a subject and an object and should make sense. Spelling errors can be ignored	N/A
Spatial orientation	Draw a triangle and ask patient to draw the same shape upside down	N/A
Visuospatial skills and executive functions	Ask the patient to draw a clock face, fill in numbers, and draw a watch needle at the specified time	"Draw a clock face, fill in numbers, and draw a watch needle at 10:00."
Abstract reasoning	Ask the examinee to identify a unifying theme of 3 or 4 objects (e.g., all the objects are fruit, vehicles of transportation, or musical instruments)	"Can you put the following items (an apple, a banana and an orange) into one group?"
Judgment	Give the patient a hypothetical scenario and ask him to judge what to do	"What will you do if you see an uncontrolled car on the street?"

3.2 Cranial Nerve Examination

Cranial nerves have more complicated and specific functions, which requires individual tests (Tab. 3.4). Olfactory cranial nerve (1st): Ask the examinee to recognize odors (perfume, vinegar) near each naris while occluding the opposite. Optic cranial nerve (2nd): Visual fields are tested by asking the examinee to follow the wiggling fingers of examiner in 4 visual quadrants. Examiners use Snellen chart to test visual acuity for distance vision or a handheld chart for near vision. Color perception is test using standard pseudoisochromatic ishihara or hardy-rand-ritter plates that have numbers or figures embedded in a field of specifically colored dots. Direct and consensual pupillary responses should be tested. Oculomotor, trochlear and abducens cranial nerve (3rd, 4th, 6th): Direct and consensual pupillary responses should also be tested for parasympathetic function. Ask the examinee to follow a target with eyes only, without turning the head. The pupillary light response is tested for symmetry and briskness. Ptosis, position and nystagmus are observed about the extraocular movements. Trigeminal cranial nerve (5th): Use a cotton swab to test facial sensation (the ophthalmic division is for the forehead, the maxillary division is for the cheeks, and the mandibular division is for the chin) and brush a cotton swab against the lower or lateral cornea to evaluate the corneal reflex. Be careful not to test the mandibular division too laterally, as the mandibular angle is innervated by the great auricular nerve (C2 and C3). Trigeminal motor function is tested by palpating the masseter muscles and temporalis. If a pterygoid muscle is weak, the jaw deviates to that side when the mouth is open. Facial cranial nerve (7th): Let the examinee raise and frown the eyebrows (epicranius), close eyes tightly (orbicularis oculi), show both upper and lower teeth (muscles surround the eyes), smile puff out both cheeks. Test the taste sense of 2/3 of tongue for the special visceral sense. Vestibulocochlear cranial nerve (8th): Hearing is tested by whispering something to one ear while blocking the other ear. Vestibular function can be evaluated by testing for nystagmus. The presence and characteristics of nystagmus help identify vestibular disorders. Glossopharyngeal and vagus cranial nerves (9th, 10th): They are usually evaluated together. Let the examinee say "ah" to see whether the palate elevates symmetrically. If one side is paretic, the uvula is lifted away from the paretic side. Gag reflex is observed when pharynx is touched. Simple hoarseness with normal gag and palatal elevation need a search for compressing the recurrent laryngeal nerve. Accessory cranial nerve (11th): For the upper trapezius, the examinee is asked to shrug the shoulders or turn the head against resistance. Hypoglossal cranial nerve (12th): Evaluate by asking the examinee to extend the tongue and inspecting it for atrophy or weakness.

Tab. 3.4 Cranial nerve examination

No.	Function	Examination
I	Sense of smell	Odor test
II	Afferent pathway for vision	Pupillary light reflex, swinging light test, menace response
III	Pupillary constriaion; extraocular muscles (other)	Pupillary light reflex, inward and upward movement of globe

Continued

No.	Function	Examination
IV	Extraocular muscle (superior oblique)	Ventrolateral rotation of globe
V	Sensory to side of head and face; motor to muscles of mastication	Corneal reflexes, pain perception from head septum, chewing, jaw tone, muscle mass
VI	Extraocular muscle (lateral rectus)	Eyeball retraction (corneal reflex), outward movement of globe
VII	Motor to muscles of facial expression	Corneal reflexes, ear, eyelid and lip (facial) tone reflexes, movement, facial symmetry, taste test
VIII	Afferent branch of vestibular system; sense of hearing	Head posture, induced eyeball movement, nystagmus, normal gait, blindfold test response to noise
IX/X/XI	Sensory and motor to pharynx, larynx	Swallowing, gag reflex, endoscopy, slap test
XII	Motor to tongue	Tongue size and symmetry

3.3 Motor System Examination

Motor system examination includes observing muscle volume, muscle tone, muscle strength, involuntary movement, coordination movement, posture and gait, etc. It can detect the patient's ability to actively exercise or resist resistance, and observe the movement amplitude and duration of muscles.

Muscle strength **Muscle tone**

3.3.1 Muscle Volume

Muscle bulk examination is to observe and compare the muscle volume of bilateral symmetrical parts, if there is muscular atrophy or pseudohypertrophy, observe its distribution range. In addition to naked eye observation, we can also compare the circumference of the same part of limbs on both sides, and those with a difference greater than 1 cm are abnormal. Observe whether there is bundle fibrillation, and tap the muscle abdomen with a percussion hammer to induce bundle fibrillation. Muscular atrophy can be seen in lower motor neuron damage and muscle diseases. Common in gastrocnemius and deltoid muscles, progressive muscular dystrophy can be seen as false hypertrophy of muscles, which is characterized by hypertrophy in appearance, hard touch, and weak muscle strength.

3.3.2 Muscle Tone

Muscle tone is the tension of muscle relaxation and the resistance encountered during passive exercise. During the examination, the patient is instructed to relax his muscles, feel muscle hardness by touching, and passively flex and stretch his limbs to sense resistance.

a. Hypomyotonia is characterized by muscle relaxation and softness, decreased passive movement resistance and expanded joint range of motion. It can be seen in lower motor neuron lesions (such as polyneuropathy and poliomyelitis of anterior horn of spinal cord), cerebellar lesions, some myogenic lesions and shock stage of acute lesions of brain and spinal cord.

b. Hypermyotonia is characterized by hard muscles, increased passive motion resistance and reduced range of joint motion, which can be seen in cone system and extrapyramidal system diseases. The former is characterized by spastic hypertensive muscle, obvious hypertensive upper limb flexor muscle and lower limb extensor muscle, large resistance at the beginning of passive exercise and small at the end, which is called folding knife-like hypermyotonia; the latter is characterized by tonic hypermyotonia, increased tension of extensor and flexor muscles, and uniform resistance when passively moving in all directions, which is also called lead tube-like hypermyotonia (without tremor) or gear-like hypermyotonia (with tremor).

3.3.3 Muscle Strength

Muscle strength refers to the contractile force of muscles. Generally, the functions of muscle group, such as extension, flexion, abduction, adduction, pronation and supination are examined with joints as the center. It is suitable for paralysis caused by upper motor neurondisease and peripheral nerve damage. However, for single nerve damage (such as ulnar nerve, median nerve, radial nerve and common peroneal nerve) and local spinal anterior horn lesions (such as poliomyelitis of spinal anterior horn), it is necessary to examine the corresponding single muscle separately. Muscle strength testing is graded according to the Medical Research Council's scale for muscle power (Tab. 3.5). Grade 4 is often subdivided into 4−, 4, and 4+ to indicate movement against slight, moderate, and strong resistance, respectively. When the six-level (0~5-level) muscle strength recording method is examined, the patient is asked to do muscle contraction exercises in turn. When the examiner gives resistance or tells the patient to maintain a certain posture, the examiner changes the patient's posture to judge the muscle strength.

Tab. 3.5 Medical Research Council's scale for assessment of muscle power

Scale	Description
0	No muscle contraction visible
1	Flicker or trace of contraction, but no movement
2	Active joint movement when effect of gravity is eliminated
3	Active movement against gravity
4	Active movement against gravity and resistance, but weaker than normal
5	Normal power

The following exercises can be selected for muscle strength measurement. Shoulder: abduction and adduction. Elbow: flexion and extension. Wrist: flexion and extension. Finger: flexion and extension. Hip: flexion, extension, abduction and adduction. Knee: flexion and extension. Ankle: dorsiflexion and plantar flexion. Toes: dorsiflexion and plantar flexion. Pet-name ruby neck: flexion and extension. Attending trunk: head up and shoulder in supine position, the examiner gives resistance and observes the contraction force of abdominal muscles;

patients raise head and shoulder in prone position, and the examiner check the contractility of paraspinal muscles. Tab. 3.6 illustrates the examination methods of muscle strength of major muscles.

Paresis that cannot be determined by routine paresis examination can be examined by the following methods.

a. Upper limb horizontal extension test: Both upper limbs are lifted horizontally, palms are upward, and the upper limbs on the paresis side gradually droop and pronate (palms are inward).

b. Barre's finger division test: The fingers of both hands are relatively separated and straightened, and the fingers on the paralyzed side gradually closed and flexed.

c. Little finger sign: The upper limbs are raised horizontally, the palms are down, and the little finger on the paralytic side is often slightly abducted.

d. Jackson's sign: The legs are straight in supine position, and the lower limbs on the paralytic side are often in external rotation position.

e. Lower limb paresis test: Prone position, both knee joints are flexed at right angles, and the calf on the paresis side gradually falls down.

Tab. 3.6 Test methods of main muscle strength

Muscle	Segment	Nerve	Function	Examination method
Deltoid muscle	C5 ~ C6	Axillary nerve	Abduction of upper arm	The upper arm is horizontally outward, and the examiner presses down the elbow
Biceps brachii muscle	C5 ~ C6	Musculocutaneous nerve	Forearm flexion and external rotation	Maintain elbow flexion and forearm rotation position, and the examiner makes it straight and applies resistance
Brachioradialis muscle	C5 ~ C6	Radial nerve	Forearm flexion, pronation	Forearm pronation, then elbow flexion, and the examiner adds resistance
Triceps brachii muscle	C7 ~ C8	Radial nerve	Straightened forearm	The elbow is straightened, and the examiner adds resistance
Extensor carpi muscle	C6 ~ C8	Radial nerve	Straightening of wrist	Maintain the wrist dorsiflexion position, and the examiner presses down from the back of the hand
Flexor carpi	C6 ~ T1	Median nerve, ulnar nerve	Wrist flexion	Maintain the wrist palm flexion position, and lift the examiner from the palm
Muscle extensor digitorum communis	C6 ~ C8	Radial nerve	2 ~ 5 fingers metacarpophalangeal joints are straightened	Keep fingers straight, and the examiner presses at the proximal knuckles
Extensor muscle of thumb	C7 ~ C8	Radial nerve	Straightening of thumb joint	Stretch the thumb, and the examiner adds resistance
Musculus flexor pollicis	C7 ~ T1	Median nerve, ulnar nerve	Flexion of thumb joint	Bend the thumb, and the examiner adds resistance

Continued

Muscle	Segment	Nerve	Function	Examination method
Flexor digitorum	C7~T1	Median nerve, ulnar nerve	Flexion of knuckles	Fingers are flexed, and the examiner lifts up at the knuckles
Flexor carpi radialis	C6~C7	Median nerve	Wrist flexion and abduction	To maintain wrist flexion, the examiner pressurize the radial palm
Flexor carpi ulnaris	C7~T1	Ulnar nerve	Carpal flexion and adduction	To maintain wrist flexion, the examiner pressurizes the ulnar palm
Iliopsoas muscle	L2~L4	Lumbar plexus, femoral nerve	Hip flexion	Lie on back, bend knees, maintain hip flexion, and push thighs toward feet
Quadriceps femoris	L2~L4	Femoral nerve	Knee straightening	Lie on back, stretch knees, and the examiner flexes it
Adductor femoris	L2~L5	Obturator nerve, sciatic nerve	Femoral adduction	Lie on back, lower limbs straight, knees together, the examiner separates the patient's knees to assess strength
Biceps femoris	L4~S2	Sciatic nerve	Knee flexion	Lie prone, maintain knee flexion, and the examiner adds resistance
Gluteus maximus muscle	L5~S2	Inferior gluteal nerve	Hip straightening	Lie on back, knees flexed 90°, knees raised, and the examiner adds resistance
Tibialis anterior muscle	L4~L5	Deep peroneal nerve	Dorsiflexion of foot	Foot dorsiflexion, and the examiner adds resistance
Gastrocnemius muscle	L5~S2	Tibial nerve	Plantar flexion of foot	Knee straighten, plantar flexion foot, and the examiner adds resistance
Female extensor muscle	L4~S11	Deep peroneal nerve	Straightening of toes and dorsiflexion of feet	Dorsiflexion of toes, and the examiner adds resistance
Flexor muscle	L5~S2	Tibial nerve	Metatarsal flexion of toes	Toes plantar flexion, and the examiner adds resistance
Extensor digitorum muscle	14~S1	Deep peroneal nerve	Dorsiflexion of 2 ~ 5 toes of foot	Straighten your toes, and the examiner adds resistance
Flexor digitorum	L5~S2	Tibial nerve	Plantar flexion of toes	Toes plantar flexion, and the examiner adds resistance

3.3.4 Involuntary Movement

Involuntary movement examination is to observe whether the patient has dance-like movements, hand and foot creep, muscle bundle tremor, muscle spasm, tremor (rest, movement and posture) and dystonia, etc., as well as the location, scope, degree and law of occurrence, and the relationship with emotion, movement, cold, drinking, etc., and pay attention to asking about past history and family history.

3.3.5 Coordination Movement

Coordination movement examination is to observe the patient's daily activities first, such as eating, dressing, fastening buttons, taking things, writing, speaking, standing and gait. If there is movement tremor and language setback, etc., then perform the following tests.

a. In the finger-to-nose test, the patient is asked to touch the indicator finger of the examiner 0.5 m away from him with the indicator finger tip, and then touch his own nose tip, and repeat it in different directions at different speeds with eyes open and eyes closed, and compare performance on both sides. Cerebellar hemisphere lesions can be seen as inaccurate finger nose, slow movement or action (intention) tremor when approaching the target, which often exceeds the target (over-finger), which is called dysmetria. Sensory ataxia has no difficulty in pointing nose with eyes open, but obstacles occur when eyes are closed.

Finger to nose test

b. Counterattack sign is also called Holmes rebound test. Ask the patient to fold his shoulder and bend his elbow, supinate his forearm, clench his fist, put his elbow joint on the table or hang close to his body, pull his wrist hard, bend his elbow to resist, and suddenly let it go. Under normal circumstances, the elbow flexion stops immediately and will not hit oneself. Patients with cerebellar diseases lose the ability to adjust quickly, and the elbow flexion force causes the forearm or palm to hit their shoulders or face.

Holmes rebound test

c. In heel-knee-shin test, the patient is asked to take supine position, lift one lower limb up, touch the opposite knee with heel, and then move down along the anterior edge of tibia. Patients with cerebellar damage have poor distance discrimination and intentional tremor when lifting legs and touching knees, and they shake unsteadily when moving down; it is difficult for patients with sensory ataxia to find knees in heels when their eyes are closed.

Heel-knee-shin test

d. In the rotation test, the patient is instructed to pronate and supinate quickly with the forearm or beat the opposite palm continuously and alternately with the palm and back of the hand of one hand, or tap the ground repeatedly and quickly with the toes. Patients with cerebellar ataxia are clumsy, slow and uncoordinated, which is called disdiadochokinesia.

Rotation test

e. Take the supine position in the sit-up test, put hands across chest, and try to sit up without support. Normal people can keep their pelvis and lower extremities still during sit-ups, with the knees straight. Patients with cerebellar lesions present with bilateral lower limb elevation, which are called combined flexion sign positive.

f. In Romberg sign test, patients stood with their feet together, their hands stretched forward and their eyes closed. In Romberg sign test, patients stood with their feet together, their hands stretched forward and their eyes are closed. Patients with sensory ataxia can maintain a stable standing posture when they open their eyes, but they are unstable when they close their eyes. When they close their eyes, they sway back and forth or left and right, which is called Romberg sign positive. Patients with cerebellar ataxia perform standing unstable either with eyes open or closed. The patient tilts to the affected side in the case of a lateral cerebellar lesion or vestibular lesion, and posteriorly in the case of a cerebellar earthworm lesion.

Romberg sign test

3.3.6 Posture and Gait

During posture and gait examination, the examiner should observe the patient's posture, gait, starting condition, stride length and speed from the front, back and side respectively. Ask the patient to stand up quickly from the sitting position, walk normally at a slower and then faster speed, and then turn around. The patient is required to walk on their heels or toes, and walk in a straight line in tandem. When walking in a straight line, the patient can open his eyes first and then close eyes to see if he can keep balance. The wide base when standing and the wide distance between feet when walking indicate balance disorder, which can be seen in cerebellar and sensory ataxia, diffuse cerebrovascular diseases and frontal lobe diseases.

3.4 Sensory System Examination

Sensory system examination is subjective and should be carried out in a quiet environment and stable mood of patients. Examiners should be patient and meticulous, and try their best to make patients fully cooperate. During the examination, look from the sensory loss part to the normal part, from the distal end to the proximal end of the limb, pay attention to the comparison between the left and right, the far and near ends, repeat the examination when necessary, and avoid suggestive questions to obtain accurate data.

3.4.1 Superficial Sensation

During pain examination, alternately gently prick the skin with the tip and blunt end of the pin to ask if it hurts.

During tactile examination, ask the patient to close his eyes, twist cotton into thin strips and touch the skin lightly, ask about the touching part, or let the patient say "1,2,3,…" with the number of touches of the examiner.

Use glass test tubes filled with cold water (0 ~ 10 ℃) and hot water (40 ~ 50 ℃) to contact the patient's skin respectively to distinguish the cold and hot senses. If there is pain and no change in touch, it is generally unnecessary to check the temperature sense. If there is sensory disturbance, the location, scope and bilateral symmetry should be recorded.

3.4.2 Deep Sensation

Let the patient with motion sense close his eyes, the examiner gently clamps both sides of the patient's finger or toe tip with his thumb and indicator finger, and moves up and down by about 5 degrees, so that the patient can distinguish between "upward" and "downward" movement. If the feeling is not obvious, the range of movement can be increased or larger joints can be tested.

The position-aware patient close his eyes, and the examiner puts the patient's limbs in a certain posture and makes the patient describe the posture or imitate it with the opposite limb.

Vibration sense place the sound handle of vibration at bone bulges, such as fingers, styloid process of radius and ulna, olecranon, clavicle, toe, internal and external malleolus, tibia, knee, anterior superior iliac spine and ribs, etc., ask whether there is vibration feeling and duration, and compare them on both sides.

3.4.3 Synthesia Sensation or Cortical Sensation

Position awareness: The patient closes his eyes, the examiner touches the patient's skin lightly with fingers or cotton swabs, and lets him point out the contact area.

Two-point discrimination: The examiner asks the patient to close his eyes and touches his skin with a blunt double foot gauge separated by a certain distance. If the patient feels two points, the distance should be reduced until he feels one point. The two points should be stimulated at the same time and the force should be equal. Normal values of the distance are 2~4 mm at fingertip, 2~3 cm at back of hand and 6~7 cm at trunk.

Graphic awareness: The examiner asks the patient to close his eyes and draws simple figures on the skin with blunt needles, such as triangles, circles or numbers such as 1, 2, 3, etc., so that the patient can distinguish them and compare them bilaterally.

Entity awareness: Let the patient close his eyes and touch common items, such as keys, buttons, pens and coins with one hand, to see if the patient can tell the shape and name of the items, and pay attention to the comparison between the two hands.

3.5 Reflex

Reflex examination includes deep reflex, shallow reflex, clonus and pathological reflex. The examination of reflex is objective and less affected by conscious activities, but the patient should keep quiet and relaxed during the examination. The intensity of reflex activity varies greatly among normal individuals, but it is basically the same up and down on both sides of the same body, so it is necessary to compare the left and right sides or upper and lower limbs when checking reflex. If one side or a single reflex is weakened, disappeared or enhanced, the clinical significance will be greater. The disappearance, attenuation or enhancement of the universality of reflex is not necessarily the manifestation of nervous system damage. According to the change of reflex, it can be divided into hyperactivity, activity (or enhancement), normal, attenuation and disappearance.

3.5.1 Deep Reflection

(1) Biceps reflex

Biceps reflex is innervated by C5~C6 and transmitted through musculocutaneous nerve. In the patient's sitting or lying position, the elbow is flexed at right angles. The examiner's left thumb (sitting position) or left middle finger (lying position) is placed on the tendon of biceps brachii at the patient's elbow, and the right hand holds a percussion hammer to tap the left thumb or middle finger, which reflects the contraction of biceps brachii and causes elbow flexion.

(2) Triceps reflex

Triceps reflex is innervated by C6 ~ C7 and transmitted through radial nerve. In sitting or lying position, the patient's upper arm is abducted and the elbow is half flexed. The examiner holds the patient's upper arm and directly taps the triceps tendon above the olecranon with a percussion hammer, which reflects the contraction of triceps brachii and causes forearm extension.

(3) Radial periosteal reflex

Radial periosteal reflex is innervated by C5 ~ C8 and conducted through radial nerve. In sitting or lying position, the patient's forearm is half flexed and half pronated, and the lower end of radius is tapped during examination, which reflects the contraction of brachioradialis muscle, causing elbow flexion and forearm pronation.

(4) Knee reflex (knee jerk)

Knee reflex is innervated by L2 ~ L4 and conducted through femoral nerve. When the patient takes the sitting position, the knee joint flexes 90°, and the calf naturally droops at right angles to the thigh; in supine position, the examiner lifts the joint from behind the knees with his left hand and flexes at 120°. With his right hand, he taps the quadriceps femoris tendon under the patella with a percussion hammer, and the reflex is calf extension.

(5) Ankle reflex

Ankle reflex is innervated by S1 ~ S2 and conducted through tibial nerve. The patient takes the supine position, bends his knees about 90°, and presents an external booth. The examiner bends the back of the patient's foot at right angles with left hand, taps the Achilles tendon, and the reflection is plantar flexion; or prone position, bend the patient's knees 90°, press his feet with left hand, and then tap the Achilles tendon; or the patient kneels by the bed with his feet hanging outside the bed and the examiner taps the Achilles tendon.

Deep reflection

(6) Clonus

Clonus is a manifestation of high hyperreflexia of tendon, which is seen in pyramidal tract damage. Common ones are as follows. a. Patellar clonus: The patient lies on his back and his lower limbs are straight. The examiner pinches the upper edge of the patella with his thumb and fingers, and suddenly and rapidly push it downward, resulting in continuous rhythmic up-and-down vibration of the patella. b. Ankle clonus: It is more common. The examiner holds the popliteal fossa of the patient with his left hand to make the knee joint semi-flexed, holds the front of the foot with his right hand, exerts force quickly and suddenly to make the dorsiflexion of the foot, and continuously presses the sole with his hand, resulting in rhythmic contraction of Achilles tendon, resulting in alternate flexion and extension of the foot.

(7) Hoffmann sign

Hoffmann sign is innervated by C7 ~ T1 and transmitted through median nerve. The patient's finger is slightly flexed, the examiner holds the patient's wrist with his left hand, clamps the patient's middle finger with his right index finger and middle finger, and quickly moves the nail of the patient's middle finger down with his thumb. The positive reaction is thumb flexion adduction

Hoffmann sign

and other finger flexion.

(8) Rossolimo sign

Rossolimo sign is innervated by L5 ~ S1 and transmitted through tibial nerve. The patient lies on his back, his lower limbs are straight, and the examiner plucks or taps the plantar surface of the toe with his fingers or percussion hammer. The positive reaction is that the toe flexes to the plantar surface. In the past, this sign and Hoffmann sign were included in pathological reflex, which is actually stretch reflex. Positive can be regarded as hyperreflexia of tendon, which can be seen in pyramidal tract damage and normal people with active tendon reflex.

Deep reflex is weakened or disappeared. Damage to any part of the solitary reflex path can cause deep reflex to weaken or disappear, such as peripheral nerve, anterior root, posterior root, posterior root ganglion, anterior horn, posterior horn and posterior cord of spinal cord. Attenuation or disappearance of deep reflex is an important sign of lower motor neuron paralysis, which can make deep reflex disappear during the period of disconnection shock of brain and spinal cord injury; the deep reflex is also affected by the pathological changes in the muscle itself or the joint of the muscles. For example, patients with myasthenia gravis or periodic paralysis who are nervous or pay attention to the examination site may also have deep reflex inhibition; sedative sleeping pills, deep sleep, anesthesia or coma may also cause deep reflex to weaken or disappear.

Deep reflex is enhanced. When the cortical motor area or pyramidal tract is damaged and the reflex arc is complete, the reflex arc of tendon below the damage level is manifested as strong tendon reflex or diffusion phenomenon. Hyperreflexia is an important sign of upper motor neuron damage. In patients with neurosis, hyperthyroidism, tetanus and so on, where the excitability of nervous system is generally increased, tendon reflex may also be enhanced. The essence of Hoffmann sign and Rossolimo sign should belong to stretch reflex (Tab. 3.7).

Tab. 3.7 Deep reflex positioning

Reflex	Inspection method	Reaction	Muscle	Nerve	Segment
Mandibular reflex	Tap the slightly open middle jaw	Mandibular lift	Chewing muscle	Mandibular branch of trigeminal nerve	Pons
Shoulder blade reflex	Tap between two shoulder blades	The scapula moves inward	Teres major and scapula	Subscapular nerve	C5 ~ C6
Biceps reflex	Tap the patient's finger placed on the biceps tendon	Elbow flexion	Biceps brachii	Musculocutaneous nerve	C5 ~ C6
Triceps brachii reflex	Tap the triceps tendon above the eagle's mouth	Elbow extension	Triceps	radial nerve	C6 ~ C8
Radial membrane reflex	Tap the styloid process of radius	Elbow flexion, pronation and finger flexion	Radial muscle, brachial head muscle, pronator muscle, biceps brachii	Median nerve, radial nerve, musculocutaneous nerve	C5 ~ C8
Knee jerk	Tap the ligament of inferior cloth of knee	Knee joint extension	Quadriceps femoris	Femoral nerve	L2 ~ L4

Continued

Reflex	Inspection method	Reaction	Muscle	Nerve	Segment
Achilles tendon reflex	Tap Achilles tendon	The foot flexes toward the plantar surface	Gastrocnemius	Sciatic nerve	S1 ~ S2
Hoffmann sign	Scrap the middle finger cover	Other fingers flex	Flexor digitorum profundus	Median nerve	C7 ~ T1
Rossolimo sign	Tap the plantar surface of the base of the toe	The toes flex toward the metatarsals	Plantar muscle	Tibial nerve	L5 ~ S1

3.5.2 Shallow Reflection

Abdominal reflex

a. Abdominal reflex is innervated by T7 ~ 12 and transmitted through intercostal nerve. The patient lies on his back, slightly flexes his lower limbs to relax his abdominal muscles, and gently scratches the skin of abdominal walls on both sides from outside to inside along the parallel directions of the lower edge of costal arch (T7 ~ 8), umbilical hole level (T9 ~ 10) and upper groin (T11 ~ 12) with blunt needles or bamboo sticks. The reaction is that the abdominal muscles on this side contract, and the umbilical hole shifts to the stimulated part, which are upper, middle and lower abdominal wall reflexes respectively. Obese people and multiparous women cannot be led out.

b. Cremasteric reflex is innervated by L1 ~ 2 and transmitted through genitofemoral nerve. Gently stroke the inner skin of the upper thigh with a blunt needle from top to bottom, and the reaction is that the lateral cremaster muscle contracts to lift the testis. Old and frail patients cannot be led out.

c. Plantar reflex is innervated by S1 ~ 2 and conducted through tibial nerve. Gently stroke the lateral plantar with a bamboo stick, and turn to the medial side from the heel forward to the foot palm at the root of the little toe, reflecting the plantar flexion of the toe.

d. Anal reflex is innervated by S4 ~ 5 and conducted through anococcygeal nerve. The skin around anus is gently scratched with bamboo sticks, and the normal reflex is the contraction of external anal sphincter.

Shallow reflex decreases or disappears. It can be found in both upper motor neuron paralysis and lower motor neuron paralysis. Attention should be paid to coma, anesthesia, deep sleep, baby shallow reflex can disappear within one year old, and abdominal wall reflex of puerpera, obese people and the elderly is often difficult to lead out. Each type of shallow reflex has reflex arc equivalent to the segment, so the weakening or disappearance of shallow reflex has a certain role in locating the segment clinically.

3.5.3 Pathologic Reflex

Babinski sign is a classic pathological reflex, suggesting that pyramidal tract is damaged. The examination method is the same as plantar reflex, and the positive reaction is dorsiflexion of toe, which can be accompanied by fan-shaped expansion of other toes, also known as extensional plantar reflex.

Babinski's allelic sign are as follows. a. Gordon's sign: from the lower part of the lateral malleolus to the lateral side of the dorsal foot; b. Oppenheim's sign: using thumb and indicator finger to slide down from top to bottom along the anterior edge of tibia; c. Scheffer sign: squeezing Achilles tendon with hand; d. Gordon sign: squeeze gastrocnemius muscle with hand; e. Gonda sign: press the 4th and 5th toes hard and suddenly relax after a few minutes; f. Pussep sign: gently stroke the lateral edge of dorsal foot. Positive reactions are dorsiflexion of toes. As for the pathological significance of the positive reaction of these alleles, it is generally considered that they are the same as Babinski's sign.

Babinski sign and allelic sign

Pathological reflex is the exact indication of pyramidal tract damage. Babinski sign is the most important pathological sign, which can be produced by stimulating different parts of lower limbs. Sometimes babinski sign is negative, but it can lead to the other forms of pathological reflex, commonly used are Chaddock sign, Oppenheim sign, Cordon sign, Schaeffer sign and Gonda sign.

3.5.4 Automatic Spinal Reflex

Automatic spinal reflex can occur when the spinal cord is completely transected, which is also called defensive response or retraction response. Spinal cord autonomic reflex in transverse spinal cord lesions, acupuncture on the skin below the lesion plane causes unilateral or bilateral hip, knee and ankle flexion (three short reflex) and Babinski sign is positive. If bilateral flexion is accompanied by abdominal muscle contraction, bladder and rectum emptying, vertical hair, sweating and skin redness below the lesion, it is called total reflex.

References

[1] GLICK T H. Neurologic skills: examination and diagnosis[M]. Boston: Blackwell Scientific Publications, 1993.

[2] SPILLANE J A. Bickerstaff's neurological examination in clinical practice[M]. Oxford: Blackwell Science, 1996.

[3] AMINOFF M J, GREENBERG D A, SIMON R P. Clinical neurology[M]. New York: McGraw-Hill Education, 2002.

[4] ROWLAND L P, PEDLEY T A. Merritt's neurology[M]. 12th ed. New York: Lippineott Williams and Wilkins, 2010.

[5] ROPPER A H, SAMUELS M A, KLEIN J P. Adams and Victor's principles of neurology[M]. 10th ed. New York: McGraw-Hill Education, 2014.

[6] LOUIS E D, MAYER S A, ROWLAND L P. Merritt's neurology[M]. Alphen aan den Rijn: Wolters Kluwer, 2015.

(Wang Xiaoshan, Xu Yuhao)

Chapter 4
Diagnosis Thinking for Neurological Disorders

Determining whether a disease is a nervous system disease or whether a lesion primarily affects the nervous system is the first problem that neurologists need to solve. Many neurological symptoms are caused by diseases of other systems, and some neurological diseases may also manifest symptoms of other systems or organs. Therefore, when diagnosing neurological diseases, clinicians should emphasize the holistic concepts, avoid the one-sided view that only pays attention to one part while ignoring the whole, and comprehensively understand the disease and the organs and systems that may be involved in the disease and lesion, and determine the direction of diagnosis, so as to make a correct diagnosis.

So clinical diagnosis in neurology requires several steps: a. Recognition of the presence and origin of impaired function. b. Identification of what site of the nervous system has been affected, that is, localization. c. Definition of the most likely etiology, often resulting in a differential diagnostic list. d. Use of ancillary procedures to determine which etiology is present in the given patient.

4.1 General Principles of Neurological Disorders

Localization is the diagnostic exercise of determining from the signs or symptoms of the patient what site of the nervous system has been affected by a disease process. Characteristics of dysfunction often pave the way for a relatively precise diagnosis. Localization refers to the determination of where the damage has occurred in the nervous system. The process of localization is commonly divided into three steps: first, to determine whether the lesion is located in the nervous system or skeletal muscle; second, to determine whether the lesion distribution is focal, multifocal, diffused or systemic; third, to determine the specific location of the lesion.

After the primary speculation of the clinical localization, the targeted ancillary procedures will be performed for further confirmation and identification of the primary clinical localization. Qualitative diagnosis is to determine the nature of the disease, also known as etiological diagnosis. There are various categories and symptoms of neurological diseases, and the qualitative diagnosis is one aspect can best reflect the basic clinical skills of Neurology. Qualitative diagnosis requires repeated practice and accumulation.

The word "MID-NIGHTS" is helpful for inexperienced medical students. Of this word, M refers to "malnutrition", I refers to "inflammation", D refers to "degeneration", N refers to "neoplasm", I refers to "infection", G refers to "gland", H refers to "hereditary", T refers to "toxication" or "trauma", and S refers to "stroke". Using this word, the common causes of neurological diseases are evaluated stepwise to avoid omission. Additionally, several principles of qualitative diagnosis should be noted: a. one cause principle, i.e., a single lesion or cause is commonly used to explain all the clinical manifestations and processes of one patient; b. auxiliary procedures should be in accordance with clinical thinking, instead of dominating clinical thinking; c. pseudo sign of the patient should be excluded, e.g., abducens nerve paralysis of patients with intracranial hypertension symptoms has no significance for localization; d. comorbidities should be noted.

4.2 Localization Diagnosis

4.2.1 Localization of the Motor System

Patients with motor deficits may present with plegia or paresis. Plegia denotes complete paralysis; paresis denotes a lesser degree of weakness.

Common patterns of weakness include monoplegia (single limb weakness), hemiplegia (loss of motor function for one side of the body), paraplegia (bilateral loss of lower limb motor function), quadriplegia or tetraplegia (loss of motor function in all four extremities), brachial diplegia (loss of motor function of both upper extremities), or facial diplegia (loss of motor function of both halves of the face).

When examining patients with any of these patterns of weakness, one should have three fundamental questions in mind: a. Where is the lesion? b. Is the lesion focal, multifocal, or diffuse? c. What is the likely underlying cause?

The clinical presentation of the upper motor neuron syndrome following cortical lesions is somewhat different from that of lower motor neurons. Damage to the upper motor neurons results in muscles that are initially weak and flaccid but eventually become spastic exhibiting hypertonia and hyperactive muscle stretch reflexes. Spasticity predominates in antigravity muscles (flexors of the upper extremities and extensors of the lower extremities). Evaluation of muscle tone shows a clasp-knife character. Weakness of upper extremity muscles is most marked in the deltoid, triceps, wrist extensors, and finger extensors; this predilection for involvement of the extensors and supinators explains the pronation and flexion tendencies of the upper limb. Weakness of lower extremity muscles is most marked in hip flexors, knee flexors, foot dorsiflexors, and foot evertors. When the lower motor neurons or their axons are damaged, the innervated muscles will show some combination of the following signs: weakness or paralysis of involved muscles, flaccidity, hypotonia, decreased or absent muscle stretch reflexes (hyporeflexia or areflexia), and eventually muscle atrophy.

Facial weakness may result from an upper or lower motor neuron lesion. Muscles of the upper half of the face, which have bilateral cortical innervation, are not affected in supranuclear lesions, or at least not to the same extent as to the lower facial musculature. Thus, if there is an upper motor neuron type of facial paresis (involvement of the lower half of the face with relative sparing of muscles of the upper half, such as the frontalis and orbicularis oculi) on the same side of the hemiplegia, the lesion is generally localizable above the upper pons. However, a lesion on the cerebral peduncles and upper pons can also cause a hemiplegia or hemiparesis with an associated upper motor neuron type of facial paresis.

Alternating hemiplegia, results in "crossed" signs, with cranial nerves (CN) involvement ipsilateral to the lesion, and contralateral hemiparesis or hemiplegia. For example, a cerebral peduncle lesion may damage the pyramidal fibers and fascicle of CN Ⅲ, causing an ipsilateral oculomotor paresis with pupillary involvement and a contralateral hemiparesis including the lower portion of the face (Weber syndrome).

Single limb weakness may result from an upper motor neuron lesion (e. g., anterior cerebral artery territory infarction or paracentral lobule mass) or an extramedullary spinal cord lesion (e. g., Brown-Séquard syndrome, characterized by ipsilateral lower motor neuron paralysis at the segmental lesional level; ipsilateral spastic paralysis below the level of the lesion due to interruption of the descending corticospinal tract; ipsilateral loss of proprioceptive function below the level of the lesion due to interruption of ascending fibers in the posterior column; and contralateral loss of pain and temperature sensation due to interruption of the crossed spinothalamic tract). However, in patients presenting with isolated monoplegia and no involvement of the homogeneous limb or face, a lower motor neuron type of syndrome (attributable to root, plexus, or nerve lesion) must always be considered.

4.2.2 Localization of Postural and Gait Disorders

(1) Localization

Neurologic disorders of gait and posture can be localized using two main approaches.

1) Characterization of gait disorder

Some types of gait, such as the hemiparetic gait, are highly stereotypic and define the cause as damage to a specific structure (e. g., the corticospinal tract in the case of hemiparesis). Other types of gait, such as the cautious gait or central disequilibrium, may have many different etiologies and the lesion causing it is more difficult to localize.

2) Identification of accompanying neurologic signs

Many lesions causing neurologic gait disorders also cause other neurologic findings that may be helpful in localizing the lesion. In the case of the hemiparetic gait, a Babinski sign pointing to a lesion may be found in the corticospinal tract.

(2) Classification of gait disorders

1) Spastic gait

Corticospinal tract lesions give rise to a spastic gait, unilateral or hemiparetic when the lesion is unilateral and paraparetic when the lesion is bilateral. The leg is externally rotated at the hip. The knee is extended and stiff, so the patient walks as if on a stilt. The foot is plantar flexed and inverted; for this reason, the patient tends to scrape the floor with the outer edge of the foot; the patient turns slowly. With each step the affected leg is rotated away from the body, then toward it (circumduction, Fig. 4.1a). There is also difficulty picking up the toes on the hemiparetic side, when the patient is instructed to walk on the heels and decrease cadence of gait. The lesion can be anywhere along the corticospinal tract.

2) Scissors gait

Patients walk with two legs crossed and adducted. The gait is stiff, and the posture of both lower limbs is like the walking gait of scissors cutting objects. This gait is often caused by injury of bilateral corticospinal tract, e.g., spinal cord or brainstem disorders (Fig. 4.1b).

3) Parkinsonian gait

The patient with Parkinson disease walks with a rigid trunk, reduced arm swing, slow and short steps, and a tendency for the knees to be flexed. The gait of patients with classical

Parkinson disease differs from that with atypical Parkinsonian syndromes, such as progressive supranuclear palsy. Festination, a tendency for the patient to begin running after taking a few steps, may be present with classical Parkinson disease, but seldom with atypical Parkinson syndromes (Fig. 4.1c).

4) Waddling gait

The waddling gait is seen with severe proximal muscle weakness. Weakness of the hip muscles, particularly the gluteus medius, results in an excessive drop of the hip and trunk tilting to the side opposite the foot placement. The hips oscillate up and down with every step, making the patient seem to waddle (Fig. 4.1d).

5) Cerebellar ataxic gait

Lesions of the anterior lobe of the cerebellum can also be accompanied by a discrete impairment in gait, and those affecting the flocculonodular lobe affect equilibrium. Cerebellar lesions may affect gait by causing disequilibrium and by altering limb and trunk kinematics and interlimb coordination. Disturbances of gait and balance are primarily caused by lesions of the vestibulocerebellum and spinocerebellum or their connections. Patients with alcoholic cerebellar degeneration have a widened base, instability of the trunk, slow and halting gait with irregular steps and superimposed lurching. The gait abnormalities are accentuated at the initiation of gait, on turning, and with changes in gait speed (Fig. 4.1e).

6) Steppage gait

Severe deafferentation or a bilateral foot drop may result in an excessive flexion of the hips and knees with every step. With sensory loss, the heel tends to strike the ground heavily. Patients use a greater foot clearance to prevent them from tripping on the toes or on floor irregularities that are poorly felt. The most common cause of this problem is severe thick-fiber neuropathy of the kind encountered with the Guillain-Barré syndrome (Fig. 4.1f).

7) Vestibular ataxia

Acute vestibular lesions cause instability and a tendency for the patient to veer or even fall to the side of the lesion. The base of support is widened and performance is markedly degraded by the Romberg maneuver or when the patient is asked to walk with eyes closed (Fig. 4.1g).

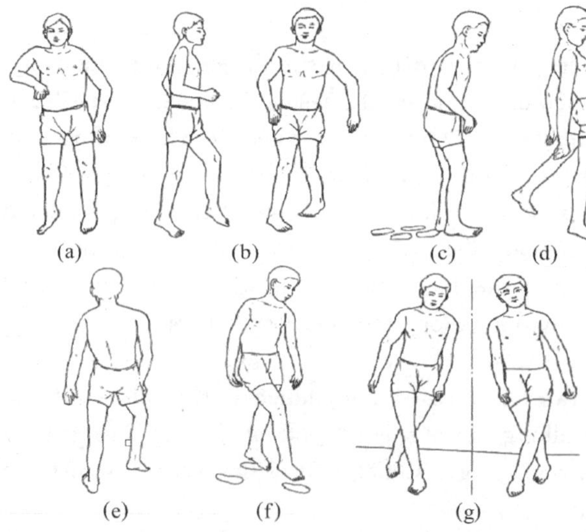

Fig. 4.1 Abnormal gaits

4.2.3 Localization of Cerebral and Cerebellar Lesions

The main clinical manifestations include disorders of conscious level and content, mental disturbance, hemiplegia, partial sensory disorders, hemianopia, seizures and so on. Each lobe lesion also has its own different characteristics, for example, frontal lobe lesion mainly manifests voluntary motor disorder, local epilepsy, motor aphasia, cognitive dysfunction and other symptoms; parietal lobe damage manifests cortical sensory disorders, dyslexia, apraxia and so on; temporal lobe damage manifests mental symptoms, sensory aphasia, psychomotor epilepsy and so on; occipital lobe damage manifests visual field impairment, cortical blindness and so on.

Cerebellar vermis damage mainly induces ataxia of the trunk, cerebellar hemisphere damage induces ataxia of ipsilateral limbs. Sometimes it induces poor cerebellar language and distance discrimination.

4.2.4 Localization of Brain-stem Lesion

One side of the brain-stem lesions manifest ipsilateral peripheral cerebral nerve palsy and contralateral limb central hemiplegia, that is, cross paralysis, or cross sensory disorders of pain and temperature hypoxia at lateral part and contralateral partial of lesions, the specific location of the lesions should be determined according to the damaged brain nerve plane. Bilateral or diffuse damage of the brainstem often results in bilateral damage to most of the cranial nerves and bilateral long tracts.

4.2.5 Localization of Spinal Cord Lesion

Spinal cord transversal injury often manifests motor, sensory and sphincter dysfunction below the site of injury, revealing complete or incomplete paraplegia or quadriplegia, conduction band type sensory disorders and urinary and stool dysfunction. The range of spinal cord damage can be roughly determined according to the highest level of sensory disorders, motor disorders, changes of deep and shallow reflex and autonomic nerve dysfunction. Unilateral damage of the spinal cord may result in spinal cord hemi-ectomy syndrome, which is characterized by loss of contralateral pain and temperature sensation below the lesion level, ipsilateral superior motor neurone paralysis and deep hypoesthesia or loss. Partial lesions of the spinal cord, can only manifest pyramidal tract and anterior horn damage symptoms, such as muscle atrophy amyotrophic lateral sclerosis, as well as pyramidal tract and cable damage symptoms, such as subacute spinal joint degeneration.

4.2.6 Localization of Peripheral Nerve Lesion

Since the spinal nerve is a mixed nerve, there are motor, sensory and autonomic symptoms in its innervated area when it is damaged. Dyskinesia can be seen in inferior motor neurone paralysis, and the extent of sensory impairment is consistent with the damaged peripheral innervation area. The damage of anterior root and posterior root shows motor and sensory disturbance with root distribution respectively. Polyneuropathy presents motor and sensory disturbances of the distal extremities.

4.2.7 Localization of Muscle Lesion

The most common symptom of lesions that damage muscles or nerve-muscle joints is muscle weakness, as well as pathological fatigue, myalgia and tenderness, muscle atrophy, muscle pseudohypertrophy, muscle rigidity and so on. There are no obvious sensory disorders.

4.3 Qualitative Diagnosis

Qualitative diagnosis is the diagnosis to determine the etiology (nature) of the disease, which is based on the localization diagnosis and analysis under the combination of age, gender, medical history, physical examination and various neuroimaging and other auxiliary examinations together. Special attention should be paid to the information of symptom onset and history. Generally, if acute onset rapidly reaches the peak of the disease, vascular lesions, inflammation, trauma and poisoning should be considered; slow onset shows insidious and progressive aggravation without obvious remission during the course of disease, then tumors or degenerative diseases should be considered. If the onset attacks intermittently, epilepsy, migraine or periodic paralysis should be considered.

Herein, the clinical characteristics of several major diseases of the nervous system are listed as follows for reference for clinical qualitative diagnosis.

(1) Vascular disease

The symptom onset is sudden and the symptoms reach peak in a short time (seconds, minutes, hours or days). It is more common in middle-aged and elderly people who has a history of hypertension, atherosclerosis, heart disease, diabetes or hyperlipidemia. Neurological symptoms include headache, dizziness, vomiting, paralysis of limbs, disturbance of consciousness, aphasia and so on. CT, MRI, DSA and other imaging examinations can obtain relatively accurate evidence of central nervous system damage, such as various cerebrovascular diseases.

(2) Infectious disease

The onset of the disease is acute or subacute, and the symptoms reach peak in a few days, or a few weeks. It is accompanied with chills, fever, increased peripheral blood leukocyte or rapid erythrocyte sedimentation rate and other systemic infection poisoning symptoms, nervous system symptoms and the signs are extensive. Specific microbiological, immunological and parasitological examinations of blood and cerebrospinal fluid can further clarify the nature and cause of infection.

(3) Degenerative disease

The onset and course of the disease are slow and progressive. The disease can occur at all ages, for example, Alzheimer's disease usually starts after the age of 60, but some degenerative diseases can also occur in young adults, such as motor neurone disease. Clinical symptoms vary, such as Alzheimer's disease mainly manifests cognitive dysfunction, Parkinson's disease mainly manifests increased muscle tone and motor disorders, motor neurone disease mainly manifests bulbar palsy, limb weakness and muscle atrophy.

(4) Trauma

It has a history of trauma and acute onset. However, some cases also have light trauma, start after a period of time, such as chronic subdural hematoma. A detailed examination of the trauma history is required to distinguish whether the onset is followed by trauma, such as head trauma after an epileptic seizure or stroke. X-ray and CT examinations are helpful for diagnosis.

(5) Tumor

The onset of the disease is slow, the condition shows progressive aggravation. However, some malignancies or metastases develop rapidly and have a short course. In addition to the localized symptoms, such as epileptic seizure, paralysis and numbness, intracranial tumors also show signs of increased intracranial pressure, such as headache, vomiting and apparent papilledema. Cerebrospinal fluid examination may manifest increased protein content and sometimes may find tumor cells. CT, MRI and other examinations can find the source of metastatic tumor.

(6) Demyelinating disease

The symptom onset is acute or subacute, there is tendency of remission and reoccurrence, some cases show slow onset and progressive aggravation. Common related diseases include multiple sclerosis and acute disseminated encephalomyelitis. MRI, cerebrospinal fluid and evoked potential tests are helpful for diagnosis.

(7) Metabolic and nutritional disease

The symptom onset is slow, the course of disease is relatively long. Most of the clinical manifestations are non-specific, and most of them show signs of neurological dysfunction on the basis of systemic symptoms. Diagnosis can be made based on abnormalities of corresponding enzymes, proteins and lipids in tissues and body fluids.

(8) Others

Others include poisoning, genetic diseases and so on. The toxic disease onset of nervous system is acute or chronic, its reasons include chemical, poisonous gas, biological toxin, food, drug poisoning and so on, diagnosis of toxic diseases need to combine medical history and necessary laboratory examination. Genetic diseases of the nervous system are more common in children and young adults, and the same diseases can be found in families with various symptoms and signs, some of which are characteristic.

4.4 Clinical Thinking Methods

Cultivation of clinical thinking of neurologists could be exercised according to the following steps:

a. Cultivate comprehensive and detailed habits, collect full and reliable clinical data through detailed interrogation, physical examination and laboratory examination and exclude some irrelevant signs and unreliable clinical data to avoid disturbance of our attention on clinical judgment.

b. Analyze the above data comprehensively by using the basic knowledge of neuroanatomy and physiology as reasonable as possible to explain the location of the lesion, determine the abnormality of the functional and anatomical structure related to the disease for location diagnosis.

c. According to the lesion location, medical history and physical signs and related laboratory examination results, the final analysis and judgment of the cause of the disease can be determined to make qualitative diagnosis.

d. After defining the nature of the disease, formulate a reasonable treatment plan.

e. According to the nature of the disease, the site of the disease, the comprehensive state of the patient and other factors, the impact of the disease can be evaluated on the patient's physiological function, psychological status, social adaptability and other aspects to judge the patient's prognosis.

References

[1] MARSDEN C, THOMPSON P. Toward a nosology of gait disorders: descriptive classification[M]//MASDEU J, SUDARSKY L, WOLFSON L. Gait disorders of aging, falls and therapeutic strategies. Philadelphia, PA: Lippincott-Raven, 1997:135–146.

[2] GILMAN S. Cerebellum and motor dysfunction[M]//ASBURY A K, MCKHANN G M, MCDONALD W I. Diseases of the nervous system, clinical neurobiology. 2nd ed. Philadelphia, PA: WB Saunders, 1992:319–341.

[3] DIENER H, NUTT J. Vestibular and cerebellar disorders of equilibrium and gait [M]//MASDEU J, SUDARSKY L, WOLFSON L. Gait disorders of aging, falls and therapeutic strategies. Philadelphia, PA: Lippincott-Raven, 1997:261–272.

(Yu Ming, He Yue)

Chapter 5
Clinical Techniques

After thorough medical history inquiry and physical examination, the clinician can determine clinical diagnosis of some diseases. However, laboratory tests are required sometimes to verify the history and physical examination. These auxiliary examinations are of great worth for clinical diagnosis and differential diagnosis of diseases. Selecting reasonable and appropriate auxiliary examination is beneficial to the localization and qualitative diagnosis of neurological diseases. However, it must be clearly recognized that any auxiliary examination has its limitations and should never be applied as a substitute for a thorough medical history and a comprehensive and careful physical examination, as well as clinical thinking. Clinicians must be familiar with or understand the indications, advantages and disadvantages of various auxiliary examination methods to correctly select the examination items, identify the reliability and significance of the examination results, and make a reasonable explanation for the examination results.

5.1 Lumbar Puncture

Cerebrospinal fluid (CSF) is a kind of clear, colorless liquid that fills the cerebral ventricles, subarachnoid space, and central spinal canal. It provides protection, support and nutrition to the brain and spinal cord (Fig. 5.1). Most CSF are absorbed through the superior sagittal sinus by the arachnoid granulation of the brain dome, and few is absorbed through the spinal nerve root space. The average amount of CSF in adults is 130 mL, and the formation rate is 0.3 ~ 0.5 mL/minutes, among which, about 500 mL are generated daily. The changes of physiological and biochemical characteristics of CSF are of great worth in the diagnosis, differential diagnosis, evaluation of curative effect and prognosis of central nervous system infection, subarachnoid hemorrhage, meningeal carcinoma, demyelination and so on. CSF is usually collected through lumbar puncture. In special cases, cerebellomedullary cistern puncture or lateral ventricle puncture are also performed. Diagnostic puncture can also inject contrast agent and air for imaging; therapeutic puncture is mainly used for injecting drugs or internal and external drainage and so on.

Lumbar puncture is a common auxiliary examination in neurology, which has great value in the diagnosis of diseases. Its indications, contraindication and complications should be correctly mastered.

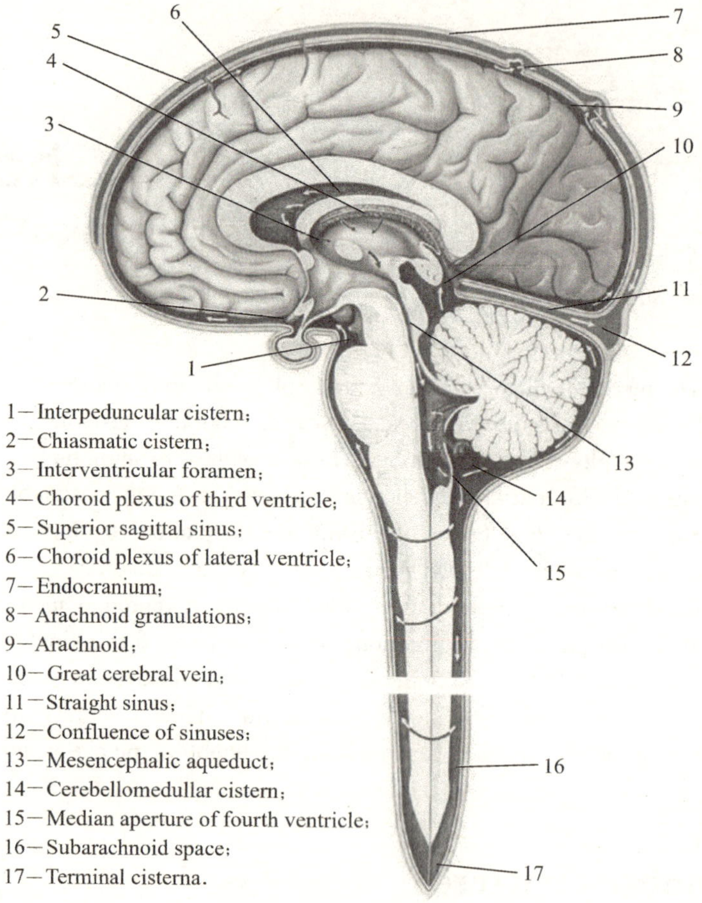

Fig. 5.1 Anatomy of CSF

(1) Indications

a. Retain CSF for various tests to help the diagnosis of central nervous system diseases.

b. Suspection of abnormal intracranial pressure.

c. Observe the changes of CSF dynamically to help judge the condition, prognosis and guide the treatment.

d. Radionuclide injection to scan the brain and spinal cord.

e. Inject fluid or release CSF to maintain or adjust the intracranial pressure balance, or inject drugs to treat the corresponding disease.

(2) Contraindications

a. Intracranial pressure is significantly increased, or there are signs of cerebral hernia, especially space occupying lesions in the posterior fossa are suspected.

b. The puncture site has infection, spinal tuberculosis or patulous injury.

c. It is not suitable to move due to obvious bleeding tendency or in critical condition.

d. The spinal cord function of spinal cord compression is at a critical state of imminent loss.

5.1.1 Operation Steps

a. Take the bent decubitus position (more left decubitus position), the patient with flexed neck hugs knees, his back should be perpendicular to the examination bed and the spine is parallel to the bed.

b. The puncture site is determined by making a line along the highest point of bilateral iliac spines, and the fourth lumbar spinous process is the intersection of the line with the midline of the spine, and then select the 4th~5th or 3rd~4th intervertebral space for the puncture.

c. After local routine disinfection and towel laying, 2% lidocaine is chosen to perform local intradermal and subcutaneous anesthesia at the puncture point, then the needle is stabbed into the ligament, next the needle is drawn back without blood, and the anesthetic is injected into the patient while the needle is removing.

d. After the anesthesia takes effect, the skin of the puncture site is fixed with one hand and the needle is slowly pierced along the direction of the spinous process with the other hand. When the adult needle is inserted about 4~6 cm, the dural membrane can be penetrated to the subarachnoid space, and the core of the needle can be extracted to drain the cerebrospinal fluid.

e. After measuring the pressure and collecting the cerebrospinal fluid, the core of the needle can be inserted and then pulled out.

f. The puncture point is applied with sterilized gauze and fixed with adhesive tape. Ask the patient to lie supinely for 4~6 hours after operation. (Fig. 5.2)

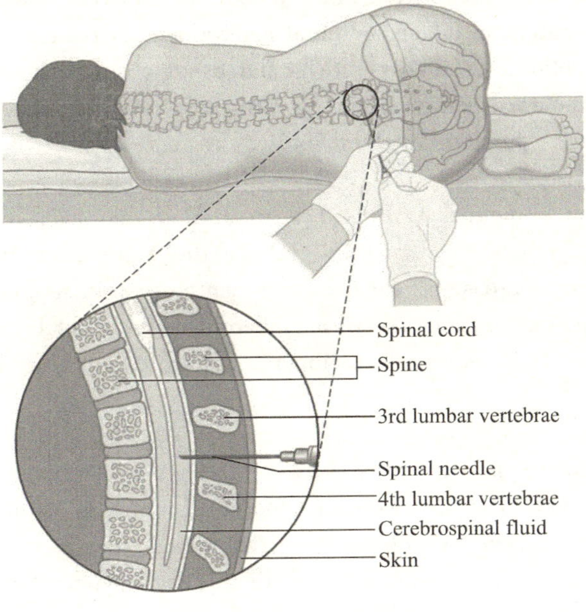

Fig. 5.2 Lumbar puncture operation

5.1.2 Cerebrospinal Fluid Analysis

(1) Characteristics

Normal CSF is colorless and transparent. If the CSF is bloody or pink, the three-tube test method can be used to distinguish, that is, using three test tubes to collect CSF continuously. Blood color is uniform and consistent in three tubes, indicating subarachnoid hemorrhage. The color of the anterior and posterior tubes decreased in order, indicating puncture injury and bleeding. Hemorrhagic CSF becomes colorless after centrifugation, indicating fresh bleeding or injury. The color is yellow after centrifugation, indicating old bleeding. CSF is cloud shape, suggesting bacterial infection leading cell number to increase, which can be seen in all types of suppurative meningitis, severe one can show rice soup sample. Fibrin membrane formation after CSF placement can be seen in tuberculous meningitis. When the CSF protein is too high, it is yellow in appearance and automatically solidifies soon after isolation, which is called Froin syndrome and can be seen in spinal canal obstruction and so on. Greenish cerebrospinal fluid can be seen in pseudomonas aeruginosa meningitis and streptococcus meningitis.

(2) Cell count

The leukocyte count in normal CSF is $(0 \sim 5) \times 10^6$ g/L, most of which are monocytes. Leukocyte increase is more common in the inflammatory lesions of the meninges and parenchyma of the brain; significant leukocytes increase with mostly multiple nuclear cells is mainly found in acute suppurative meningitis; mild or moderate leukocytes increase with mostly mononuclear cells is often seen in viral encephalitis; a large number of lymphocytes or monocytes increase is mainly seen in subacute or chronic infections; relative eosinophils increase is seen in parasitic infections of the brain.

(3) Protein

The protein content in normal CSF is 0.15~0.45 g/L. Significant increase of CSF proteins are common in suppurative meningitis, tuberculous meningitis, guillain-Barre syndrome, central nervous system malignant tumor, cerebral hemorrhage, subarach noid cavity hemorrhage and spinal canal obstruction, especially with spinal canal obstruction increased significantly. Decreased CSF proteins are seen in patients with loss of CSF, extreme weakness, and malnutrition due to lumbar puncture or dural injury.

(4) Sugar

The level of sugar in normal CSF is 1/2 to 2/3 of the level of blood glucose, and the normal value is 2.5 ~ 4.4 mmol/L (45 ~ 60 mg/dL), the abnormal value is less than 2.25 mmol/L. Significant decreases of sugar content can be seen in suppurative meningitis, and mild or moderate decreases can be seen in tuberculous or fungal meningitis (especially cryptococcal meningitis) and meningeal carcinomatosis. Increased sugar levels can be seen in diabetes.

(5) Chloride

The level of chloride in normal CSF is 120~130 mmol/L, which is about 1.2~1.3 times higher than that in blood. The decrease of chloride content is common in patients with electrolyte disturbances caused by tuberculous, bacterial, fungal meningitis and systemic diseases, especially tuberculous meningitis. Patients with hyperchloremia may also have increased levels of chloride in their CSF.

(6) Special examination

In recent years, the research on immune related diseases has made great progress, which has promoted new clinical testing projects. For example, the detection of ganglioside antibodies is helpful in the diagnosis of acute Guillain-Barre syndrome and ganglioside antibody spectrum diseases. The detection of aquaporin antibody is helpful to the diagnosis of neuromyelitis optica spectrum disease. Hu, Yo, Ri and other paraneoplastic-associated antigen and antibody indicators have important significance in tumor-associated central damage. Detection of *N*-methyl-D-asparticacid (NMDA) receptor antibodies has been used in clinical diagnosis of anti-NMDA receptor encephalitis.

(7) Pressure

Pressure is generally measured when the patient keep fully relaxed. Cerebrospinal fluid rises to a certain height in the pressure tube until it no longer continues to rise, the pressure at this time is initial pressure. The final pressure is measured after released a certain amount of cerebrospinal fluid. The normal pressure in the decubitus position generally is 80~180 mmH_2O in adults, the value greater than 200 mmH_2O indicates increased intracranial pressure and the value less than 80 mmH_2O indicates decreased intracranial pressure. Pressure increase can be seen in intracranial space-occupying lesions, brain trauma, intracranial infection, subarachnoid hemorrhage, venous sinus thrombosis, benign intracranial pressure increase and so on. The main causes of pressure decrease are hypotensive cranial pressure, dehydration, shock, spinal subarachnoid obstruction, cerebrospinal fluid leakage and so on.

5.2 Imaging Examination

5.2.1 Computed Tomography

Computed tomography (CT) is a medical imaging technology, which combines digital imaging technology with X-ray tomography technology. Its scanning inspection is convenient, rapid, and its safe density resolution is obviously better than traditional X-ray image, which can significantly improve the accuracy of diagnosis and has important diagnostic value for central nervous system diseases. There are many technology of CT used widely now, including plain CT scan, contrast-enhanced CT, spiral CT, computerized tomography angiography (CTA), CT perfusion imaging, etc.

For neurological diseases, CT scanning is mainly applied for the diagnosis of cerebral hemorrhage, cerebral infarction, brain tumor, hydrocephalus, brain atrophy and some diseases in the spinal canal. In special cases, iodic contrast medium can be used to enhance tissue imaging to confirm the diagnosis.

5.2.2 Magnetic Resonance Imaging

Magnetic resonance imaging (MRI) is a biomagnetic nuclear spin imaging technique firstly used in clinic in the early 1980s. Compared with CT, MRI can manifest the anatomical structure of any section of the human body, with high resolution of soft tissue, bony artifact-free, and can clearly show the lesions areas in the spinal cord, brain stem and posterior fossa. In addition, MRI has no ionizing radiation, thus it has no radioactive damage to the human body. However, the inspection time of MRI is relatively long, and patients with magnetic metal implants cannot be inspected by MRI.

(1) MRI techniques introduction

In recent years, except conventional MRI, a variety of new MRI techniques have emerged, including magnetic resonance angiography (MRA), magnetic resonance venography (MRV), MR-perfusion weighted imaging (MR-PWI), diffusion-weighted imaging (DWI), magnetic resonance spectroscopy (MRS), diffusion tensor imaging (DTI), sensitivity weighted imaging (SWI), high resolution magnetic resonance imaging (HMRI), functional magnetic resonance imaging (FMRI) and so on, which have greatly promoted the development of neuroscience.

(2) Clinical applications of MRI in diagnosis of neurological diseases

1) Cerebral infarction

Signal changes in different stages are shown in Tab. 5.1.

Tab. 5.1 Signal changes of cerebral infarction in different stages

No.	Time	Characteristic
1	Within 12 hours	Normal vascular flow disappears, T_1WI and T_2WI signal changes are not obvious, the cerebral sulcus disappears, gyri swells, gray matter boundary disappears, DWI appears high signal
2	12~24 hours	Infarction lesions show equal T_1 or slightly longer T_1 and long T_2 signal, and DWI appears high signal
3	1~3 days	Infarction lesions show long T_1 and T_2 signals, DWI appears high signal and edema and mass effect, complicated with post-infarction hemorrhage
4	4~7 days	Edema and mass effect are obvious, T_1 and T_2 signals are significantly longer and DWI signal begins to decrease
5	1~2 weeks	The lesion shows long T_1 signal, increasing long T_2 signal, DWI signal continuous to decrease, T_2WI signal is stronger than DWI signal
6	Over 2 weeks	T_1 is longer than T_2, with clear boundaries and fancy-shaped shapes, showing signs of local brain atrophy, such as enlarged ventricles and widened sulci

2) Intracerebral hemorrhage

MRI signals are different at different stages of intracerebral hemorrhage, which depend on the changes of oxygenated hemoglobin, deoxygenated hemoglobin, methemoglobin and hemosiderin. Generally speaking, within 7 days after bleeding, T_1WI shows equal signal and T_2WI shows slightly lower signal. 1~4 weeks after bleeding, both T_1WI and T_2WI show high signal; one month after bleeding, T_1WI shows low signal, T_2WI shows high signal in the center and low signal in the periphery. MRI is not recommended for the diagnosis of early intracerebral hemorrhage due to the lack of characteristic manifestation. However, recent researches have found that magnetic resonance gradient echo (GRE) can detect intracerebral hemorrhage at early stage, and the diagnostic accuracy of acute intracerebral hemorrhage is similar to that of CT, and the detection of new or old microhemorrhage lesions is better than that of CT.

3) Brain tumors

MRI is superior to CT in the detection of poorly differentiated and relatively small tumors and metastases. The characteristics of signal intensity are associated with the water content of the tumor, but the intratumoral and periatumoral hemorrhage, edema, necrosis, cystic degeneration, calcification and other changes can affect the signal intensity and characteristics of the tumor. Enhanced scan is of great help in the diagnosis of tumors, especially pia, dural, and meningeal metastases.

4) Cerebrovascular diseases

MRA can identify a variety of cerebrovascular abnormalities, using the flow cavity effect to find arterio-venous malformations can not only show the location and size of vascular malformations, sometimes also show its supply artery and drainage veins.

5) Leukodystrophy and demyelination

MRI is very sensitive in observing white matter structures, such as leukodystrophy and multiple sclerosis.

6) Intracranial infection

Head MRI scan is very sensitive in the diagnosis of herpes simplex encephalitis, whose typically characteristics are long T_2 signals in the temporal lobe, hippocampus, and limbic system.

7) Neurodegenerative diseases

MRI is superior to CT in the diagnosis of dementia. It can observe the degree of hippocampal atrophy by hippocampus volume measurement, which is associated with the severity of Alzheimer's disease.

5.2.3 Digital Subtraction Angiography

Digital subtraction angiography (DSA) is an imaging technique derived from the combination of traditional angiography and electronic computer. It has significant practical value, especially in the diagnosis and treatment of cerebrovascular diseases. The optical images are obtained by X-ray casting into the human body, after image enhancement video scanning and digital-to-analog conversion, the images of bone and brain tissue can be removed by subtraction finally after digital processing, and the vascular images filled with contrast agent are retained to produce real-time dynamic vascular images.

5.2.4 Electroencephalography

Electroencephalography (EEG) is an examination technology of biological electrical activity of the brain, which is the most objective means of diagnosis and classification of epilepsy by measuring spontaneous and rhythmic biological electrical activity to understand the functional state of the brain.

EEG is mainly used for diagnosis, classification and location of epileptic lesions, which has auxiliary diagnostic value to distinguish organic or functional brain lesions from diffuse or localized lesions, encephalopathy caused by various reasons, such as encephalitis, toxicity and metabolism.

(1) Normal adult EEG

The basic rhythm of the EEG is the α rhythm at 8~13 Hz, and the amplitude of 20~100 μV is mainly distributed in the occipital and apical regions in the awake, quiet and relaxed state; the frequency of β activity ranges from 14 Hz to 25 Hz and the amplitude of 5~20 μV is mainly distributed in the frontal and temporal lobes; a small amount of θ wave at 4~7 Hz can be seen in front of cerebral hemisphere of certain normal people; the frequency below 4 Hz is called δ wave, which is almost absent in normal awake people, but can appears when they are asleep, and gradually increases from shallow to deep. Brainwaves with frequencies below 8 Hz are called slow waves.

(2) Sleep EEG

According to eye movement, it can be divided into non-rapid eye movement (NREM) and rapid eye movement (REM). (Tab. 5.2)

Tab. 5.2 **The characteristic of sleep EEG in different stages**

Stage	Characteristic
NREM 1	A transient stage from awake state to asleep state, the α rhythm gradually disappears and is replaced by low amplitude slow waves, a transient high amplitude bilateral symmetric negative phase wave called "V" wave appears at the top
NREM 2	Sleep spindles (12~14 Hz) appears on the basis of low-amplitude brainwaves
NREM 3	High amplitude slow wave (δ wave) appears on the basis of sleep spindles in the third stage, but the proportion is less than 50%
NREM 4	The sleep spindles gradually decrease to disappear, and its proportion reaches more than 50%
REM	EEG changes from the main δ waves with high amplitude in NREM stage 4 to the θ waves with mixed frequency and interval low amplitude, the α wave is 1~2 Hz slower than that in waking state, and a small amount of fast waves are mixed

(3) Common abnormal EEG

Diffuse slow wave: The background activity is diffuse slow wave, which is a common abnormity without specificity.

Focal slow wave: Mainly caused by local brain parenchymal dysfunction. It is mainly seen in focal epilepsy, herpes simplex encephalitis, brain abscess, focal subdural or epidural hematoma and so on.

Triphasic wave: It usually refers to a negative-positive-negative or positive-negative-positive wave with medium to high amplitude and frequency at 1.3~2.6 Hz. It is mainly seen in Creutzfeldt-Jakob disease (CJD), hepatic encephalopathy and toxic metabolic encephalopathy caused by other factors.

Spike wave: The waveform is a sudden transient wave with a sharp tip, lasting for 20~70 ms. Its main component is negative phase, and its amplitude is variable, showing typical spinous wave with steep ascending branch and acclive descending branch. It is mainly seen in epilepsy.

Sharp wave: The waveform is similar to the spike wave, but the time limit is wider than that of spike wave, which is 70~200 ms. It is usually negative phase and its amplitude is 100~200 μV. It is mainly seen in epilepsy.

3 Hz spike and ware complex: A spinous wave followed by a slow wave, which is easily induced by hyperventilation. It is often seen in typical absence seizure.

Multiple spike wave: Two or more high-amplitude biphasic spike waves appear rhythmically. It is often seen in myoclonic and tonic-clonic seizures.

Sharp and slow wave complex: It consists of a sharp wave and the following slow wave. It is mainly seen in epileptic seizures.

Multiple spike and slow wave complex: More than one spinous wave and a following slow wave, whose frequency is 2~3 Hz. It often appears in a single form or bilateral synchronous symmetry form. It is often seen in myoclonic epilepsy.

Hypsarrhythmia: Refers to the discharge of the spike wave and spike wave with high amplitude, and then there is a period of static electrical activity. It is often seen in infantile spasm, phenylketonuria and other patients.

5.2.5 Magnetoencephalography

Magnetoencephalography (MEG) is a record of spontaneous neural magnetic fields of brain tissue. The magnetic field of brain tissue that is detected and recorded under stimulation of sound, light and electricity is called induced brain magnetic field. This technology began in the 1970s, with the development of computer technology and imaging information processing technology, especially the application of superconducting quantum interference devices (SQUID), the design and performance of magnetoencephalography have been fundamentally changed. It has been applied in clinical research since the 1990s, but has not been applied in clinical practice as a routine auxiliary examination method due to high price and other reasons.

MEG works by using a SQUID multi-channel sensor system to detect bio-electromagnetic fields generated by excitatory postsynaptic potentials of neurons. Compared with EEG, the former has good spatial resolution and can detect epileptic foci with a diameter less than 3.0 mm, with small error of localization and high sensitivity. In addition, it can be applied to locate brain functional areas and epileptic discharge foci by combined with anatomical image information, such as MRI and CT, which is helpful for surgical treatment to refractory epilepsy. However, only a few hospitals use it presently due to expensive cost.

5.2.6 Evoked Potential

Evoked potential (EP) is a biological electrical activity produced by the nervous system when affecting by external or internal stimulation. The amplitude of most evoked potentials (also known as signals) is very small, only 0.1 ~ 20 μV, which is drowned in spontaneous brain electrical activity (amplitude at 25 ~ 80 μV) or various artifacts (collectively called noise). The average technique and superposition technique must be adopted, that is, repeat the same stimulus several times to increase the induced electrical activity and expose it. At present, sensory pathways, such as somatosensory, visual and auditory pathways, as well as motor pathways and cognitive functions can be examined.

5.2.7 Electromyography and Nerve Conduction Velocity

Electromyography (EMG) and nerve conduction velocity (NCV) are important auxiliary examinations of the nervous system. They are usually used in combination, and their indication is lesions of spinal cord anterior horn cells, mainly used for diagnosis of lesions of peripheral nerve, neuromuscular junction and muscle. EMG includes conventional EMG, motor unit count, single fiber EMG and so on.

(1) Electromyography

Electromyography or conventional EMG, is a technique, which uses concentric needle electrodes to record the electrical activity of muscles at rest and in varying degrees of voluntary contraction.

(2) Nerve conduction velocity

Nerve conduction velocity is a diagnostic technique to assess the conduction function of peripheral nerves, usually including motor nerve conduction velocity (MNCV) and sensory nerve conduction velocity (SNCV).

Clinical application of NCV: The detection of NCV is applied in the diagnosis and differential diagnosis of peripheral neuropathy caused by various reasons. It can detect the subclinical lesions of peripheral neuropathy and distinguish the axonal damage from myelinoclasis. Combined with EMG, it can distinguish anterior horn cells, nerve roots, peripheral nerves, myogenic lesions and so on.

5.2.8 Carotid Ultrasonography

Carotid artery ultrasound is a noninvasive method widely applied in clinic, which can objectively detect and evaluate the structure, functional status or hemodynamic changes of the carotid artery. It is of great significance to the diagnosis of head and neck vascular diseases, especially ischemic cerebrovascular diseases.

5.2.9 Transcranial Doppler

Transcranial doppler (TCD) is a noninvasive technique that uses weak areas of the skull as acoustic windows and use doppler shift effect to study hemodynamics of the main subcerebral arteries. In 1982, Rune Aaslid first established the TCD diagnosis method. Due to the advantages of real-time, portable, non-invasive, repeatable and long-range monitoring, TCD is widely applied in clinic and plays a significant role in the diagnosis of neurological diseases.

5.2.10 Radionuclide Examination

Nuclear medicine imaging, that is, radionuclide imaging, is a kind of imaging method reflecting function and metabolism, which includes single photon emission computed tomography (SPECT) and position emission tomography (PET). SPECT mostly uses radiopharmaceutics that can pass through the blood-brain barrier to manifest the local distribution of cerebral blood flow. PET mainly uses positron radionuclides and their labeled compounds to manifest the local brain glucose metabolism, the distribution and number of cerebral receptors and the distribution of cerebral blood flow.

(1) Single photon emission computed tomography

The 3D imaging method of SPECT provides a relatively accurate, safe and inexpensive method for the display and measurement of cerebral blood flow changes, which can assist in the diagnosis of some neurological diseases. Compared with the structural images, such as CT and MRI, SPECT imaging can get the cerebral function data, which cannot be obtained by the former two methods, and has relative advantages in the diagnosis of some diseases.

(2) Position emission computed tomography

PET is an image manifesting brain metabolism and function, such as local cerebral glucose metabolism, amino acid metabolism, oxygen metabolism and cerebral blood flow, as well as the location, density and distribution of nerve receptors. With the advent of advanced instruments, such as PET/CT and PET/MRI that can simultaneously manifest the anatomical structure and functional metabolism and the successful application of multimodal imaging and new imaging agents, PET can provide more accurate location and quantification, and display the cerebral physiological and pathological changes from the molecular level.

PET makes up for the deficiency of simple anatomic morphological imaging. It can reflect the changes of local brain function, and can find the abnormalities of local brain metabolism before the occurence of structural changes of the brain caused by the disease, which has significant clinical application.

5.2.11 Biopsy of Brain Tissue

Biopsy of brain tissue is a method for pathological examination by sampling local brain tissue, which can provide significant evidence for the diagnosis of some brain diseases.

Brain biopsy is a traumatic examination, which may lead loss of brain function. Sometimes, it is difficult to determine the diagnosis even if the biopsy is performed, thus the advantages and disadvantages should be considered and the indications should be strictly mastered.

5.2.12 Nerve Biopsy

Sural nerve biopsy is the most commonly used nerve biopsy, which is helpful to determine the nature and degree of peripheral nerve lesions and is a significant basis for diagnosis of the etiology of peripheral nerve diseases.

The causes of peripheral neuropathy are very complex, and sural nerve biopsy also has limitations. Some toxic, metabolic and inherited peripheral neuropathy lack specific pathological changes, thus the diagnosis of peripheral neuropathy needs to be considered in combination with clinical and other laboratory results.

5.2.13 Muscle Biopsy

Muscle biopsy is a commonly used pathological examination method in clinic, its main clinical indications contain: a. diagnosis and differential diagnosis of muscle diseases; b. distinguishing neurogenic or myogenic muscle damage; c. determine whether there is muscle tissue involvement, vascular inflammation or abnormal substance deposition in muscle mesenchyme in systemic diseases (such as secretory myopathy) with muscle weakness.

Due to the limitation of sampling and methodology, although muscle pathological examination can provide great help for clinical diagnosis, it still has some limitations. Only by combining the results of family history, clinical manifestations and other examinations, can the final diagnosis be determined.

5.2.14 Gene Diagnosis Technique

Gene diagnosis, also called molecular diagnosis, refers to the use of molecular biology techniques to analyze whether the structure (DNA level) or function (RNA level) of a specific gene of the client are abnormal, so as to diagnose the corresponding disease, which is one of the important etiological diagnosis techniques. Genetic diagnosis can not only make an exact diagnosis of some diseases, but also determine the status related to the disease, such as the susceptibility, type and stage of disease. The methods of gene diagnosis mainly include DNA detection, gene linkage analysis and mRNA detection. Common techniques for gene diagnosis include nucleic acid hybridization, polymerase chain reaction (PCR), gene sequencing, gene chip and so on.

Genetic diagnosis can make up for the deficiency of clinical (phenotype) diagnosis of genetic diseases of nervous system, help early diagnosis, provide a new method and basis for the classification of genetic diseases, and provide a new method for the treatment of genetic diseases. At the same time, we should also note that the basis of genetic diagnosis is still clinical diagnosis, many genetic diseases cannot be diagnosed until the gene mutation type and its distribution pattern are clear. Only on the basis of correct clinical diagnosis can the genetic diagnosis methods be reliable.

References

[1] ROPPER A H, SAMUELS M A, KLEIN J, et al. Adams and Victor's principles of neurology[M]. New York: McGraw-Hill Education/Medical, 2019.

[2] ALBERT M S, DEKOSKY S T, DICKSON D, et al. The diagnosis of mild cognitive impairment due to Alzheimer's disease: recommendations from the National Institute on Aging-Alzheimer's Association workgroups on diagnostic guidelines for Alzheimer's disease [J]. Alzheimer's & Dementia, 2011, 7(3):270-279.

[3] MEYERS P M, SCHUMACHER H C, HIGASHIDA R T, et al. Indications for the performance of intracranial endovascular neurointerventional procedures. A scientific statement from the American Heart Association Council on Cardiovascular Radiology and Intervention, Stroke Council, Council on Cardiovascular Surgery and Anesthesia, Interdisciplinary Council on Peripheral Vascular Disease, and Interdisciplinary Council on Quality of Care and Outcomes Research[J]. Journal of NeuroInterventional Surgery, 2010, 2(2):177-188.

[4] POWERS W J, RABINSTEIN A A, ACKERSON T, et al. 2018 guidelines for the early management of patients with acute ischemic stroke: a guideline for healthcare professionals from the American Heart Association/American Stroke Association[J]. Stroke: A Journal of Cerebral Circulation, 2018, 49(6):E233-E234.

(Li Jingwei, Chen Siyuan)

SECTION II

Common Clinical Diseases

Chapter 6

Cerebrovascular Diseases

Cerebrovascular disease (CVD), also called stroke, is a general term of brain dysfunction caused by cerebrovascular diseases. Localized or diffuse brain dysfunction is caused by vascular cavity occlusion or stenosis, vascular rupture, vascular malformation, vascular wall damage or permeability changes, except for global cerebral ischemia or hypoxia is caused by factors, such as hemodynamic abnormalities and diffuse brain dysfunction. Stroke is the third most common cause of human fatal diseases following heart disease and cancer, and is also the leading disabling disease in adults.

6.1 Cerebrovascular Anatomy

6.1.1 Arterial System

(1) Anterior circulatory system

Anterior circulatory system, which supplies blood to the front brain, consists of the common carotid artery, the external carotid artery, the internal carotid artery, the anterior cerebral artery, the middle cerebral artery and various branches. The blood supply area accounts for about 3/5 of the brain, including the eyes, frontal lobe, temporal lobe, insula, parietal cortex, white matter, basal ganglia and so on.

a. Common carotid artery (CCA) has different starting points on both sides, the right side originates from the brachiocephalic trunk behind the sternoclavicular joint, and the left side originates from the autonomous arterial arch. The bifurcation of the common carotid artery is the prone site of atherosclerotic plaque formation.

b. The external carotid artery (ECA) is generally emitted by the common carotid artery at the superior margin of thyroid cartilage, which is anterior to the medial side of the internal carotid artery, and then transferred to the lateral side through its front, ascending and issuing superior thyroid artery, lingual artery, facial artery, ascending pharyngeal artery, posterior auricular artery, occipital artery, superficial temporal artery and maxillary artery.

c. The internal carotid artery (ICA) is the larger one of the two terminal branches of the common carotid artery. Its starting part is located in the posterior lateral of the external carotid artery, then turned to the posterior medial side, through the carotid artery tube into the skull, then through the cavernous sinus, ending above the anterior clinoid process. It emits the anterior cerebral artery from the middle cerebral artery.

d. Anterior cerebral artery (ACA) is one of the terminal branches of internal carotid artery. It runs above the optic nerve, walks forward and inwardly, enters the longitudinal fissure of the brain, connects with the opposite homonymous artery by the anterior communicating artery (AComA), and then moves backward along the corpus callosum sulcus. It mainly supplies blood to the medial side of frontal parietal lobe, caudate nucleus, basal ganglia, corpus callosum and basal frontal lobe.

e. Middle cerebral artery (MCA) can be considered as a direct continuation of the internal carotid artery. It originates from the deep part of the lateral fissure of the brain and runs on the surface of the insula posteriorly to the external part, including the temporal lobe, anterolateral frontal lobe, insula, parietal lobe, and basal ganglia.

(2) Posterior circulation system

Posterior circulation system, also called vertebrobasilar artery system, is composed of vertebral artery, basilar artery, posterior cerebral artery (PCA) and their branches. It covers about 2/5 of the brain, including the brainstem, cerebellum, occipital lobe, posterior temporal lobe, thalamus and so on. (Fig. 6.1)

a. Vertebral artery (VA) contains two branches on both sides, it is the largest branch of the subclavian artery. Generally, both vertebral arteries merge into one basilar artery. The branches include the posterior meningeal artery, anterior spinal artery, posterior spinal artery, and posterior inferior cerebellar artery.

b. Basilar artery (BA) is formed by the convergence of bilateral vertebral arteries at the lower margin of the pons. It runs along the basilar sulcus of pons to the superior margin of the pons and is divided into two terminal branches including the left and right posterior cerebral arteries. The main branches are pontine perforating branch, anterior inferior cerebellar artery, superior cerebellar artery and posterior cerebral artery.

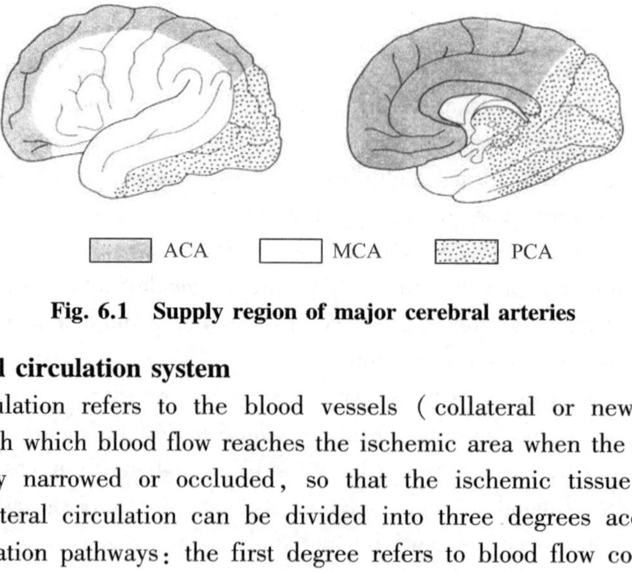

Fig. 6.1 Supply region of major cerebral arteries

(3) Collateral circulation system

Collateral circulation refers to the blood vessels (collateral or newly formed vascular anastomosis) through which blood flow reaches the ischemic area when the supposed supplying arteries are severely narrowed or occluded, so that the ischemic tissue can get perfusion compensation. Collateral circulation can be divided into three degrees according to different blood flow compensation pathways: the first degree refers to blood flow compensation through circle of Willis; the second degree refers to blood flow compensation between ocular artery through meningeal anastomotic branch and other relatively small collateral anastomotic branches; the third degree belongs to neovascularization, that is capillaries, which can only form after a period of ischemia in some cases. Among them, the circle of Willis is the main collateral circulation pathway of cerebrovascular.

Q: What is circle of Willis?

A: Circle of Willis (cerebral arterial circle or circulus arteriosus) is an anastomotic ring of arteries located at the base of the brain. This arterial anastomotic circle connects the two major arterial systems to the brain, the internal carotid arteries and the vertebrobasilar systems. It is formed by a single unpaired anterior communicating artery and paired anterior cerebral arteries, internal carotid arteries, posterior communicating arteries, posterior cerebral arteries.

6.1.2 Intracranial and Extracranial Venous System

(1) Extracranial venous system

It mainly includes scalp vein, conducting vein, barrier vein, orbital vein, facial vein, internal jugular vein, external jugular vein, vertebral vein and so on.

(2) Intracranial venous system

The intracranial venous system includes venous sinuses and brain veins, of which brain veins include cerebral veins and cerebellar veins.

a. Venous sinus: The main venous sinuses include superior sagittal sinus, inferior sagittal sinus, straight sinus, transverse sinus, sigmoid sinus, cavernous sinus, superior petrosal sinus and subpetrosal sinus.

b. Cerebral veins: Venous blood from cortical and subcortical white matter is collected in superficial veins and injected directly into adjacent venous sinuses. Deep veins collect venous blood from deep cerebral white matter, basal ganglia, diencephalon and ventricular choroid plexus, and finally form the Galen vein, which is discharged backward into straight sinus. There was extensive anastomosis between shallow and deep groups on the brain surface or in white matter.

c. Cerebellar veins: They are located in the soft membrane of the cerebellar surface, and divided into upper and lower groups. The superior cerebellar veins are formed by the confluence of small veins above the cerebellar, some of which are injected forward and inward into the straight sinus and the intracerebral vein, and some outward into the transverse sinus and subpetrosal sinus. Inferior cerebellar veins are larger and injected into sigmoid and occipital sinuses.

6.1.3 Etiology of Cerebrovascular Diseases

Various causes such as arteriosclerosis, vasculitis, congenital vascular disease, trauma, drugs, blood diseases, and various emboli and hemodynamic changes can lead acute or chronic cerebrovascular disease. The etiology of cerebrovascular diseases can be classified into several categories according to different anatomical structure and pathogenesis: a. Vascular wall lesion caused by hypertensive arteriosclerosis and arteritis caused by tuberculosis, syphilis, connective tissue disease and leptospirosis. Other vascular injury reasons cover congenital cardiovascular disease (such as aneurysms, vascular malformations, and congenital stenosis), trauma, brain surgery, insert the catheter, piercing, drugs, poisons, malignant tumors, etc. b. Heart disease and hemodynamic changes, such as hypertension, hypotension or arrhythmias, especially atrial fibrillation (AF). c. Changes in blood composition and hemorheology, including increased blood clotting and bleeding tendency due to various causes. The abnormal coagulation mechanisms caused by the application of anticoagulants, antiplatelet drugs, disseminated intravascular coagulation and various blood system diseases. d. Other causes include emboli such as air, fat, cancer cells and parasites, cerebrovascular compression and trauma.

6.1.4 Risk Factors and Prevention of Stroke

(1) Risk factors of CVD

Risk factors of CVD can be divided into two categories: non-interventionable risk factors and interventionable risk factors. Non-interventionable risk factors include age, gender, genetic factors and race. Interventionable risk factors are as follows: hypertension, smoking, diabetes mellitus or obesity, atrial fibrillation, dyslipidemia, carotid artery stenosis, sickle cell anemia, and other risk factors. Hypertension is the most important risk factor for stroke. Increased systolic and diastolic blood pressure are positively and linearly associated with the risk of stroke. Atrial fibrillation can increase the risk of stroke by 3 to 4 times after adjustment for other vascular risk factors; other heart diseases, such as heart valve repair, myocardial infarction, dilated cardiomyopathy, perioperative heart disease, cardiac catheterization and endovascular therapy, pacemakers, and radiofrequency ablation, increase the incidence of embolic stroke. Asymptomatic carotid artery stenosis is a distinct independent risk factor for stroke. Sickle cell anemia may give homozygous patients a cumulative incidence of prestroke of more than 11% by age 20, mostly in childhood. Other risk factors include the metabolic syndrome, oral contraceptives, substance abuse, sleep apnea disease, migraine, high lipoprotein hematic disease, high coagulation, inflammation, infection, hemodynamic abnormalities, elevated fibrinogen and platelet aggregation function, etc.

(2) Prevention of stroke

The prevention of stroke actually includes primary and secondary ones.

1) Primary prevention

Hypertension: Prevention and treatment measures include limiting salt intake, reducing dietary fat content, weight loss, appropriate physical exercise, reducing alcohol consumption and long-term adherence to antihypertensive medication.

Smoking: Smokers should quit smoking with nicotine replacement and oral smoking cessation pills.

Hyperlipidemia: Patients with dyslipidemia have lipid targets based on their risk stratification. Low density lipoprotein cholesterol (LDL-C) is mainly used as the target of lipid regulation to reduce LDL-C below 2.59 mmol/L or reduce LDL-C level by 30% ~ 40% from baseline.

Diabetes: Diabetes patients should improve their lifestyle, control diet, strengthen physical exercise. Ideal blood glucose control is HbA1c, fasting blood glucose, postprandial blood glucose and blood glucose fluctuations are well controlled, the general goal is HbA1c less than 7%.

Atrial fibrillation: Decisions on antithrombotic therapy should be made based on stroke risk stratification, bleeding risk assessment in patients with atrial fibrillation, patient willingness, and availability of necessary anticoagulant monitoring at local hospitals.

Asymptomatic carotid stenosis: Carotid endarterectomy should be considered for patients at high risk of stroke in eligible hospitals; however, it is not clear whether CAS can replace CEA. For patients at high risk of CEA, CAS can be considered.

Aspirin: Low-dose aspirin (50~150 mg daily) is recommended for primary prevention of cardiovascular and cerebrovascular disease in individuals who have high risk of stroke.

Diet and nutrition: The types of daily diet should be diversified, so that the intake of energy and nutrition tends to be reasonable; adopting a balanced diet includes fruits, vegetables and low-fat dairy products and saturated fat.

Exercise: Using tailored physical activity to reduce the risk of stroke.

Excessive drinking: We do not advocate the use of a small amount of alcohol to prevent cardiovascular and cerebrovascular diseases. Drinkers should drink in moderation and avoid excessive drinking.

Others: The person who has cerebral vascular disease risk factor, such as myocardial infarction, carotid artery stenosis, obesity, should take corresponding measures for intervention and processing.

2) Secondary prevention

Regulating risk factors for intervention: It is the same as primary prevention.

Antiplatelet therapy: Antiplatelet therapy is recommended for noncardiogenic stroke.

Anticoagulant therapy: Warfarin is generally recommended for patients with a definite diagnosis of cardiogenic cerebral embolism or cerebral infarction with AF.

Intervention of TIA: Patients with recurrent TIA are at great risk of stroke, and the etiology of TIA should be actively sought and treated.

6.1.5 Diagnosis and Management Principles

Stroke can be initially considered based on the symptoms and signs of sudden onset, rapidly onset of localized or diffuse brain damage. It is easy to diagnose combining with vascular lesions of the brain shown by brain CT, MRI, MRA, DSA examinations, as well as the associated stroke risk factors, such as age, high blood pressure, heart disease, hyperlipidemia, diabetes and smoking. Stroke is an emergency. Whether patients are sent to hospital in time and received early diagnosis and treatment after the onset of stroke is the key point for the best treatment effect. Hospitals should open a "green passage" for patients to supply thrombolytic therapy of acute ischemic stroke. The "stroke unit" is a multidisciplinary, organized ward management system with a core staff of clinicians, professional nurses, physiotherapists, occupational therapists, speech trainers and social workers. At present, "stroke unit" has been proved by evidence-based medicine to be the best approach for stroke treatment. All patients with acute cerebrovascular disease should be admitted to the "stroke unit" for treatment.

6.2 Cerebral Infarction

Cerebral infarction refers to the cerebral blood supply disorders caused by various cerebrovascular lesions, leading to local cerebral tissue ischemia, hypoxic necrosis, and rapid emergence of the corresponding neurological defects. TOAST classification denotes five subtypes: large artery atherosclerosis (LAA); cardioembolism; small-artery occlusion; stroke of other determined cause; stroke of undetermined cause.

6.2.1 Cerebral Thrombosis

(1) Etiology and pathogenesis

Atherosclerosis is the key cause of this disease. Atherosclerosis is aggravated with age, advanced age, hypertension, hyperlipidemia, diabetes, smoking and other risk factors. Large atherosclerotic cerebral infarction has a variety of pathogenesis.

a. Thrombosis *in situ*: It is the main pathogenesis of large atherosclerotic cerebral infarction. Thrombotic obstruction leads to acute occlusion or severe stenosis of the artery, which develops relatively slowly. Its symptoms often progress in a few hours or days, and the clinical manifestations are similar to those of large cerebral infarction.

b. Embolism from artery to artery: A thromboembolus on the atherosclerotic vessel wall breaks off and blocks the distal artery. Cerebral infarction locates in the blood supply area of the main vascular lesions, the infarction foci are small, the symptoms are more limited.

c. Rupturing and bleeding within the plaque: Rupturing and bleeding within the plaque is rare, it's often associated with local thrombosis leading to cerebral infarction, or leading to severe stenosis, there is a core infarct of local cerebral ischemia in combination with hypoperfusion, or the borderline watershed infarction occurred at the same time.

d. Hypoperfusion: Severe vascular stenosis does not change significantly because of atherosclerosis, but it develops into watershed infarction combined with hypoperfusion at the vascular junction.

e. Perforator artery blocking of carrier artery disease: There are atherosclerotic lesions or thrombosis in the carrier artery branch opening, which results in perforator artery occlusion and leads to cerebral infarction.

(2) Clinical feature

1) Clinical manifestation

Atherosclerotic cerebral infarction is more common in middle-aged and elderly people. It occurs in quiet or sleep state, and some cases have prodromal symptoms such as limb numbness and weakness. The focal signs mostly reach their peak in more than 10 hours or 1~2 days after onset. Clinical manifestations depend on the size and location of infarct foci, as well as collateral circulation and vascular variation.

① Appearance of internal carotid artery occlusion

Symptomatic occlusion may present with ischemia of the middle cerebral artery and (or) anterior cerebral artery. Internal carotid artery ischemia may show monocular transient amaurosis, and permanent blindness occasionally or Horner's sign.

② Appearance of middle cerebral artery occlusion

Occlusion of trunk: It shows three partial symptoms, the lesions of the contralateral hemiplegia, and hemidysesthesia and hemianopsia, gaze with both eyes toward the lesion. Aphasia occurred in dominant hemisphere injury and body dysmorphic disorder occurred in non-dominant hemisphere injury. Large area cerebral infarction can lead to severe cerebral edema, cerebral hernia, or even death.

Occlusion of cortical branch: Occlusions of the upper branches lead to paralysis of the lateral face and lateral limbs and anaesthesia, but paralysis of the lower limbs is more serious than that of the upper limbs. Occlusion of the lower branch occurs rarely, resulting in contralateral homogenous upper quarter field defect.

Occlusion of deep perforating branch: Striatal body sac infarction is common. The performances are the opposite side of the central light hemiplegia, sensory disturbances of hemilateral body, homonymous hemianopia. Subcortical aphasia occurs in dominant hemisphere lesions, which is characterized by spontaneous speech limitation, low volume, low intonation, and short duration.

③ Appearance of anterior cerebral artery occlusion

Anterior and medial infarction of bilateral cerebral hemispheres results in paraplegia of both lower limbs, erectoral incontinence, loss of will, motor aphasia and personality change. In occlusion of the anterior artery after anterior communicating artery, sensorimotor impairment of the contralateral feet and lower limbs, paralysis of the upper and shoulder limbs is mild and the face and hands are not involved. Urinary incontinence, indifference, lethargy, euphoria and muteness, contralateral grip and sucking reflex and twofold rigidity may occur. In occlusion of cortical branch, contralateral central limb palsy, sensory disturbances, contralateral temporary ataxia, grip reflex, and psychiatric symptoms may occur. Patients with occlusion of deep perforating branch present with contralateral central facial and lingual palsy and proximal upper limb paresis.

④ Appearance of posterior cerebral artery occlusion

Unilateral cortical branch: Contralateral hemianopsia, but the macular vision is not involved. Dyslexia, nomenclative aphasia and agnosia may occur when the dominant hemisphere is involved.

Bilateral cortical branch: Completely cortical blindness, sometimes it accompanied by shapeless visual hallucinations, impaired memory, etc.

Interfoot branch at the beginning: Central brain and hypothalamus syndrome, including vertical gaze paralysis, lethargy, and even coma. Paramedian artery syndrome, which is characterized by ipsilateral oculomotor nerve palsy and ipsilateral hemiplegia, or Weber syndrome. Claude syndrome presents with psilateral oculomotor palsy, contralateral ataxia and tremor. Benedikt syndrome presents with ipsilateral oculomotor nerve palsy, contralateral involuntary movement and tremor.

Deep perforating branch: Thalamic perforating artery occlusion produces red nucleus thalamic syndrome, which is characterized by dance-like involuntary movement on the focal side, intentional tremor, cerebellar ataxia, and contralateral partial sensory disturbance. Thalamic geniculate artery occlusion produces thalamic syndrome, which is characterized by contralateral deep sensory disturbance, spontaneous pain, hypersensory, mild hemiplegia, ataxia, hand distemper and foot asthenia, etc.

⑤ Occlusion of vertebrobasilar artery

Basilar or bilateral vertebral artery occlusion is a serious life-threatening cerebrovascular disease, resulting in brain stem infarction, dizziness, vomiting, quadriplegia, ataxia, pulmonary edema, gastrointestinal bleeding, coma and high fever. Pons lesions show needle-point holes. Locked-in syndrome, Millard-Gubler syndrome, Foville syndrome, basilar syndrome, Wallenberg syndrome may occur because of different vessels lesions.

⑥ Particular types of cerebral infarction

Massive cerebral infarction: It is caused by internal carotid artery, middle cerebral artery or cortical branch occlusive. It shows complete hemiplegia, hemidysesthesia and gaze toward focus opposite side paralysis. The course of disease shows progressively, it shows obviously brain edema and intracranial pressure heighten.

Cerebral watershed infarction (CWSI): It is caused by adjacent blood vessels. It's also known as border zone cerebral infarction, which is caused by hemodynamic reasons.

Hemorrhagic cerebral infarction: Ischemia leads to arterial blood vessel injury and necrosis. If blood flow restoration, blood will leak from the damaged vessel, causing hemorrhagic cerebral infarction, it's common in large area cerebral infarction.

Multiple infarction: Infarction is caused by occlusion of cerebral vessels in two or more different blood supply systems.

2) Diagnostic investigation

All patients should have auxiliary examination items: brain CT scan or MRI; blood sugar; full blood count, PT, INR and APTT; liver and kidney function, electrolyte, blood lipid; markers of myocardial ischemia, such as troponin and myocardial enzyme; oxygen saturation; ECG; chest X-ray examination. Patients with normal ECG but suspected paroxysmal atrial fibrillation can be monitored by dynamic electrocardiogram. Echocardiography and transesophageal ultrasonography can detect suspected cardiac emboli, such as mural thrombus of heart, atrial stem fluid tumor, mitral valve prolapse and patent foramen ovale. Assays for protein C, protein S, and antithrombin E can be used to screen for hereditary hypercoagulability. Other laboratory tests, such as glycosylated hemoglobin, homosorosine and anti-lectin antibody are helpful in identifying risk factors for cerebral infarction. Patients can choose the following examinations when necessary: toxicological screening; blood alcohol level; arterial blood gas analysis (if hypoxia is suspected); lumbar puncture (suspected subarachnoid hemorrhage but not shown by CT, or suspected stroke secondary to infectious diseases); EEG (suspected seizure of epilepsy), etc.

CT is the first step to identify intracranial bleeding and distinguish non-vascular lesions. In most cases, brain CT gradually shows low-density infarct focal 24 hours after onset, and obvious low-density focal are observed after 2~15 days (Fig. 6.2). Large scale cerebral infarction has cerebral edema and mass effect, and hemorrhagic infarction shows mixed density. It is the infarction absorption period after 2~3 weeks, it is difficult to distinguish on CT because of the disappearance of the edema and the infiltration of phagocytes, it is called "fuzzy effect". Multimodal CT examinations, such as perfusion CT, can distinguish reversible ischemia from irreversible ischemia and identify ischemic penumbra.

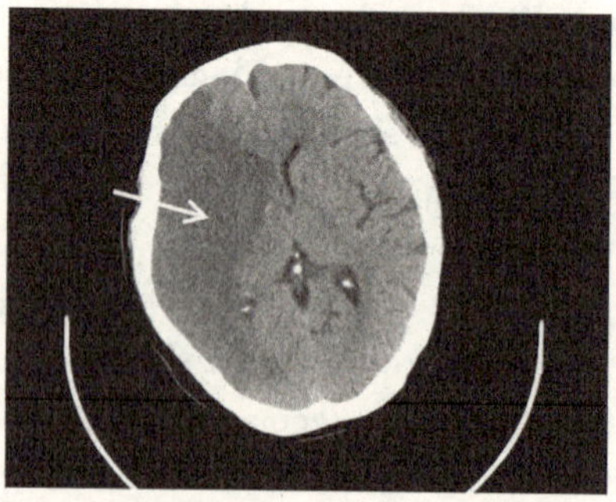

Fig. 6.2 Low-density infarction

MRI can clearly show early ischemic infarction, with low signal in T_1 and high signal in T_2. Diffusion-weighted MRI (DWI) can show focal ischemia within minutes of symptom onset (Fig. 6.3). Common vascular examination methods include carotid duplex ultrasound, transcranial doppler (TCD), MRA, CTA and DSA.

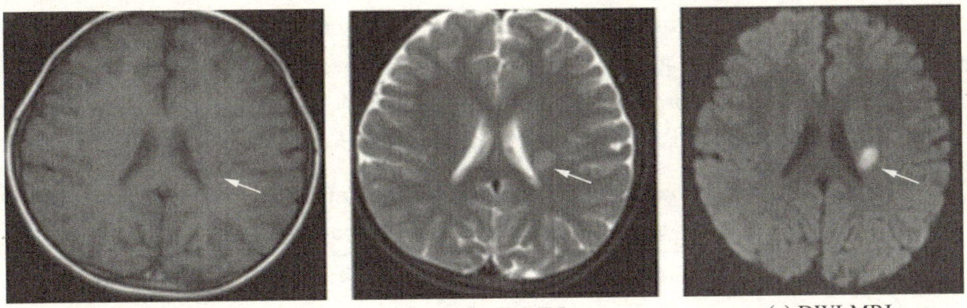

(a) T_1-MRI (b) T_2-MRI (c) DWI-MRI

A focal ischemia (arrow) near the lateral ventricle present with low signal in T_1-MRI, high signal in T_2-MRI, and high signal in DWI-MRI.

Fig. 6.3 Cerebral infarction in MRI

(3) Diagnosis and differential diagnosis

The first step is to determine whether it is stroke. Middle-aged patients have rapid occurrence of focal brain damage symptoms and signs, the symptoms and signs can be explained by the functional injury of an arterial blood supply area, excluding non-vascular causes, acute stroke should be considered. The second step is to determine whether it is ischemic or hemorrhagic stroke. CT or MRI can rule out cerebral hemorrhage and other lesions, it is helpful to make a differential diagnosis. The third step is to determine whether it is suitable for thrombolytic therapy. Differential diagnosis should be made with the following diseases: cerebral hemorrhage, cerebral embolism, intracranial space occupying disease.

(4) Treatment

1) General processing

Oxygen can be given when necessary to maintain oxygen saturation greater than 94%. ECG examination should be carried out within 24 hours after cerebral infarction, and ECG monitoring for 24 hours or longer can be carried out according to conditions. Antipyretic measures should be given to patients with body temperature greater than 38 ℃. Blood pressure decreases within 24 hours after stroke spontaneously. In patients with stable condition and without intracranial hypertension or other serious complications, the blood pressure level can reflect the pre-disease level after 24 hours. When blood glucose exceeds 10 mmoL/L, insulin treatment should be given, and blood glucose monitoring should be strengthened to avoid hypoglycemia. Blood glucose target can be 7.7 ~ 10 mmol/L. Hypoglycemia (less than 3.36 mmol/L) can be corrected by oral or intravenous administration of 10% ~ 20% glucose. Enteral nutrition should be initiated within 7 days for acute stroke, and nutritional supplements may be used for patients with malnutrition or risk of malnutrition. Nasal feeding can be used for those who cannot eat normally, but for longer duration (greater than 2 ~ 3 weeks), percutaneous endoscopic gastrostomy (PEG) tube feeding can be used for supplement nutrition.

2) Specific therapy

① Intravenous thrombolysis

It is the most important measure to restore blood flow by rtPA-intravenous thrombolysis. Patients should be strictly screened according to indications and contraindications and given rtPA venous thrombolysis as soon as possible within 4.5 hours of onset (Tab. 6.1). The dose of rtPA is 0.9 mg/kg (maximum dose 90 mg/kg) intravenously, 10% of rtPA is given intravenously within 1 minute and the rest is given continuously in 1 hour. Patients should be monitored during 24 hours of intravenous thrombolysis, and blood pressure and neurological function should be examined regularly. In case of severe headache, hypertension, nausea and vomiting, or significant deterioration of neurological symptoms and signs, thrombolytic drugs should be stopped and brain CT examination should be performed immediately.

Tab. 6.1 Indications and contraindications for intravenous thrombolysis of rt-PA within 4.5 hours window

Indications	1	Symptoms of neurological impairment caused by acute cerebral infarction
	2	Symptoms appear less than 4.5 hours
	3	Age is equal to or greater than 18 years
	4	Informed consent is signed by patients or their family members
Contraindications	1	Previous history of intracranial hemorrhage
	2	History of major head trauma or stroke in the last 3 months
	3	Suspected subarachnoid hemorrhage
	4	Intracranial tumors, arteriovenous malformations or aneurysms
	5	Arterial puncture at the site of hemostasis is not easy to compress in the past 1 week
	6	Increased blood pressure: systolic pressure is equal to or greater than 180 mmHg, or diastolic pressure is equal to or greater than 100 mmHg
	7	Active internal bleeding
	8	Propensity for acute bleeding, including platelet count below 100×10^9/L or other conditions, such as heparin treatment within 48 hours
	9	Oral anticoagulant with INR greater than 1.7 or PT greater than 15 seconds
	10	Using of thrombin inhibitors or factor Xa inhibitors for various sensitive laboratory abnormalities at present
	11	Blood sugar is equal to or less than 2.7 mmol/L
	12	Multilobular infarction suggested by CT
	13	Recent history of intracranial or spinal surgery
Relative contraindications	Within 3 hours window	Mild stroke or stroke with rapid improvement of symptoms
		Pregnancy
		Neurological impairment symptoms after epilepsy
		Major surgery or severe trauma within the last 2 weeks
		Gastrointestinal or urinary bleeding within the last 3 weeks
	3~4.5 hours window	Age is greater than 80 years
		Severe stroke (NIHSS is greater than 25)
		Oral anticoagulants
		History of diabetes mellitus and ischemic stroke

② Endovascular interventional therapy

Endovascular interventional therapy includes arterial thrombolysis, bridging, mechanical thrombectomy, angioplasty and stenting.

③ Antiplatelet therapy

Antiplatelet therapy includes aspirin and clopidogrel. Patients who do not receive thrombolytic therapy should take aspirin (150 ~ 325 mg/d) as early as possible within 48 hours, and clopidogrel may be used instead when patients are allergic to aspirin or aspirin is unavailable. Generally, antithrombotic drugs and dosage are selected according to secondary prevention plan after 2 weeks of stroke. If the patient's NIHSS score is ≤3 within 24 hours of onset, aspirin combined with clopidogrel should be given as soon as possible for 21 days to prevent the early recurrence of stroke.

④ Anticoagulation treatment

Prophylactic doses of anticoagulant therapy may be used in patients with hypercoagulant status, and the patient who is at high risk for developing deep vein thrombosis and pulmonary embolism. Patients with acute ischemic stroke and atrial fibrillation can start oral anticoagulant therapy between 4 and 14 days after onset.

⑤ Brain protection treatment

Brain protective agents include free radical scavengers, opioid receptor blockers, voltage-gated calcium channel blockers, excitatory amino acid receptor blockers, speculum ions and statins, which can reduce ischemic brain injury by reducing brain metabolism and interfering the mechanism of ischemia-induced cytotoxicity.

⑥ Dilatation therapy

Correction of hypoperfusion is suitable for cerebral infarction caused by hemodynamic mechanisms.

3) Management of acute complications

① Cerebral edema and increased intracranial pressure

It is recommended to raise the head of the bed by 20° ~ 45° to avoid and deal with factors causing increased intracranial pressure, such as excessive twisting of the head and neck, excitement, force, fever, epilepsy, respiratory tract obstruction, cough, constipation, etc. 20% mannitol can be used in intravenous drops every 6 ~ 8 hours. For patients who have cardiac and renal insufficiency, 20 ~ 40 mg furosemide can be injected intravenously every 6 ~ 8 hours. Glycerol fructose can be used at the same time, 1 ~ 2 times a day. Albumin can also be used as adjuvant therapy. Decompressive craniectomy is an effective lifesaving measure for patients under the age of 60 with malignant middle cerebral artery infarction and severe intracranial hypertension within 48 hours after onset.

② Hemorrhage after infarction

Antithrombotic therapy and other hemorrhagic drugs should be discontinued for symptomatic hemorrhage transformation, while general antithrombotic therapy for meta-symptomatic intracerebral hemorrhage transformation can continue to be used. When antithrombotic therapy is needed, the advantages and disadvantages should be weighed. Generally, antiplatelet therapy can be started a few days or weeks if symptomatic bleeding is stabilized. For those patients who have a low risk of recurrent thrombosis or poor systemic condition, antiplatelet agents may be used instead of warfarin. Anticoagulant therapy should be avoided for at least 4 weeks after symptomatic ich unless mechanical heart valves are involved.

③ Epilepsy

Prophylactic use of antiepileptic drugs is not recommended. It is not recommended to use antiepileptic drugs for a long time after isolated attack or acute epilepsy attack.

④ Infection

Patients are prone to respiratory tract and urinary tract infections in the acute phase, and infection is an important cause of aggravation of the condition. Oral health care should be administered to reduce the risk of pneumonia after stroke. It is an important measure to prevent pneumonia to adopt appropriate body position, turn over and knock back frequently and prevent aspiration. The treatment of pneumonia mainly includes respiratory support and antibiotic treatment. Urinary tract infection is mainly secondary to urinary incontinence and indwelling catheterization. Intubation and indwelling catheterization should be avoided as far as possible.

⑤ Upper gastrointestinal bleeding

Elderly patients and patients with severe cerebral apoplexy are prone to stress ulcerative carcinoma in the acute stage. Routine intravenous anti-ulcer drugs are recommended. For patients with gastrointestinal bleeding, gastric lavage with frozen saline and local application of hemostatic agents (such as oral or nasal feeding of Yunnan Baiyao, thrombin, etc.) should be performed. If the amount of blood loss is large enough to cause shock, transfusion of fresh whole blood or red blood cell components should be necessary, and hemostasis under gastroscope or surgical hemostasis should be performed.

⑥ Deep vein thromhosis (DVT) and pulmonary embolism (PE)

For elderly patients, both severe paralysis and atrial fibrillation increase the risk of DVT, and DVT increases the risk of PE. Patients should be encouraged to move as early as possible, raise the lower extremities, and avoid intravenous fluids in the lower extremities. Patients with high risk of DVT and PE can be given prophylactic anticoagulant therapy with low dose of anticoagulant drugs, such as low molecular weight heparin 4000 IU, subcutaneous injection once a day.

⑦ Dysphagia

In order to prevent and treat poststroke pneumonia and malnutrition, attention should be paid to the evaluation and management of dysphagia. Patients should be screened for dysphagia and identified as high risk of aspiration before starting eating, drinking, or taking medications orally.

⑧ Heart injury

Stroke combined with heart injury is one of the manifestations of brain-heart syndrome, which includes acute myocardial ischemia, myocardial infarction, arrhythmia and heart failure. The condition of the heart should be closely observed, and dynamic electrocardiogram monitoring and myocardial enzyme spectrometry should be carried out to find the heart injury in time and treat it in time if necessary. Reducing cardiac load, using drugs that increase cardiac burden with caution, paying attention to infusion speed and volume, reducing the amount of mannitol in elderly patients or patients with original heart disease by half or use other dehydrating agents, and dealing with heart injury.

4) Early rehabilitation

It is given priority to make short-term and long-term rehabilitation treatment plans according to local conditions. Early, heavy exercise should not be performed within 24 hours of stroke onset. When the condition is stable, activities such as sitting, standing and walking should be started as soon as possible. Bedridden people should persist in good limb placement, minimize skin friction and skin compression, maintain good skin hygiene, prevent skin cracking, and use specific mattresses, wheelchair cushions or seats until restoring the ability. Attention should be paid to language, motor and psychological rehabilitation training, routine screening of post-stroke depression, and antidepressant treatment for patients with post-stroke depression without contraindications, in order to restore patients' self-care ability in daily life as far as possible.

Early initiation of secondary prevention: The convalescence period usually begins 2 weeks after the onset of stroke. For patients with stable acute stroke, secondary prevention of stroke should be safely started as early as possible, and health education should be given to patients.

(5) Prognosis

Within 30 days of onset, the fatality rate is about 5%~15%, and the disability rate is over 50%. More than 40% of the survivors may relapse. And the mortality and disability rate usually increase with recurrence. The prognosis is influenced by age, underlying diseases and complications.

6.2.2 Cerebral Embolism

Cerebral embolism refers to a variety of emboli along with the blood flow into the cerebral artery, resulting in local brain tissue ischemia, hypoxic necrosis, and rapid emergence of the corresponding neurological defects of a group of clinical syndromes. Cerebral embolism can be divided into cardiogenic, non-cardiogenic and unknown sources.

(1) Etiology and pathogenesis

The emboli of cardiogenic cerebral emboli comes from atria, ventricular wall thrombus, and heart valve vegetations, and a few of embolus come from atrial stover tumor. The etiology of cerebral embolism is as follows: non-valvular atrial fibrillation (AF), rheumatic heart disease, acute myocardial infarction, left ventricular thrombosis, congestive heart failure, artificial heart valve, dilated cardiomyopathy, and other rare causes, such as infective endocarditis, non-bacterial thrombotic endocarditis, pathological sinus syndrome, left atrium Mongolian fluid tumor, atrial septal defect, patent foramen ovale, atrial flutter, mitral valve prolapse, mitral annulus calcification and endocardial fibrosis.

AF is the most common cause of cardiac embolism. Emboli comes from the left atrial appendage. The main pathogenesis is the slow stagnation of blood flow caused by atrial fibrillation, which activates the coagulation cascade under the action of low shear rate and other factors, and finally it forms erythrocyte fibrin thrombus, leading to cerebral embolism. Rheumatic valvular heart disease is often comlicated with atrial fibrillation, which causes the atria and ventricles to dilate, these lesions increase the likelihood of thrombosis. Cardiogenic cerebral embolism accounts for about 10% of acute myocardial infarction and about 20% of infective endocarditis. Nonbacterial thrombotic endocarditis is an important cause of cerebral embolism, which mainly occurs in hypercoagulable diseases such as cancer, systemic lupus erythematosus and antiphospholipid antibody syndrome.

(2) Clinical feature

1) Clinical manifestation

Cardiogenic cerebral embolism can occur at any age. The cerebral embolism caused by rheumatic heart disease is mostly in young women, while the cerebral embolism caused by acute myocardial infarction is mostly in middle-aged and elderly people. Typical cerebral embolism usually occurs suddenly in the activity, and the signs of primary prodrome and focal nerve function defect reach their peak in a few seconds to a few minutes.

The neurological deficits and brain parenchyma imaging findings are basically the same as those of large atherosclerotic cerebral infarction, but multiple vascularized areas of brain damage may occur simultaneously.

Cardiogenic cerebral embolism is prone to recurrence and bleeding. The disease is serious at the beginning with unconsciousness when the main artery is blocked. The clinical symptoms of some cases can relieve quickly because of the recirculation of blood vessels and deteriorate rapidly due to concurrent bleeding.

Infective endocarditis is common in patients with valvular heart disease, congenital heart disease, obstructive hypertrophic cardiomyopathy, and rheumatic immune diseases who take glucocorticoid for a long time. Cerebral embolism occurs before antibiotic treatment or within the first week. Cerebral embolism can be complicated with intracranial infection, headache, fever and diffuse brain symptoms. Sometimes infective endocarditis can lead to intracerebral hemorrhage or subarachnoid hemorrhage, and intracerebral hemorrhage can occur hours or days before TIA or ischemic stroke.

2) Diagnostic investigation

The routine and identified examinations are similar to cerebral infarction. When the patient has fever and leukocyte increase, blood culture should be performed to exclude infective endocarditis. When nonbacterial thrombotic endocarditis is suspected, immunological autoantibodies such as antiphospholipid antibodies should be tested. In the case of patent foramen ovale and cerebral infarction of unknown cause, venous embolus sources such as deep vein thrombosis of lower limbs should be explored, and protein C, protein S and antithrombin E should be tested to screen for hypercoagulability. Transthoracic echocardiography (TTE), transesophageal echocardiography (TEE), and transcranial Doppler ultrasound foaming tests can be used to explore patent foramen ovale and right-to-left shunt channels. ECG examination can be used to determine myocardial infarction, atrial fibrillation, and other arrhythmias. Paroxysmal AF may require long-term continuous electrocardiogram monitoring to detect.

(3) Diagnosis and differential diagnosis

The diagnosis of cardiogenic cerebral embolism can be made according to the sudden onset of the disease, the peak within seconds to minutes, the occurrence of focal neurological defects such as hemiplegia and aphasia, the previous history of embolic underlying diseases, such as atrial fibrillation and rheumatic heart disease, and CT or MRI examination excluding cerebral hemorrhage and other lesions. The diagnosis is more supported by the presence of consciousness disturbance at the onset of cerebral infarction or the rapid improvement of the symptoms of major neurological deficits at the early stage of the onset. Vascular imaging examination confirms that there is no atherosclerotic stenosis of intracranial or extracranial large vessels corresponding to nerve function defect of cerebral infarction (>50%), or multiple infarction areas dominated by blood vessels at the same time, or combined with embolism of other organs of the body.

(4) Treatment

The treatment principles are the same as those of atherosclerotic cerebral infarction. Anticoagulant therapy is generally not recommended in the acute stage. For most patients of ischemic stroke caused by cardiogenic cerebral embolism, oral anticoagulant therapy can be started within 4 ~ 14 days of onset to prevent stroke recurrence and it is recommended to maintain PT-INR between 2.0 and 3.0 with warfarin. In patients with high risk of bleeding transformation, anticoagulation is generally delayed to 14 days later. Targeted treatment of the primary disease is controlling cerebral embolism and preventing recurrence. Arrhythmia should be corrected. Antibiotics should be used for infectious embolism, and thrombolytic and anticoagulant treatment should be prohibited to prevent the spread of infection. For nonbacterial thrombotic endocarditis, oral anticoagulants are less effective in treating hypercoagulability and heparin or low molecular weight heparin may be used. Atrial myxoma can be surgically resected. In the case of patent foramen ovale and deep vein thrombosis, transcatheter foramen ovale closure can be considered for abnormal embolism.

Cardiogenic cerebral embolism has a worse prognosis and higher disability rate than other types of cerebral infarction. It is related to larger thrombus from the atrium and ventricular lumen.

6.2.3 Lacunar Ischemic Stroke

A small artery occlusion stroke, known as a lacunar ischemic stroke, occurs when a small artery blocked after a prolonged period of high blood pressure and other risk factors. Lacunar infarct refers to arteriolar occlusive cerebral infarction, involving deep white matter, basal ganglia, thalamus and pons.

(1) Etiology and pathogenesis

Arteriosclerosis is considered to be the main cause. Age, hypertension, diabetes mellitus, smoking and family history are the main risk factors for this disease, while hyperchloremia, excessive drinking, history of stroke and other factors have little correlation with this disease. Small deep or subcortical infarcts of the brain are caused by occlusion of a single small perforating artery. Microatherosclerotic plaque is the main cause of occlusion or stenosis of small perforating artery. Other mechanisms include carrier atherosclerotic lesions or thrombosis involving small perforating arterial openings.

(2) Clinical feature

According to clinical and pathological data, Fisher classified the disease into 21 clinical syndromes, 5 common syndromes are as follows.

1) Pure motor hemiparesis (PMH)

PMH is one of the most common type, accounting for about 60%. Lesions are mostly located in the inner capsule, radiative corona or pons. Performance shows opposite face and limbs light hemiplegia, without feeling obstacle, visual obstacle and cortical function obstacle. It usually shows no vertigo, tinnitus, nystagmus, diplopia and cerebellar sex ataxia.

2) Pure sensory stroke (PSS)

It is characterized by partial sensory loss. It can be accompanied by paresthesia, such as numbness, burning or heavy feeling, tingling and stiffness. The lesions are mainly located in the ventral posterior lateral nucleus of the contralateral thalamus.

3) Ataxic-hemiparesis

It shows light hemiplegia with cerebellar ataxia, and lower limb is heavier than upper limb. Ataxia cannot be explained with weakness, it can be accompanied by pyramidal bundle sign. The lesions are located at the base of pons, inner capsule or subcortical white matter.

4) Dysarthric-clumsy hand syndrome (DCHS)

It shows dysarthria, dysphagia, the opposite side of the central facial palsy, facial palsy lateral hand weakness and clumsy fine movements, finger nose test is not accurate. The lesion is located at the base of pons, forelimb of inner capsule or knee.

5) Sensorimotor stroke (SMS)

The disease starts with partial sensory disturbance, followed by mild hemiplegia. The lesions are located in the posterior ventral nucleus of thalamus and the posterior limb of the adjacent inner sac, and they are caused by occlusion of thalamic geniculate artery branch or thalamic branch of posterior choroid artery. Lacunar state refers to multiple lacunar infarction caused by repeated attacks of this disease, involving bilateral corticospinal tracts and cortical brainstem tracts, and presenting severe mental disorders, cognitive decline, pseudobulbar paralysis, bilateral pyramidal tracts, Parkinsonian syndrome, urinary and fecal incontinence, etc.

(3) Diagnosis and differential diagnosis

Auxiliary examination is the same as cerebral infarction with large atherosclerotic. Neuroimaging examination is the main basis of diagnosis. Middle-aged and elderly patients with chronic hypertension, diabetes and other risk factors, acute onset, focal neurological defects, clinical manifestations show lacunar syndrome and can be preliminarily diagnosed. If CT or MRI examination confirms the presence of cerebral lacunar lesions consistent with neurological dysfunction, infarcts with diameter less than 1.5 ~ 2.0 cm, and infarcts locate in deep white matter, basal ganglia, thalamus, pons and other regions of the brain, the diagnosis can be confirmed. It can be distinguished from small cerebral hemorrhage, infection, cysticercosis, moyamoya disease, brain abscess, extracranial carotid artery occlusion, pons hemorrhage, demyelinated encephalopathy, and metastasis.

(4) Treatment

The treatment of this type of cerebral infarction is similar to that of atherosclerotic cerebral infarction. Arteriolar occlusive cerebral infarction generally has a better prognosis of lower mortality and disability. Nearly 70% ~ 80% of these patients recovered totally, while only 50% of other types of cerebral infarction recovered well.

6.3 Transient Ischemic Attack

Transient ischemic attack (TIA) describes neurologic symptoms of ischemic origin that last less than 24 hours. Most attacks last only a few minutes to an hour and the event that leaves no clinical or imaging trace of infarction.

(1) Etiology and pathogenesis

Reduced blood flow or embolic particles are likely the causes of TIA. Some TIAs tend to be brief if transient thrombosis come from severe large carotid or vertebrobasilar stenosis. Some TIAs, especially vertebrobasilar, may have a hemodynamic basis, including transient hypotension and cardiac arrhythmia. Those TIAs responsive to calcium-channel blockers suggest vasospasm. Attacks without severe stenosis tend to last longer and often are associated with distal branch occlusion, suggesting embolism from an ulcerated plaque or a more proximal source. Other TIAs may be a consequence of primary intraparenchymal vascular disease, anemia or polycythemia.

(2) Clinical feature

TIAs may present themselves as transient spells of hemiparesis, aphasia, numbness, or tingling on one side of the body, dysarthria, diplopia, ataxia, obscuration of a visual field, or combinations of those replicate the stroke syndromes. Even limb shaking can represent a TIA. Symptoms vary with the arterial territory involved. Carotid territory TIAs that involve the brain produce varying combinations of limb weakness and sensory loss, aphasia, hemineglect, and homonymous hemianopia. Posterior circulation TIAs cause symptoms referable to the cerebrum, brainstem, and cerebellum. Blood routine and biochemical tests are necessary. CTA/MRA/DSA shows vascular stenosis and atherosclerosis. CT or MRI is mostly normal.

(3) Diagnosis and differential diagnosis

TIAs have focal neurologic episodes that correspond to a vascular territory, appear abruptly and cease in matter of minutes or last less than 24 hours without clinical or imaging trace of infarction. TIAs must be distinguished from other brief neurologic attacks that are from seizures, migraine, and its variants, transient global amnesia, syncope, vertigo from labyrinthine disease, and psychogenic episodes, as emphasized further on.

(4) Treatment

TIA is an emergency. The high-risk period for stroke is 2~7 days after the onset of TIA. Emergency assessment and intervention of patients can reduce the incidence of stroke. A common TIA risk stratification tool is the $ABCD^2$ score (Tab. 6.2). Hospitalization is recommended if symptoms occur within 72 hours and one of the following conditions exists: $ABCD^2$ score>3; $ABCD^2$ score 0~2, the outpatient department cannot complete TIA system examination within 2 days; $ABCD^2$ score 0~2, and other evidence suggest that symptoms are caused by ischemia.

Tab. 6.2 $ABCD^2$ score

	Clinical character	Score
Age	>60	1
Hypertension	SBP>140 mmHg or DBP>90 mmHg	1
Clinical manifestation	Unilateral limb weakness	2
	Language disorders without limb weakness	1
Duration of symptoms	>60 minutes	2
	10~59 minutes	1
Diabetes	Yes	1

1) Medicine treatment

① Antiplatelet therapy

Antiplatelet therapy is recommended for noncardiogenic embolic TIA. Within 24 hours of onset, there is a high risk of stroke recurrence. Patients ($ABCD^2$ score ≥4) with acute non-cardiogenic TIA or mild ischemic stroke (NIHSS ≤3) should be treated with aspirin in combination with clopidogrel for 21 days as soon as possible. Patients with TIA with symptomatic severe intracranial artery stenosis within 30 days of onset should be treated with aspirin in combination with clopidogrel for 90 days as soon as possible. Other TIA or minor stroke generally use: a. aspirin (50~325 mg/d); b. clopidogrel (75 mg/d); c. aspirin (25 mg bid) + dipyridamole (200 mg bid).

② Anticoagulant therapy

Anticoagulant therapy is generally recommended for cardiogenic embolic TIA as soon as possible after cerebral hemorrhage is ruled out by neuroimaging. Heparin, low molecular weight heparin, warfarin and new oral anticoagulants are included.

③ Dilatation therapy

Correction of hypoperfusion is appropriate for hemodynamic TIA.

④ Thrombolytic therapy

For a recent occurrence of TIA, patients are not contraindicated for thrombolytic therapy, even if neuroimaging findings show a clear responsibility for cerebral infarction. If TIA occurs again, the diagnosis of cerebral infarction may be clinically possible, and thrombolysis should be actively performed according to the guidelines instead of waiting.

⑤ Others

TIA patients with hyperfibrinogen can be treated with defibrase.

2) Surgery treatment

For those who are suitable for carotid endarterectomy or carotid angioplasty and stent implantation, surgery should be performed within 48 hours.

3) Control risk factors

See 6.1.4(1) of this chapter.

(5) Prognosis

Patients with TIA have a high risk of early stroke, and the incidence of cerebral infarction is 4% ~ 10% within 7 days and 10% ~ 20% within 90 days. A progressive TIA with short intervals between episodes, prolonged episodes, and progressively worsening clinical symptoms is a strong warning sign of impending cerebral infarction.

6.4 Cerebral Hemorrhage

Intracerebral hemorrhage (ICH) is non-traumatic bleeding within the brain parenchyma. The most common etiology is hypertension with parvosclerosis, other etiologies include arteriovenous malformation, cerebral amyloidosis vascular diseases, blood disorders (e.g., leukemia, aplastic anemia, thrombocytopenia epilepsy, hemophilia, polycythemia and sickle cell disease), anticoagulant or thrombolytic therapy, etc. The main pathogenesis of hypertensive intracerebral hemorrhage is small arteries ruptured under the action of long-term hypertension. Chronic hypertension can cause hyaline degeneration, fibrinoid necrosis, and even the formation of microaneurysms or dissecting aneurysms, and the small cerebral arteries are prone to rupture when the blood pressure elevates. Deep perforating branches, such as the pisoline artery and the paramedian artery, arise at right angles from the artery at the base of the brain and endure high pressure blood flow impact, leading to blood vessel rupture bleeding easily, so it is also called bleeding artery. The pathogenesis varies in non-hypertensive intracerebral hemorrhage because of different etiologies.

(1) Clinical feature

1) Clinical manifestation

ICH is more common in patients over 50 years old, especially in male. The incidence is higher in cold season. Hypertension is the most common cause of ICH. The blood pressure of ICH patients increased significantly after onset. Headaches, vomiting and varying degrees of unconsciousness are common due to elevated intracranial pressure. The putamen is the site most frequently affected. When the expanding hematoma involves the adjacent internal capsule, there is a contralateral hemiparesis, usually with hemianesthesia and hemianopia, aphasia or impaired awareness of the disorder in large hematomas. However, small self-limiting hematomas close to the capsular region may occasionally mimic lacunar syndromes featuring pure motor or sensory deficits. When the hemorrhage arises in the thalamus, hemianesthesia precedes the hemiparesis. Once contralateral motor, sensory, and visual field signs are established, the main points that distinguish the two sites are conjugate horizontal ocular deviation in putaminal hemorrhage and impaired upward gaze in thalamic hemorrhage. Pontine hemorrhage usually plunges the patient into coma with quadriparesis and grossly disconjugate ocular motility disorders, although small hemorrhages may mimic syndromes of infarction. The cerebral lobes hematomas often result from arteriovenous malformations, amyloid angiopathy, tumors, or other causes that rarely affect the basal ganglia, thalamus and pons. Cerebellar hemorrhages' syndrome usually begins abruptly with vomiting and severe ataxia; it is occasionally accompanied by dysarthria, adjacent cranial nerve affection, and paralysis of conjugate lateral gaze to one side.

2) Diagnostic investigation

Blood routine, blood biochemistry, coagulation function, ECG and chest X-ray examination shoud be done first to find the etiology. But CT scan of the brain is the preferred method for the diagnosis of ICH, which can clearly show the bleeding site, the bleeding volume, the morphology of the hematoma, whether it penetrates into the ventricle, and whether there is low-density edema zone and mass effect around the hematoma. (Fig. 6.4)

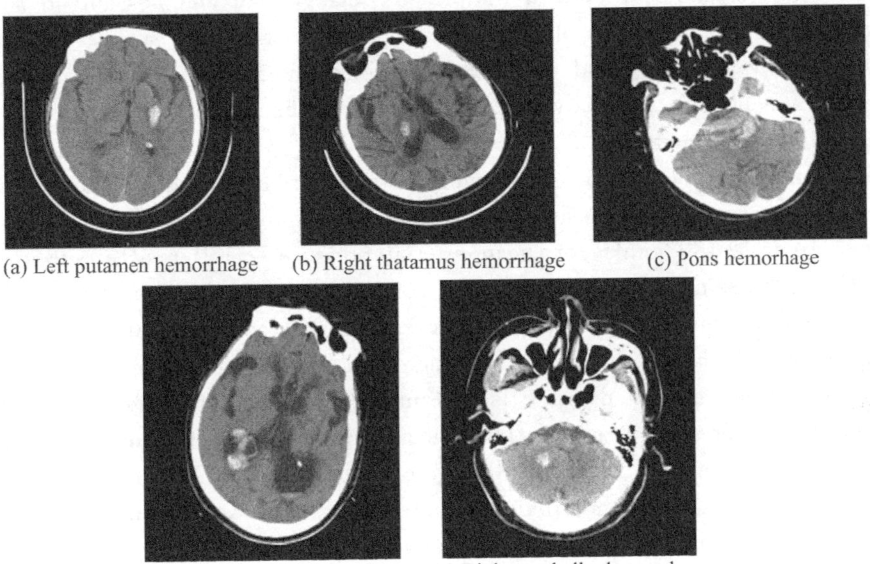

(a) Left putamen hemorrhage (b) Right thatamus hemorrhage (c) Pons hemorhage

(d) Intraventricular hemorrhage (e) Right cerebellar hemorrhage

Fig. 6.4 Diversified ICH

MRI shows its' advantages in finding structural abnormalities and identifying the cause of cerebral hemorrhage. MRI changes during intracerebral hemorrhage, the law of transformation shows as follows. The hyperacute phase (<24 hours) shows long T_1 and long T_2 signals, which could not be differentiated from cerebral infarction and edema. The acute phase (2~7 days) shows isoT_1 and short flight signal. The subacute phase (8 days to 4 weeks) shows short T_1 and long T_2 signal. Long T_1 and long T_2 signals are observed in chronic stage (>4 weeks). MRA can find cerebrovascular malformation, hemangioma and other lesions.

(2) Diagnosis and differential diagnosis

For middle-aged and elderly patients with sudden onset of activity or emotional, rapid onset of focal neurological deficits and headache, vomiting and other symptoms of intracranial hypertension, the possibility of cerebral hemorrhage should be considered, it can be diagnosed combined with head CT scan.

(3) Treatment

The treatment principles include quiet rest, dehydration, intracranial pressure reduction, blood pressure adjustment, bleeding cessation and complications nursing. So the whole target is reducing the rates of mortality, disability and recurrence.

1) General treatment

It is reasonable to keep the patient at rest for 2~4 weeks, avoid emotional agitation and higher blood pressure. Patients with conscious disorder or chemotract hemorrhage should fast for 24~48 hours and empty stomach contents if necessary. Pay attention to water and electrolyte balance, preventing aspiration pneumonia and controlling infection. Patients with obvious headache can be appropriately given sedative analgesic, and patients with constipation can be given laxative.

2) Reducing intracranial pressure

Controlling cerebral edema and reducing intracranial pressure (ICP) are important for the treatment of acute cerebral hemorrhage. For patients with progressive ICP due to hematoma or edema, and with worsening of clinical findings associated with compression on surrounding tissues, intravenous administration of intravenous hypertonic glycerol, such as mannitol, may be considered. Elevating head and upper body position by 30° is also recommended. Mild hypothermia treatment is the auxiliary treatment of cerebral hemorrhage.

3) Adjusting blood pressure

When systolic blood pressure is ≥200 mmHg or mean arterial blood pressure ≥150 mmHg, continuous intravenous antihypertensive drugs should be initiated to lower blood pressure. When systolic pressure is ≥180 mmHg or mean arterial pressure ≥130 mmHg with evidence of increased ICP at the same time, intermittent or continuous intravenous anti-hypertensive drugs can be used, but ICP monitoring should be started to ensure cerebral perfusion pressure more than 60~80 mmHg. If there is no evidence of increased ICP, the target blood pressure is 160/90 mmHg or the mean arterial pressure is 110 mmHg. Intensive anti-hypertensive therapy to reduce systolic blood pressure is not recommended as cerebral hypoperfusion can be caused by rapidly blood pressure decline. Early switching to oral anti-hypertensive drugs, if possible, may be reasonable. In the convalescence period of cerebral hemorrhage, blood pressure should be controlled within the normal range as far as possible.

4) Hemostatic treatment

In patients with hypertensive ICH, administration of tranexamic acid may be considered. If there is coagulation dysfunction, hemostatic drug therapy can be used, such as heparin can be neutralized with protamine, vitamin K_1 can be used to treat warfarin.

5) Mild hypothermia treatment

It is the auxiliary treatment of cerebral hemorrhage.

6) Surgical treatment

When severe intracerebral hemorrhage is life-threatening, medical treatment is usually ineffective, while surgical treatment may be life-saving. However, surgical treatment usually increases the risk of severe disability over medical treatment. Major surgical procedures include: decompression of the bone flap surgery, small bone window craniotomy hematoma removal, drilling hematoma aspiration and ventricular puncture drainage. The surgery should be performed at an early stage. Surgical treatment is usually considered for the following conditions: a. more than equal amount of hemorrhage in the basal ganglia area. b. cerebellar hemorrhage greater than or equal to 10 mL or diameter greater than or equal to 3 cm, or combined with obvious hydrocephalus. c. severe ventricular hemorrhage. d. with the complications of cerebrovascular malformation, aneurysm and other vascular lesions.

7) Rehabilitation treatment

It should be carried out as soon as possible when patient's vital signs are stable and the symptoms do not deteriorate.

(4) Prognosis

The prognosis of cerebral hemorrhage is poor. Cerebral edema, increased ICP and brain eggplant formation are the main death causes of ICH. Prognosis is related to the amount of bleeding, bleeding site, state of consciousness and complications.

6.5 Subarachnoid Hemorrhage

Intracranial blood vessels rupture and the blood flows into the subarachnoid space is called subarachnoid hemorrhage (SAH). Intracranial aneurysm is the most common cause. Most of them are cystic aneurysms, and there are also fusiform aneurysms caused by hypertension atherosclerosis, dissecting aneurysms and aneurysms caused by fungal infection. Vascular malformation accounts for approximately 10% of SAH causes, arteriovenous malformation (AVM) accounts for 80% of vascular malformations. Besides, SAH can be caused by moyamoya disease, intracranial tumor, pituitary apoplexy, blood system diseases, intracranial veins systemic thrombosis and anticoagulant treatment complications.

(1) Clinical feature

1) Clinical manifestation

The clinical manifestations of SAH vary greatly. Mild cases may have no obvious clinical symptoms and signs, while severe cases may suddenly fall into coma or even death. It is reported that most young patients have an obvious incentive before onset suddenly.

① Headache

Aneurysmal SAH is typically characterized by a sudden onset of severe total headache, which is often described as "the worst headache" they have ever experienced in their life by some patients. The headache may get worse progressively.

② Meningeal stimulation signs

The signs include nuchal rigidity, Kerning's sign and Brudzinski sign, among which nuchal rigidity is the most common one. Among senile or frail patients or patients with small amount of bleeding, meningeal irritation may be not obvious.

③ Ocular symptoms

Subvitreous bleeding, the sign of acute intracranial pressure increasing, appears within one hour of onset in 20% of patients. In addition, impaired eye movement can indicate the location of an aneurysm.

④ Mental symptoms

About 25% of patients may have mental symptoms, such as euphoria, false speech and hallucination. Some patients may develop seizures, brain-heart syndrome, gastrointestinal bleeding, acute pulmonary edema and localized neurological deficits symptoms.

⑤ Complications

Recurrence of hemorrhage is the major acute complication of SAH, which means the recurrence of headache, vomiting, painful attack, coma and even cerebral ankylosis attack, cervical ankylosis, Kerning's sign aggravation, and cerebrospinal fluid is bright red. Cerebrovascular spasm (CVS), often leading to death or disability, occured in the blood vessel surrounded by a blood clot in the subarachnoid space. The severity of the spasm is related with the amount of blood loss. The clinical symptoms depend on the vessel where the spasm occurs, which often present as fluctuating hemiplegia or aphasia. Acute or subacute hydrocephalus is another complication as blood clots block the circulation of cerebrospinal fluid in the ventricular system and subarachnoid space. In mild cases, signs such as drowsiness, dullness, impaired short-term memory, limited upper vision, abducens palsy, hyperreflexes of lower limbs may occur, and in severe cases, intracranial hypertension or even cerebral apoplexy may occur. Subacute hydrocephalus occurs several weeks after onset and it is characterized by latent dementia, abnormal gait, and urinary incontinence.

Q: What are the symptoms of various aneurysms?

A: Cavernous segment aneurysm of internal carotid artery: Patients have forehead and eye pain, vascular murmurs, eye protrusion, and Ⅲ, Ⅳ, Ⅵ, and V_1 cranial nerves damage caused by ocular movement disorders, the rupture of cavernous aneurysm of internal carotid artery can cause internal carotid cavernous sinus thinning.

Internal carotid artery and posterior communicating aneurysm: Patients have oculomotor paralysis, which suggests posterior communicating aneurysm.

Middle cerebral aneurysm: Patients have hemiplegia, aphasia and aspiration and other symptoms.

Anterior cerebral artery and anterior communicating aneurysm: Patients have psychiatric symptoms, unilateral or bilateral paralysis of the lower limbs, and disturbance of consciousness, etc.

Posterior cerebral aneurysm: Patients present with cohemianopia, Weber syndrome, and palsy of the Ⅲ cranial nerve.

Pushed-basal aneurysm: Patients may experience occipital and facial pain, facial muscle problems, facial paralysis, and brain stem compression.

2) Diagnostic investigation

Blood routine, coagulation and liver function tests can help find other causes of bleeding. Head CT scan is the first choice for suspected SAH (Fig. 6.5). SAH shows high-density hemorrhage signs in lateral cistern, anterior longitudinal cistern, suprasellar cistern, pontine cistern, circumferential cistern, and posterior longitudinal cistern. But when the amount of bleeding is low, the CT scan is not clear. When the sensitivity of CT examination decreases several days after the onset, MRI plays an important role. CTA and MRA is mainly used for screening patients with a family history of aneurysm or premonitory rupture, follow-up of aneurysm patients, and

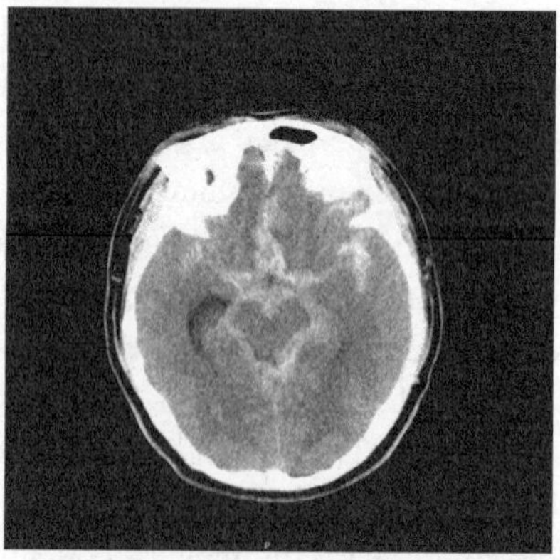

Fig. 6.5 Head CT scan of SAH

it is an alternative method when DSA cannot be timely examined.

If conditions permit, whole-brain DSA examination should be performed as soon as possible to determine aneurysm, the cause of hemorrhage, the treatment and prognosis. DSA is still the "gold standard" for clinical diagnosis of primary aneurysm, which can determine the size, location, relationship with the parent artery, and the presence of vascular blast twins and other anatomical characteristics. TCD can be used as a non-invasive technique to monitor cerebrovascular disease after SAH.

(2) Diagnosis and differential diagnosis

Sudden onset of persistent severe headache, vomiting, meningeal stimulation sign positive, with or without disturbance of consciousness, examination of no focal nervous system sign, SAH should be highly suspected. At the same time, CT can confirm the high-density signs of cistern and subarachnoid space or lumbar puncture examination shows increased pressure and bloody cerebrospinal fluid. Subarachnoid hemorrhage should be distinguished from hypertensive cerebral hemorrhage, intracranial infection and brain tumor, etc.

(3) Treatment

The treatment objective is to prevent rebleeding and minimize the risk of complications. First, to prevent the onset of subarachnoid hemorrhage, smoking cessation, blood pressure control, and alcohol savings or avoidance is recommended. Patients should be transferred to a neurosurgical centre immediately. They require frequently neurological observations, including pulse, blood pressure and Glasgow coma scale. Those confused and unconscious patients are recommended to receive an appropriate nursing care. So the management of SAH is suggested below.

a. Reducing high cranial pressure: Dehydrating agents such as mannitol, enseme, glycerin fructose, or uranium glycerin chloride are used for reducing high cranial pressure, and albumin may be another choice.

b. Symptomatic supportive treatment: Beside avoiding exertion, rage and bowel movement obstruction, relieving irritants and headaches, it is essential to maintain water and electrolyte balance, keep high-fiber and high-energy diet, operate intensive care unremittingly, prevent urinary tract infection and inhalation pneumonia.

c. Complications treatment: Rebleeding can be prevented either by clipping the aneurysm or by blocking it with a coil, which are endovascular techniques. The risk of ischemic complications caused by vasospasm can be reduced by sustained hypervolaemia and a calcium antagonist (nimodipine). Lowering blood pressure aggressively may increase ischemic complications, so strong anti-hypertensives are not recommended. Fludrocortisone or hypertonic saline can be used to treat hyponatraemia and an appropriate drainage procedure to hydrocephalus.

(4) Prognosis

The prognosis of SAH is poor, the fatality rate is up to 45%, and the survival disability rate is high. The prognosis of SAH is related to etiology, bleeding site, bleeding volume, meta-complication and proper treatment.

6.6 Other Cerebrovascular Diseases

6.6.1 Moyamoya Disease

Moyamoya refers to an extensive basal cerebral rete mirabile, which is a network of small anastomotic vessels at the base of the brain around and distal to the circle of Willis, along with segmental stenosis or occlusion of the terminal parts of both internal carotid arteries. (Fig. 6.6)

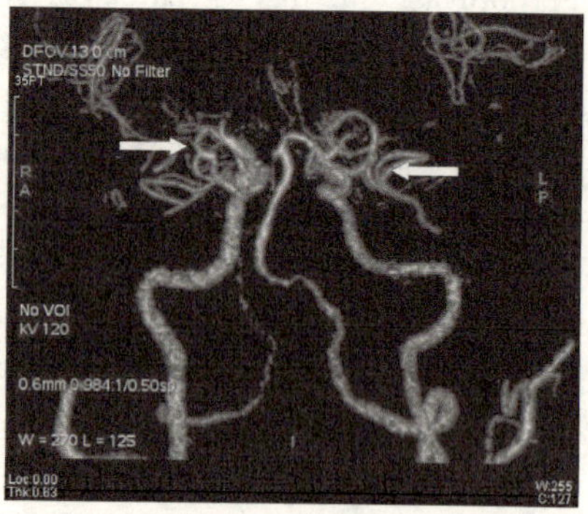

Fig. 6.6 Moyamoya Disease in CTA

The etiology is complex, although genetic factors and acquired environmental factors are related to the pathogenesis. It is more common with two peak ages of onset in children of 5 years old and young adults of 40 years old. The common clinical manifestations can be divided into defective symptoms and hemorrhagic symptoms, including TIA, stroke, headache, epilepsy and intelligent decline. The majority of children have ischemic stroke, due to a lack of blood flow, or recurrent TIAs, while hemorrhagic stroke is common in adults.

Treatment cannot cure moyamoya disease but can be very effective in preventing strokes. The goal of treatment is to reduce symptoms, improve brain blood flow, and lower risk of serious complications, such as an ischemic stroke, intracerebral hemorrhage or death. Medications may be prescribed to manage symptoms and reduce the risk of stroke, including blood thinners, calcium channel blockers or anti-seizure medications, etc. Early surgical treatment can help slow progression of moyamoya disease. Direct and indirect revascularization surgeries are operated to restore blood flow to brain. Surgeons stitch the vascular muscle flap to the superficial temporal artery to middle cerebral artery directly. The indirect revascularization is to lay over the brain surface blood-rich tissues to increase blood flow to the brain gradually over time and it is almost always combined with direct revascularization in adult patients.

6.6.2 Cerebral Amyloid Angiopathy

Cerebral amyloid angiopathy (CAA) is a cerebrovascular disease caused by the deposition of amyloid in the pia mater and the middle layer of cerebral cortex arterioles. The clinical features are multifocal spontaneous cerebral parenchymal hemorrhage caused by repeated vascular rupture at multiple sites. Elderly patients, without a history of primary hypertension, recurrent or multifocal lobar hemorrhage confirmed by CT or MRI, and excluding other causes, may be clinically prescribed diagnosis of CAA. Neuropathological examination is the most reliable auxiliary examination to diagnose CAA.

The management of CAA is generally similar to that of other causes of cerebral hemorrhage. Patients with secondary epilepsy should be treated with anti-seizure drugs. Anticoagulants should be avoided for CAA with cerebral infarction, and antiplatelet drugs should be used with caution.

6.7 Cerebral Venous Thrombosis

Intracranial venous sinus and cerebral venous thrombosis (CVT) is a group of cerebral venous system vascular diseases caused by a variety of etiology. It is common in the elderly and puerperium women. The clinical symptoms are different because of the etiology and lesion location. CVT is caused by abnormal blood coagulation, which mainly includes hypercoagulable conditions, abnormal hereditary coagulation, abnormal hemodynamics, the whole body disease, drug-induced and infection or tumor invasion.

(1) Clinical feature

1) Clinical manifestation

The clinical manifestations of CVT are varied with different locations, ranges, obstruction speeds, onset ages and etiologies. Common clinical manifestations include high cranial pressure symptoms, stroke symptoms and encephalopathy symptoms. Headache is the most common symptom of ICP and it is severe and persistent, associated with ejective vomiting, visible papilloedema. In some elderly patients, headache may be absent and may only present with paresis or seizures. Stroke symptoms include hemorrhagic, more common with multiple small bleeding, or ischemic venous infarction. Although encephalopathy symptoms are rare, they are seriously showing mental disorders, confusion, blurred consciousness, and even coma. Cerebral hernia caused by cerebral edema is the most common cause of death in patients with CVT.

Superior sagittal sinus thrombosis: The superior sagittal sinus is the most common site of non-infectious venous sinus thrombosis. It is not only usually seen in dehydrated and weakened infants, but also in patients with trauma, tumors, oral contraceptives, baby vibrations, blood disorders and immune system diseases. General symptoms include: acute or subacute onset, systemic weakness, fever, headache, and apparent papilledema. Sometimes it can be complicated with intracranial hemorrhage, epilepsy, hemiplegia, aphasia, hemianopia, etc. Sometimes there are no focal signs, and intracranial hypertension is the only symptom. Elderly patients show mild symptoms, such as headache and dizziness.

Cavernous sinus thrombosis: The orbital, sinus and upper face of the body infection or systemic infection is common, non-infectious cavernous sinus thrombosis is rare. It rapidly spread from one side to the opposite side. The symptoms include poisoning, fever and other systemic poisoning symptoms, eyeball pain and orbital tenderness. The main manifestations are cerebral nerve damage and obstruction of ocular venous reflux. If Ⅲ, Ⅳ, Ⅵ, $V_{1\sim2}$ cerebral nerve damaged, eye ptosis, limited or fixed eye movement, diplopia, enlarged sleep hole, loss of light response, loss of corneal reflex, etc. might occur. Obstruction of ocular venous reflux can cause eye danger, periorbital, bulbar conjunctival edema and eyeball herniation. Papillary edema and hemorrhage are seen in the fundus, but vision is usually not involved. Water salt metabolism disorder may present if pituitary is involved. CSF shows increased cell count, too.

Sagittal and lateral sinus thrombosis: In the case of sagittal sinus thrombosis, intracranial hypertension with headache, vomiting, and papilledema may constitute the entire syndrome or it may be conjoined with hemorrhagic infarction, paraparesis, hemiparesis, fluctuating unilateral or bilateral sensory symptoms, or aphasia only if the thrombosis propagates to surface veins.

Galen vein thrombosis: Galen venous thrombosis is common in non-infectious diseases, such as puerperium, dehydration and hematology, and it is mostly caused by venous sinus thrombosis, involving deep brain structures such as the diencephalon and basal ganglia. It shows intracranial pressure heighten and mental symptoms at the beginning, coma, high fever, epileptic seizure, even brain rigidity appear when the condition is serious. Surviving patients can live with hand and foot asthenia, chorea, etc.

2) Diagnostic investigation

The direct signs of CT include: a. Cerebral venous sinus wall shows the high density and intracavitary cavity shows the low density under the role of contrast agents. b. Dense triangle sign. The high dense triangular image of the posterior superior sagittal sinus at the unenhanced coronal level suggests fresh thrombus. c. Cord sign. High-density shadow which parallel to blood vessels suggests fresh thrombosis. Indirect signs include focal or diffuse cerebral edema, which is manifested as narrowing of ventricles and sulci, and low density of white matter. Venous infarction is characterized by low density foci, and sometimes there is high density hemorrhage foci in the infarction area, and subarachnoid hemorrhage is occasionally seen. Cerebral falx and tentorium are enhanced.

MRI behaves differently at different times. In acute stage (1~5 days), empty phenomenon of normal blood flow disappears, T_1 isometric signal and T_2 low signal can be observed. In subacute stage (1~2 weeks), T_1 and T_2 show high signal. During the convalescence period (2 weeks later), empty blood flow may reappear. The main direct signs of MRV are blood flow signal loss in cerebral veins (sinus), and the indirect signs are the formation of collateral circulation on the distal side of the lesion, deep vein dilation or other drainage veins. DSA is the "gold standard" for the diagnosis of CVT, which is characterized by the absence of venous sinus lesions.

In the early stage of cerebrospinal fluid examination, intracranial pressure is increased, cell number and biochemical indexes are usually in the normal range, and cerebrospinal fluid protein is usually mild or moderate increased in the middle and late stage. In patients with hemorrhage, erythrocytes can be seen in cerebrospinal fluid, and protein can be significantly elevated. An increase in neutrophils is seen in thrombus induced by chemical administration.

(2) Diagnosis and differential diagnosis

The diagnosis is based on typical history, symptoms of high cranial pressure, and imaging features such as CT, MRI, MRV. DSA can confirm the diagnosis. The disease needs to be distinguished from benign intracranial hypertension, central nervous system infection, intracranial tumor, and cerebral hemorrhage.

(3) Treatment

Treatment should be started as soon as the diagnosis is confirmed, it consists of reversing the underlying cause, control of seizures and intracranial hypertension, and antithrombotic therapy. Anticoagulation is the mainstay of acute and subacute treatment for CVT.

a. Etiological treatment: Etiological treatment is one of the fundamental treatments for CVT. Infectious patients should be treated with sensitive, sufficient amount and sufficient course of antibiotics as early as possible according to different pathogens. Severe dehydration patients should be carried out to maintain water and electrolyte balance. People with autoimmune diseases such as systemic lupus erythematosus can be treated with hormones. Corresponding treatment should be initiated to blood system diseases. Patients with increased blood viscosity should be treated with dilatation and reduction of blood viscosity.

b. Anticoagulant therapy: Low molecular weight heparin can be used with attention to the risk of intracranial hemorrhage, so the clotting time and partial thrombin time should be monitored during the treatment. For long-term treatment lasting for 6 ~ 12 months, oral anticoagulant warfarin can be used. INR should be detected, and the dose should be adjusted according to situation to keep the target INR between 2.0 and 3.0.

c. Thrombolytic therapy: Urokinase and RT-PA intravenous thrombolytic therapy can be used, but there is no evidence that the treatment is superior to anticoagulant therapy. But they can be used as a secondary option for deterioration due to anticoagulant therapy.

d. Interventional therapy: Mechanical thrombolytic therapy and angioplasty with intravenously interventional catheter can be an option for some severe CVT patients if the disease deteriorates further.

e. Symptomatic supportive treatment: Drugs such as mannitol, glycerin fructose, enantiome and albumin can be used in the treatment of lowering cranial pressure. For acute high cranial pressure caused by CVT, surgical treatment should be considered when drugs fail, such as ventricular drainage and vein bypass. Anti-seizure drugs can be given to epileptic patients continuously. And cerebral hernia needs more intensive care to the detection and treatment of focal space-occupying lesions.

(4) Prognosis

Most patients with CVT have a good prognosis as the treatment and diagnostic techniques have improved, more than half of patients can be cured, the mortality rate is less than 10%, and a few have recurrence. The factors of poor prognosis included advanced age, intracranial hemorrhage, coma and mental disorders, deep cerebral vein thrombosis, primary or new lesions, central nervous system infection or tumor, etc. Survivors of CVT have varying degrees of residual symptoms and are not able to return to their previous work.

References

[1] FURIE K L, KASNER S E, ADAMS R J, et al. Guidelines for the prevention of stroke in patients with stroke or transient ischemic attack: a guideline for healthcare professionals from the American Heart Association/American Stroke Association[J]. Stroke, 2011,42(1):227-276.

[2] FONSECA A C, MERWICK A, DENNIS M, et al. European Stroke Organisation (ESO) guidelines on management of transient ischaemic attack[J]. European Stroke Journal, 2021,6(2):CLXIII-CLXXXVI.

[3] KLEINDORFER D O, TOWFIGHI A, CHATURVEDI S, et al. 2021 guideline for the prevention of stroke in patients with stroke and transient ischemic attack: a guideline from the American Heart Association/American Stroke Association[J]. Stroke, 2021,52(7):e364-e467.

[4] BROWN D L, LEVINE D A, ALBRIGHT K, et al. Benefits and risks of dual versus single antiplatelet therapy for secondary stroke prevention: a systematic review for the 2021 guideline for the prevention of stroke in patients with stroke and transient ischemic attack[J]. Stroke, 2021,52(7):e468-e479.

[5] GU H Q, YANG X, WANG C J, et al. Assessment of trends in guideline-based oral anticoagulant prescription for patients with ischemic stroke and atrial fibrillation in China[J]. JAMA Network Open, 2021,4(7):517-584.

[6] GOLDSTEIN L B, BUSHNELL C D, ADAMS R J, et al. Guidelines for the management of spontaneous intracerebral hemorrhage: a statement for healthcare professionals

from the American Heart Association/American & Stroke Association[J]. Stroke, 2011,42: 517-584.

[7] CAO Y, YU S L, ZHANG Q, et al. Chinese Stroke Association guidelines for clinical management of cerebrovascular disorders: executive summary and 2019 update of clinical management of intracerebral haemorrhage[J]. Stroke Vascular Neurology, 2020,5(4):396-402.

[8] WAHAB K W, TIWARI H K B, OVBIAGELE B, et al. Genetic risk of spontaneous intracerebral hemorrhage: systematic review and future directions [J]. Journal of the Neurological Sciences, 2019,407:116526.

[9] DONG Y, GUO Z N, LI Q, et al. Chinese Stroke Association guidelines for clinical management of cerebrovascular disorders: executive summary and 2019 update of clinical management of spontaneous subarachnoid haemorrhage [J]. Stroke & Vascular Neurology, 2019,4(4):176-181.

[10] FAN Y H, YU J, CHEN H B, et al. Chinese Stroke Association guidelines for clinical management of cerebrovascular disorders: executive summary and 2019 update of clinical management of cerebral venous sinus thrombosis[J]. Stroke & Vascular Neurology, 2020,5(2):152-158.

[11] ALET M, CIARDI C, ALEMÁN A, et al. Cerebral venous thrombosis in Argentina: clinical presentation, predisposing factors, outcomes and literature review[J]. Journal of Stroke and Cerebrovascular Diseases, 2020,29(10):105145.

[12] PENG D T. Clinical practice guideline for cognitive impairment of cerebral small vessel disease[J]. Aging Medicine, 2019,2(2):64-73.

[13] QU Y, HU H Y, OU Y N, et al. Association of body mass index with risk of cognitive impairment and dementia: A systematic review and meta-analysis of prospective studies[J]. Neuroscience and Biobehavioral Reviews, 2020,115:189-198.

(Yu Ming, Jiang Ping, Zheng Qiuyue)

Chapter 7
Infectious Diseases

Infectious diseases of the nervous system include bacterial, viral, fungal, spirochetal, and parasitic infections. Similar to all types of infection of the nervous system, bacteria may involve any of the nervous system compartments: the epidural space (epidural abscess), the dura (pachymeningitis), the subdural space (subdural empyema), the leptomeninges and the subarachnoid space containing cerebrospinal fluid (meningitis or leptomeningitis), and the brain parenchyma (brain abscess). This chapter is concerned mainly with various infections of the central nervous system (CNS), particularly acute transverse myelitis, bacterial meningitis, brain abscess, HSV-1 encephalitis, tuberculosis, neurosyphilis, and certain parasitosis. Prion disease and HIV-associated infections are also discussed in detail.

7.1 Acute Bacterial Meningitis

Bacterial meningitis is a bacterial infection of the meninges, which is the protective covering for the brain and spinal cord resulting in inflammation. Common causes of community-onset bacterial meningitis include *Streptococcus pneumoniae*, *Neisseria meningitidis*, and *Listeria monocytogenes*. *Neisseria meningitidis* is still the most common cause. *Group B Streptococcus* is common in infants less than 2 months of age while *Streptococcus pneumoniae* is the most common in all other age groups with the exception of 11~17 years old. *Listeria monocytogenes*, *Escherichia coli*, *Klebsiella*, *Enterobacter* and *Pseudomonas aeruginosa* are other less common causes. Nosocomial infections are caused by pneumonia, *Staphylococcus aureus*, *Staphylococcus albus* and Gram-negative bacilli. Immunodeficient states are risk factors for pneumococcal meningitis.

(1) Pathophysiology

Bacteria requires access to the meninges to cause meningitis. There are several mechanisms for entry: a. Bacteremia, or bacteria in the blood, can result in bacteria crossing the blood-brain barrier. This can only be accomplished by certain bacteria, most notably *N. meningitidis* and *S. pneumoniae*. b. Direct extension of otitis media or sinusitis to the central nervous system (CNS) may also occur. Dural defects, either congenital or acquired, allow bacteria to enter the CNS. c. Nosocomial bacterial meningitis is the result of the manipulation of the meninges during neurosurgical procedures or cerebrospinal fluid leakage. Invasion of bacteria into the subarachnoid space results in inflammation of the meninges. Lipopolysaccharide in the walls of Gram-negative organisms and techoic acid in the walls of Gram-positive microorganisms activate brain microglia, leading to a cascade of inflammatory changes that causes cortical microvascular permeability with diffuse cerebral edema, resulting in increased intracranial pressure. Altered mental status, seizures, and focal neurologic deficits occur due to decreased perfusion.

(2) Clinical feature

1) Clinical manifestation

Fever, neck stiffness, and altered mental status are the classic triad of symptoms most commonly seen in some patients for meningitis. 70% patients present with at least one of these symptoms. Symptoms of acute meningitis may be subacute and nonspecific. In severe cases, bacterial meningitis may present with coma, seizure, and focal neurologic deficits, which are associated with an unfavorable prognosis. History should include questioning about any recent neurosurgical procedures, immunization status, and living arrangements. The fundoscopic exam may reveal papilledema due to increased intracranial pressure. A rapidly spreading petechial rash, known as purpuric rash, would suggest a meningococcal infection. A physical exam may reveal positive signs of meningeal irritation, that presents as nuchal rigidity or positive Kernig's or Brudzinski's signs. Though the absence of these does not reliably rule out the diseases. These signs are thought to be secondary to meningeal irritation.

2) Diagnostic investigation

Given the lack of specific symptoms or physical findings, the diagnosis of meningitis is based on the analysis of cerebrospinal fluid (CSF) sample. A non-contrast CT scan of the head should be performed before lumbar puncture if the patient has a risk of herniation. The CSF should be sent for Gram stain, culture, complete cell count, and glucose and protein levels. A rapidly performed Gram stain of cerebrospinal fluid can provide timely identification of the causative pathogen because the sterilization of cerebrospinal fluid can occur as quickly as 15 minutes after parenteral antimicrobial therapy. Even if the CSF culture is subsequently negative, a Gram stain of the cerebrospinal fluid may show the causative organism. Bacterial meningitis typically results in low glucose and high protein levels in the cerebrospinal fluid. As CSF glucose levels are dependent on circulating serum glucose levels, the CSF to serum glucose ratio is considered more reliable parameter for the diagnosis of acute bacterial meningitis than absolute CSF glucose levels. A neutrophil predominance on cell count can be expected. The diagnosis would be confirmed with bacteria identified on Gram stain or culture. Opening pressure is typically elevated in bacterial meningitis. Lumbar puncture should not delay initiation of antimicrobial therapy in cases in which bacterial meningitis is suspected. Blood cultures should be obtained as 53% of patients have concurrent bacteremia.

(3) Differential diagnosis

A number of nonbacterial meningitides must be considered in the differential diagnosis when the meningitis recurs repeatedly and all cultures are negative. These recurrent syndromes rarely present in the fulminant manner of acute bacterial meningitis but sometimes they do, and the CSF formulas can be similar, including a reduction in glucose concentration. Included in this group are: Epstein-Barr virus (EBV) infections; Behçet's disease, which is characterized by recurrent oropharyngeal mucosal ulceration, uveitis, orchitis, and meningitis; mollaret meningitis, which consists of recurrent episodes of fever and headache in addition to signs of meningeal irritation; Vogt-Koyanagi-Harada syndrome, in which recurrent meningitis is associated with iridocyclitis and depigmentation of the hair and skin (poliosis and vitiligo); CNS vasculitis, a fulminant case of cerebral angiitis or intravascular lymphoma will present with headache, fever, and confusion in conjunction with a meningeal inflammatory reaction.

(4) Treatment

1) Antimicrobialtherapy

Patients suspected of having meningococcal meningitis should be placed in droplet precautions until they have received 24 hours of antibiotics. Timely administration of antibiotics is essential. The choice of empiric antimicrobials should be based on those agents with activity against most likely pathogens, epidemiologic data, age, patient immune status, or other predisposing factors. Another important factor is antimicrobial penetration into the central nervous system. An approach to empirical therapy is summarized (ESCMID guideline) in Tab. 7.1. Patients who are immunocompromised or older than 50 should receive ampicillin. Patients due to head trauma or post-neurosurgical procedure should receive vancomycin and ceftazidime or cefepime. Acyclovir can also be administered for HSV coverage. Vancomycin, combined with either third-generation or fourth-generation cephalosporins or a carbapenem, are appropriate empiric antimicrobial regimens for nosocomial meningitis. Once a causative pathogen is identified, antimicrobial therapy should be modified. A repeat lumbar puncture is the most effective way for inadequate response to antimicrobial therapy.

Tab. 7.1 Empiric antibiotic in-hospital treatment for bacterial meningitis

Patient group	Standard treatment		Intravenous dose
	Reduced *S. pneumoniae* antimicrobial sensitivity to penicillin	*S. pneumoniae* susceptible to penicillin	
Neonates< 1 month old	Amoxicillin/ampicillin/penicillin + cefotaxime, or amoxicillin/ampicillin+an aminoglycoside		Age<1 week: cefotaxime 50 mg/kg q8h; ampicillin/amoxicillin 50 mg/kg q8h; genta-micin 2.5 mg/kg q12h Age 1~4 weeks: ampicillin 50 mg/kg q6h; cefotaxime 50 mg/kg q6h~q8h; gentamicin 2.5 mg/kg q8h; tobramycin 2.5 mg/kg q8h; amikacin10 mg/kg q8h
Age 1 month to 18 years old	Cefotaxime/ceftriaxone + vancomycin/rifampicin	Cefotaxime or ceftriaxone	Vancomycin 10~15 mg/kg q6h; rifampicin 10 mg/kg q12h up to 600 mg/d; cefotaxime 75 mg/kg q6h~q8h; ceftriaxone 50 mg/kg q12h (maximum 2 g/kg q12h)
Age 18~50 years old	Cefotaxime/ceftriaxone + vancomycin/rifampicin	Cefotaxime or ceftriaxone	Ceftriaxone 2 g/kg q12h or 4 g/kg q24h; cefotaxime 2 g/kg q4h ~ q6h; vancomycin 10~20 mg/kg q8h~q12h; rifampicin 300 mg/kg q12h
Age>50 years old, or 18~50 years old plus risk factors for *Listeria monocytogenes*	Cefotaxime/ceftriaxone + vancomycin/rifampicin + amoxicillin/ampicillin/penicillin G	Cefotaxime/ceftriaxone + amoxicillin/ampicillin/penicillin G	Ceftriaxone 2 g/kg q12h or 4 g/kg q24h; cefotaxime 2 g/kg q4h~q6h; vancomycin 10~20 mg/kg q8h~q12h; rifampicin 300 mg q12h, amoxicillin or ampicillin 2 g/kg q4h

2) Supportive care

Comprehensive supportive care is required in the management of meningitis. Appropriate circulatory resuscitation is essential. Periodic mental status assessment is useful for evaluation of recovery, as well as prompt recognition of new-onset focal neurologic changes or seizures.

3) Adjuvant therapy

Corticosteroids are also used for bacterial meningitis among pediatric patients or *S. pneumoniae* infections. Corticosteroids should be administered simultaneously with antimicrobial agents because the lysis of bacteria by antimicrobial agents triggers the release of inflammatory cytokine, which is felt to worsen local tissue damage. But the overall benefit of corticosteroid therapy is still not clearly understood.

(5) Prognosis

Hyponatremia and seizure are the most common complications of meningitis. Delayed therapy can result in vascular inflammation with cerebral infarction. Other long-term complications include cognitive decline, paralysis, balance and coordination difficulties, learning difficulties, speech problems, vision loss and hearing loss. The mortality for bacterial meningitis varies from 10% ~ 15%. Survival depends on early recognition of acute bacterial meningitis, followed by administration of appropriate antibiotic therapy.

7.2 Brain Abscess

Brain abscess is a localized zone of necrosis with a surrounding membrane within the brain parenchyma, usually resulting from an infectious or traumatic process. The most frequent microbial pathogens isolated from brain abscesses are *Staphylococcus* and *Streptococcus*. The incidence of brain abscess is approximately 8% of intracranial masses in developing countries and 1% ~ 2% in the western countries with approximately four cases occurring per million. The incidence of fungal brain abscesses also has increased because of the higher usage of broad-spectrum antibiotics and immunosuppressive agents like steroids. Data suggests that brain abscesses are more predominant in males with a male-to-female ratio varying between 2 : 1 and 3 : 1.

(1) Pathophysiology

Understanding the pathogenesis of brain abscesses is important in determining the most likely causative microorganisms and subsequent treatment. As a brain abscess can originate from infections in head and neck sites: otitis media and mastoiditis, paranasal sinus infection, infection from frontal or ethmoid sinuses spreads to the frontal lobes, dental infection usually causes frontal lobar abscesses. Facial trauma, even from neurosurgical procedures, can result in necrotic tissue, and brain abscesses are reported afterward. Valveless emissary veins may allow microorganism to flow into the venous system of the brain from these sites. Various conditions can cause hematogenous seeding of the brain. Some common ones include pulmonary infections or cystic fibrosis from an important encountered cause. Bacterial endocarditis, ventricular aneurysms, and thrombosis are also among the causes. Skin, pelvic and intraabdominal infections are also reported frequently as risk factors. Brain abscesses associated with bacteremia commonly cause multiple abscesses, mostly in the distribution of the middle cerebral artery and usually at the gray-white matter junction. Fungal brain abscesses caused by yeast, dimorphic fungi, and molds associated with immunocompromised states and poorly controlled diabetes.

Protozoa and helminths can cause parasitic brain abscesses. The histologic changes depend upon the acute and subacute stages of the infection: a. The acute (first 1 to 2 weeks) lesion, often called focal cerebritis, is evident by vascular congestion and localized edema. This early stage is commonly acute inflammatory change. b. Necrosis and liquefaction occur after 2 ~ 3 weeks. Lesion is then covered by a distinct capsule consisting of an inner layer of granulation tissue, a middle collagenous layer, and an outer astroglial layer, with surrounding cellular swelling.

(2) Clinical feature

1) Clinical manifestation

The course ranges from indolent to fulminant. Most manifestations of brain abscess tend to be nonspecific. Most symptoms are a direct result of the size and location of the space-occupying lesion or lesions. The triad of fever, headache, and the focal neurologic deficit is observed in less than half of patients. New-onset seizures can also be an initial symptom of brain abscess. Clinical manifestations are dependent on the location and size of the brain abscess, host immunestatus, and the virulence of the causative microorganism. The frequency of common symptoms and signs is as follows in Tab. 7.2.

Tab. 7.2 Common symptoms and signs of brain abscess

Symptom and sign	Frequency/%
Headache	69 ~ 70
Mental status changes	65
Focal neurologic deficits	50 ~ 65
Fever	45 ~ 53
Nausea and vomiting	40
Seizures	25 ~ 35
Nuchal rigidity	15
Papilledema	25

2) Diagnostic investigation

① Routine tests

Complete blood count with differential and platelet count, erythrocyte sedimentation rate, serum C-reactive protein, serologic test, blood cultures.

② Lumbar puncture

Rarely required and only should be performed after ruling out increased intracranial pressure because of the potential for herniation and death. The CSF results are mostly nonspecific, consisting of an elevated protein level, pleocytosis with the variable neutrophil count, typically a normal glucose level, and sterile cultures. A lumbar puncture in the case of rupture when white blood cell (WBC) count becomes high in addition to elevated CSF lactic acid and abundant red blood cells (RBCs) in the CSF.

③ Imaging examination

Early cerebritis often appears as an irregular low-density area that does not enhance or may show infrequent patchy enhancement. Serial CT examinations in patients with late abscesses show progressively decreasing edema and mass effect. As cerebritis evolves, CT with intravenous contrast may reveal single-ring or multiple-ring enhancing lesions, particularly in well-established or chronic brain abscess. The ring of enhancement may not be uniform in thickness and can be relatively thin on the medial or ventricular surface in the deep white matter. MRI is more sensitive for early cerebritis and satellite lesions particularly those present in the brain stem as well as estimating the necrosis and extent of the lesion. Abscesses are typically hyperintense on DWI-MR and a contrast-enhanced rim surrounding a necrotic core. (Fig. 7.1)

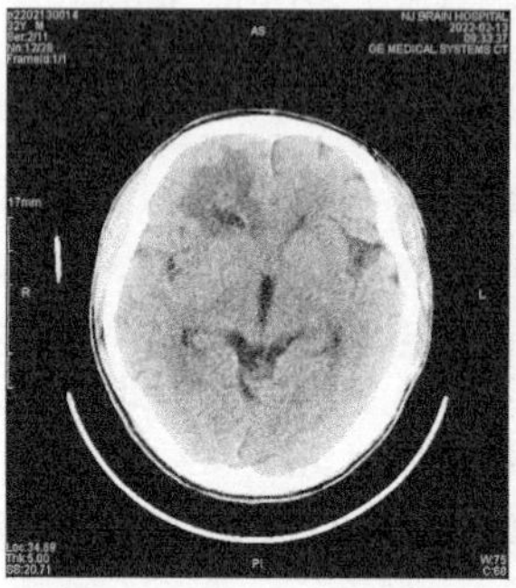
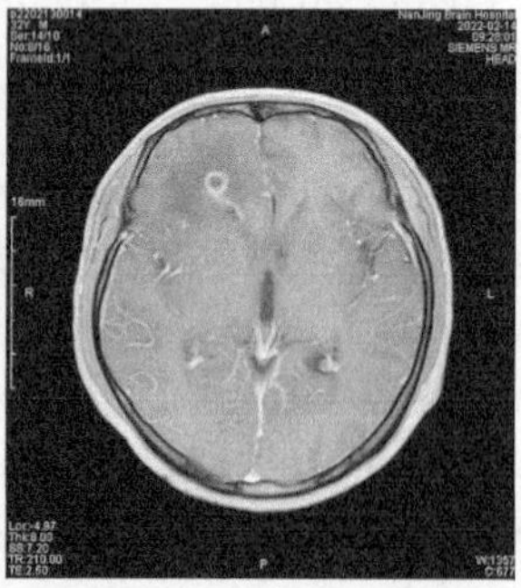

(a) CT (b) Enhanced MRI

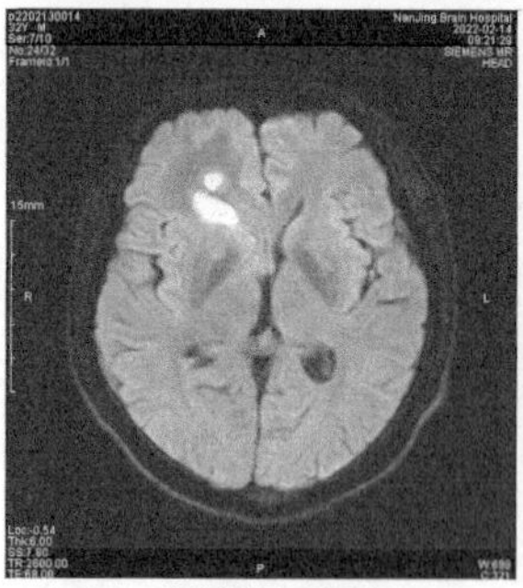
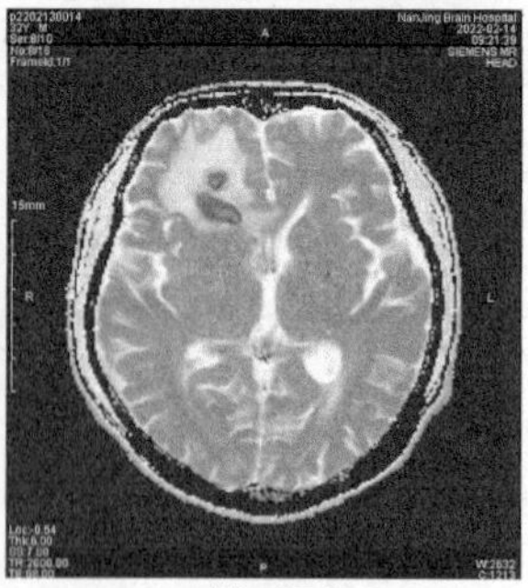

(c) MRI-DWI (d) ADC

CT image of the cranium (a) shows right frontal abscess characterized by a hypodense center, an isodense ring, and a surrounding edema. Enhanced MRI (b) shows a hypointense necrotic center with pus, ring-shaped enhancement wall, and a hypointense zone of edema. MRI-DWI shows a hyperintense signal within the abscess (c), which is hypointense on apparent-diffusion-coefficient (ADC) imaging (d).

Fig. 7.1 Imaging studies of brain abscess

MRS analysis reveals elevated succinate, elevated acetate, alanine, and lactate signals. Amino acids from neutrophil-driven protein breakdown suggest a pyogenic abscess. MRS may be used to further differentiate anaerobic from aerobic metabolism by elevated succinate and acetate peaks. Also, lactate peaks are lowest in strict anaerobes owing to metabolic lactate consumption.

(3) Differential diagnosis

① Bacterial meningitis

Fever, neck stiffness, and altered mental status are the classic triad of symptoms of patients for meningitis. Generally none space-occupying lesion can be found by CT/MRI scan rather than an evidence of meningitis with leptomeningeal enhancement.

② Brain tumors

Differentiating brain abscesses from cystic or necrotic tumors by CT or MR imaging can be difficult. MRS analysis often provides the most valuable information. MRS of brain abscess revealed multiple resonance peaks: amino acids (valine, leucine, and isoleucine), acetate, alanine, and lactate identified in patients with abscesses. Spectra in patients with cystic or necrotic tumor showed only the peak attributed to lactate, which is a nonspecific metabolite that results from anaerobic glycolysis.

③ Epidural/subdural empyema

It is defined as a purulent infection of the space between the cranial dura and arachnoid membrane, which is a neurosurgical emergency. Major symptoms include headache, altered mental status, and focal signs, similar to those of brain abscesses. CT scan of the brain usually shows a hypodense subdural lesion with medial membrane enhancement, MRI may be more sensitive to visualize subdural lesions.

④ Encephalitis

Patients with HSE typically present with headache, fever, seizures, viral prodrome, and mental status changes. The classic imaging findings are bilateral asymmetric involvement of the temporal and inferior frontal lobes with less common involvement of the insula and cingulategyri.

(4) Treatment

Treatments can be divided into medical and surgical approaches. Usually, large abscesses (more than 2 cm) are considered for aspiration or excision based on the surgical skills of the operator. The approach for multiple abscesses includes a long course (4 to 8 weeks) of high-dose antibiotics with or without aspirations, based on weekly CT scanning. Medical management can be considered for deep-seated, small abscesses (less than 2 cm), cases of coexisting meningitis, and few other selected cases. Usually, a combination of both medical and surgical approaches is considered. While empiric antimicrobial therapy should be started, particularly in patients with sepsis or impending herniation. Empiric antimicrobial therapy should cover Gram-positive, Gram-negative, and anaerobic microorganisms (Tab. 7.3). Every effort should be made to quickly obtain microbiologic or tissue diagnosis before initiating antimicrobial therapy, as selection of an antibiotic regimen should be wisely made based on microorganisms isolated from blood or CSF. Steroids can be considered in selected cases, especially to reduce the mass effect and improve antibiotic penetration and cerebral edema. As seizure occurs in 13%~25% of cases, an anticonvulsant should be prescribed to prevent seizure in early course of therapy.

Tab. 7.3 Specific antibiotic regimens according to microorganisms

Microorganism	Antibiotic regimen
Gram-positive bacteria (*streptococci*)	Third-generation cephalosporin (e. g., cefotaxime, ceftriaxone) or penicillin G
Staphylococcus aureus, *Staphylococcus epidermis* Clostridium species	Vancomycin, linezolid, trimethoprim-sulfamethoxazole, or daptomycin (if vancomycin resistance)
Fungal infections (*Candida*, *Cryptococcus*)	Amphotericin B
Aspergillus, *Pseudallescheria boydii*	Voriconazole

(5) Prognosis

The complications that can occur secondary to brain abscess are meningitis, ventriculitis, brain herniation, seizures, septicemia, neurological deficits, thrombosis of intracranial blood vessels and death. Delays in hospitalization, focal neurologic deficits at admission, impaired host immunity, uncontrolled diabetes, and Glasgow coma scale < 12 are associated with death and permanent neurologic deficits because of brain abscesses.

7.3 Viral Encephalitis

Encephalitis implies inflammation of the brain substance, parenchyma, which may coexist with inflammation of the meninges (meningoencephalitis) or spinal cord (encephalomyelitis). Causes of viral encephalitis include herpes simplex virus types 1 and 2 (HSV-1, HSV-2), Epstein-Barr virus (EBV), varicella zoster virus, enteroviruses, adenovirus, parechovirus, measles virus and HIV. Acute disseminated encephalomyelitis, Bickerstaff's encephalitis and autoimmune encephalitis exposure to antibodies factors are also indispensable parts. Age has an impact in the specific microorganism: EBV and HSV-1 are more common in young patients. Routine childhood vaccinations prevent many of the diseases that can cause encephalitis (mumps, poliomyelitis, measles and rubella). HSV encephalitis is more common than other causes of sporadic infectious encephalitis and accounts for up to 20% of all cases of acute encephalitis.

(1) Pathophysiology

HSV gains access to humans through mucous membranes or damaged skin. It then infects sensory neurons and travels by fast retrograde axonal transport to neurons in the dorsal root ganglia. It appears most plausible that HSV retrograde transports through the olfactory/trigeminal nerves or via hematogenous dissemination.

The immune response triggered by HSV appears to be crucial to the pathophysiologic changes in patients with acute encephalitis. Early in the course of the immune response to HSV, Toll-like receptors (TLRs) dimerize to activates signaling pathways that initiate the production of proinflammatory cytokines, such as interferons, tumor necrosis factor, and various interleukins. The inflammatory cascade recruits innate immune cells and primes adaptive immunity, particularly recruitment of activated leukocytes, may contribute to tissue destruction and consequent neurologic sequelae. After primary infection, the virus establishes a latent state for the life of the host, include silencing of viral lytic-phase genes, cellular apoptosis, and evasion of host immunity. Once reactivated, the virus can travel to tissues innervated by the infected dorsal root ganglia to cause recurrent disease and shed infectious viral particles that can be transmitted to others.

(2) Clinical feature

1) Clinical manifestation

Many patients present with prodromal symptoms, suggesting upper respiratory tract or other systemic infection. Signs and symptoms of encephalitis then progress over the course of several days in most cases of HSV. Patients with HSV typically present with encephalopathy (a broader term that refers to a clinical state of disorientation, confusion, behavioral, and other cognitive changes that can occur in the setting of encephalitis, as well as numerous other noninflammatory conditions), headache, fever, seizures, focal neurological deficits (aphasia, hemiparesis, abnormal sensory perception), and mental status changes. Meningeal signs are typically not presented in patients with HSV-1 encephalitis.

2) Diagnostic investigation

Blood tests are useful to exclude alternative diagnoses but cannot confirm the presence of herpes simplex encephalitis. More useful tests for the evaluation of HSV encephalitis are the CSF examination, brain MRI, and EEG.

① CSF

Lumbar puncture usually shows increased opening pressure (>30 cmH_2O), moderate lymphocytic pleocytosis ($< 50 \times 10^6$ cells/L), and a mild to moderate rise in protein with glucose >60% of that in blood. PCR testing of CSF for HSV DNA has high sensitivity and specificity at presentation. PCR and culture of CSF are usually positive for the enterovirus and meanwhile throat and stool culture should also be performed.

② Imaging

MRI is the gold standard technique for brain imaging in encephalitis, and is abnormal in 90% of cases of HSV encephalitis. The classic imaging findings are bilateral asymmetric involvement of the temporal and inferior frontal lobes with less common involvement of the insula and cingulategyri. The involved brain typically demonstrates high signal on T_2-weighted images and gyral expansion (Fig. 7.2). Diffusion restriction is a sensitive marker of the disease early in its course. Fluid-attenuated inversion recovery (FLAIR)/T_2-weighted sequences demonstrate increased signal in both the swollen cortex and subcortical white matter. Restricted diffusion occurs in the same regions in which FLAIR changes are noted, but DWI changes may precede FLAIR changes. The basal ganglia are rarely involved in HSV, which helps to distinguish this disease process from other encephalitides. Corresponding CT findings include areas of hypoattenuation and gray-white differentiation loss. Metabolic alterations are demonstrated by MRS in cases of HSV with reduced NAA, elevated choline compounds, and sometimes elevated lactate.

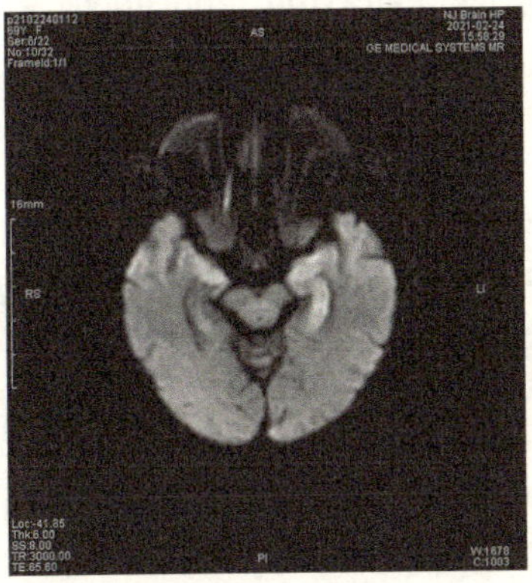

(a) MR-DWI scan showing high-signal in medial temporal lobes

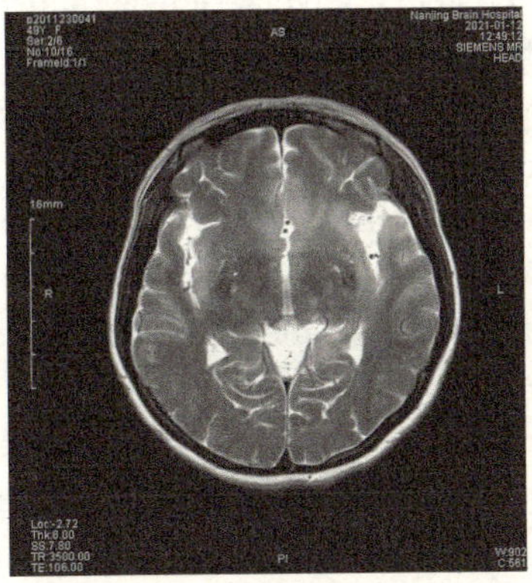

(b) T_2-weighted axial MRI from the same patient showing biateral asymmetrical signal abnormality in both limbic areas

Fig. 7.2 Brain imaging of acute HSV-1 encephalitis

③ Electroencephalogram (EEG)

Slow background with superimposed periodic discharges (unilateral, independent bilateral or generalized) are characteristic of HSV encephalitis. Frontotemporal slowing with periodic discharges may help distinguish HSV infection from other forms of encephalitis. Yet, there is no EEG pattern that can be considered pathognomonic of the HSV encephalitis.

(3) Differential diagnosis

The major differential diagnosis is meningitis or parameningeal infection, especially if meningitis is caused by atypical pathogens, such as *Listeria monocytogenes*. A combination of MRI and CSF examination narrows the broad differential diagnosis, including:

a. Metabolic disturbances (hypoglycaemia, hyponatraemia, hypocalcaemia);

b. Thiamine deficiency (Wernicke encephalopathy);

c. Drugs (including neuroleptics, non-steroidal anti-inflammatory drugs, intoxications);

d. Inflammatory disorders, such as Behçet's disease, Reye syndrome and Guillain-Barré syndrome, sarcoidosis, cerebral vasculitis, systemic lupus erythematosus (SLE) and Wegener's granulomatosis.

e. Status epilepticus and paraneoplastic syndrome may also sometimes be confused with encephalitis.

(4) Treatment

A severe case should be managed in an intensive care unit. Management may be divided into supportive and specific.

1) Supportive treatment

a. Airways, breathing, and circulation should be maintained.

b. Convulsions are best managed with intravenous anticonvulsants, such as phenytoin or valproate which does not depress the sensorium.

c. Mannitol infusion (0.25 ~ 1.0 mg/kg q4h ~ q6h) or intravenous furosemide may be needed in the presence of features of raised intracranial pressure.

d. Gastric hemorrhage (stress ulcer) is a common event and should be managed with antihistamines, antacids, ranitidine, and a blood transfusion.

e. The role of steroids in acute infectious encephalitis is debatable. It has possible attenuation of brain swelling and potential prevention of a secondary autoimmune brain disease. But it may has systemic adverse effects and possibly facilitate viral replication.

2) Specific therapy

Among the viral agents, specific therapy is recommended in encephalitis due to the herpes group of viruses.

a. Acyclovir is highly effective for treatment of HSV encephalitis, in a dose of 10 mg/kg q8h for 14~21 days. The toxicity and side effects of acyclovir include neurologic adverse effects (tremor, myoclonus, and alterations in the content and level of consciousness), bone marrow suppression, vomiting and hypotension, and occasionally renal failure in dehydrated patients.

b. Foscarnet (90 mg/kg q8h) is used for acyclovir-resistant HSV. Acyclovir is also recommended for varicella zoster encephalitis, and ganciclovir (5 mg/kg q12h) is an alternative drug. The tetracycline drug minocycline is a known neuroprotective agent with antiviral properties and excellent penetration into CSF.

c. Azithromycin or oral minocycline/doxycycline is currently recommended for rickettsial meningoencephalitis.

(5) Prognosis

Seizures are probably the most common complication and brain swelling is the gravest complications of HSV infection. Nearly a third of patients with HSV encephalitis demand intensive care unit admission and close to 20% need mechanical ventilation. Factors associated with worse outcome include older age, coma, restricted diffusion on MRI, and delay in the initiation of acyclovir. Antibodies against neuronal surface antigens are reported in some of these patients and it is becoming increasingly accepted that a secondary cerebral autoimmune disease can take place after appropriate treatment of an episode of HSV encephalitis.

7.4 Autoimmune Encephalitis

Autoimmune encephalitis (AE) is a treatable group of CNS disorders associated with auto-antibodies against neurosurface or synaptic antigens and proteins localised on the neuronal cell surface. The anti-*N*-methyl-D-aspartate receptor (anti-NMDAR) encephalitis is the most common type of AE, followed by anti-leucine-rich glioma-inactivated 1 (anti-LGI1) encephalitis and anti-γ-aminobutyric acid type B receptor (anti-GABABR) encephalitis. Other types of antibodies include anti-contactin-associated protein-like 2 (anti-CASPR2) antibody, anti-Hu or anti-Ma antibody and anti-α-amino-3-hydroxy-5-methyl-4-isoxazolepropionic acid receptor (anti-AMPAR) antibody.

Anti-NMDAR encephalitis was first described in 2007, it is an autoimmune disease mediated by antibodies against the NMDAR in the CSF from patients with non-infectious encephalitis, especially those present with rapidly progressive psychiatric symptoms or cognitive impairment, seizures, abnormal movements, or coma of unknown cause. Although the disease is rare, with an estimated incidence of 1.5 per million population per year and around 4% of adults and children presenting with an encephalitis-like disorder. It is more prevalent in females (a female to male ratio of around 8 : 2) with a median age of 21.

(1) Pathophysiology

Anti-NMDAR encephalitis is a neuroinflammatory disease mainly mediated by autoantibodies against the GluN1 subunit of the receptor. Its etiopathogenesis remains an enigma. Now two confirmed triggers of anti-NMDAR encephalitis are tumours (mostly ovarian teratomas) and herpes simplex encephalitis. In the first stage (around 3 months), patients develop severe symptoms, reports on brain biopsy or autopsy findings have shown infiltrates of B cells, plasma cells, CD4 T cells and less frequently CD8 T cells, accompanied by microglial activation, deposits of IgG, and little or no neuronal loss. In the second stage (around 6 months or longer) the presence of inflammation is minimal, when the indicated symptoms have largely resolved. In both stages, IgG antibodies against GluN1 subunit of the receptor are detected and progressively decrease during symptom improvement in CSF.

(2) Clinical feature

1) Clinical manifestation

The predominant presentation comprises autonomic dysfunction (86%), movement disorders (84%) followed by seizures (77%) and behavioural changes. It is suggested that seizures, abnormal movements, insomnia, and irritability are more frequently identified in children, whereas psychosis and abnormal behaviour are more common in adults.

a. Psychiatric features: Patients initially present with psychiatric symptoms, including visual or auditory hallucinations, acute schizoaffective episodes, depression, mania and addictive or eating disorders always are first admitted to a psychiatric institution.

b. Movement disorders: Facial dyskinesias and a large variety of abnormal movements affecting the limbs and trunk are common manifestations of anti-NMDAR encephalitis and valuable clues to recognise the disease. Oral, facial, or lingual dyskinesias, chorea, athetosis, dystonia, opisthotonus, ballismus, blepharospasm can occur in these patients.

c. Seizures and the risk of epilepsy: Seizures are a common presentation in children and young men. A prolonged follow-up (at least 1 year) before the diagnosis of epilepsy is considered in those who require antiepileptic medication. Prolonged follow-up indicates that, in most patients, the seizures resolve after the encephalitis subsides, which supports a gradual removal of antiepileptic therapy during the process of recovery.

2) Diagnostic investigation

a. CSF examination. Diagnosis relies on excluding other causes of encephalitis and undertaking the antibody screen for the NMDA receptor in serum as well as CSF, which is usually positive. Routine CSF profile may present results similar with viral encephalitis. Patients with relapsing HSE or prolonged atypical symptoms with negative CSF PCR for HSV should be tested routinely for anti-NMDAR antibodies in CSF and serum.

b. Diagnostic imaging. Brain MRI has abnormal fluid-attenuated inversion recovery sequence signals, including in the medial temporal lobe, the frontal, parietal, occipital cortices, diencephalon, cerebellum, and brainstem. EEG abnormalities manifest as extreme delta brushes (EDB), rhythmic delta activity without EDB, generalised rhythmic delta activity and excessive delta activity.

c. In 2016, a group of experts develop a set of diagnostic criteria to improve the clinical recognition of anti-NMDAR.

Diagnostic criteria of anti-NMDAR encephalitis (2016)

Probable

(1) Rapid onset (<3 months) of >4/6 major groups of symptoms:

- Abnormal (psychiatric) behaviour or cognitive dysfunction;
- Speech dysfunction (pressured speech, verbal reduction, or mutism).
- Seizures;
- Movement disorder, dyskinesias, rigidity, or abnormal postures;
- Decreased level of consciousness;
- Autonomic dysfunction or central hypoventilation.

(2) >1/3 of the laboratory studies:

- Abnormal EEG (focal or diffuse slow or disorganised activity, or extreme delta brush);
- CSF with pleocytosis or oligoclonal bands.

(3) 3 of the above groups of symptoms + identification of a systemic teratoma.

(4) Exclusion of recent history of herpes simplex virus encephalitis or Japanese B encephalitis, which might result in relapsing immune-mediated neurological symptoms.

Definite

(1) One or more of the 6 major groups of symptoms + IgG GluN1 antibodies in CSF;

(2) Exclusion of recent history of herpes simplex virus encephalitis or Japanese B encephalitis.

(3) Treatment

The treatment approach to anti-NMDAR encephalitis involves escalation of immunotherapy, starting with first-line therapies (steroids, intravenous immunoglobulins, or plasma exchange) and transition to second-line therapies (rituximab or cyclophosphamide) if needed. There is no consensus regarding the management of anti-NMDAR encephalitis. There is no clear evidence regarding when to proceed with the second line of therapy. In addition to specific management, patients require antiepileptic drugs for acute symptomatic seizures, status epilepticus and symptomatic treatment for the movement disorder. Maintenance of anticonvulsants usually depends on the seizure type and EEG changes. A multidisciplinary approach including psychiatric support is very important.

(4) Prognosis

Early diagnosis and therapeutic intervention of anti-NMDAR encephalitis usually achieve a favourable outcome. Outcome depends on early recognition and therapeutic intervention. Approximately 80% of patients improve or recover after immunotherapy and tumour removal. Within the first 2 years of the disease, 12% of patients will relapse and the symptom will be less severe than the initial episode.

7.5 Aseptic Meningitis

Aseptic meningitis is an umbrella term for various etiologies of inflammation of the brain meninges with negative CSF bacterial cultures. It is one of the most common inflammatory disorders of the meninges. It occurs at all ages but is more common in children than adults, without any particular preference for racial difference.

(1) Etiology

The etiology of aseptic meningitis can be categorized into infectious and non-infectious. In terms of infectious causes, they include viruses, bacteria, fungi, and parasites, and the most common agent is viral. More than half of the cases encompass enteroviruses (Coxsackie and ECHO viruses), followed by HSV-1, HSV-2, West Nile virus, and varicella-zoster. Bacterial, fungal, and parasitic infectious are less common than viral. Ultimately, the exact etiology can only be identified in 30%~65% of the cases, despite all the diagnostic advancements made to date. The rest cases of unknown etiology are labeled "idiopathic". For the non-infectious causes of aseptic meningitis, etiologies can be classified into some groups: a. Systemic diseases with meningeal involvement (i.e., sarcoidosis, Behçet's disease, Sjögren syndrome, systemic lupus erythematosus and granulomatosis with polyangiitis); b. Drug-induced aseptic meningitis [most commonly reported with non-steroidal anti-inflammatory drugs (NSAIDs), antibiotics (sulfamides, penicillins), intravenous immunoglobulin, and monoclonal antibodies]; c. Neoplastic meningitis related to either solid cancer metastasis or lymphoma/leukemia; d. Post-vaccine meningitis, such as measles, mumps, rubella vaccine primarily, varicella vaccine, yellow fever vaccine, rabies vaccine, pertussis vaccine, and influenza vaccine.

(2) Clinical feature

1) Clinical manifestation

History taking should include sick contacts, recent travels, substance abuse, sexual history, preceding or concurrent infections, and recent use of medications. Drug-induced aseptic meningitis, in particular, may have few lab abnormalities, so clinicians have to maintain a high level of suspicion and perform a comprehensive history regarding all medications a patient might be taking. Adults can present with a myriad of symptoms and are more likely to complain of headaches, nausea, vomiting, malaise, weakness, stiff neck, photophobia, or even altered mental status. In children, symptoms at presentation seem less specific, consisting of fever, coexisting respiratory illness, rash and irritability. Neonates and infants less than three months of age may have a bulging anterior fontanelle and irritability. It seems that nuchal rigidity and fever are common physical findings in both children and adults.

2) Diagnostic investigation

Primary evaluation should include serologic laboratory testing to look for alternative causes, including complete blood counts, erythrocyte sedimentation rate (ESR), and IgM and IgG for enterovirus, adenovirus, EBV, and HSV. Over the years, polymerase chain reaction (PCR) and next-generation sequencing have aided in identifying pathogens. A lumbar puncture (LP) should be performed to collect CSF to make a definitive diagnosis. On CSF analysis, cell count, glucose, Gram stain, protein, culture, bacterial PCR can be gained and viral PCR studies can be selected. Other tests can also be taken into consideration, such as syphilis serology, tuberculosis testing, serum human immunodeficiency virus (HIV) testing. Typical CSF results in patients with aseptic meningitis include: opening pressure either normal or slightly elevated, glucose normal to mildly decreased, protein normal to mildly elevated, cell count of 10 ~ 1 000 cells per microliter (initially neutrophils gradually shift toward lymphocytes).

(3) Differential diagnosis

The signs and symptoms (headache and fever) of aseptic meningitis are often vague and nonspecific, therefore, the differential is quite broad.

a. Bacterial meningitis is the most concerning and common alternative cause and should be the default diagnosis until ruled out.

b. Intracranial hemorrhage, especially subarachnoid hemorrhage, should be considered in patients with appropriate clinical presentation.

c. Neoplastic disorders (leukemia, tumors of the brain), other types of headaches (migraine), inflammation of brain structures (brain abscess, epidural abscess) should also be considered.

d. Systemic diseases: Viral syndromes, in particular, often demonstrate headaches, muscle aches, weakness, and fever; anemia, carbon monoxide exposure, tick-borne illness, and TB demonstrate headaches and weakness classically.

(4) Treatment

Early recognition of the most plausible cause of meningitis is crucial to begin treatment as soon as possible. If bacterial meningitis is suspected, prompt initiation of empiric antibiotics is recommended. Obtaining CSF would be ideal before starting antibiotics. If the CSF results are more consistent with aseptic meningitis, antibiotics should then be discontinued. Steroids are used as adjunctive therapy to reduce the inflammatory response. Evidence supports the use of dexamethasone 10 ~ 20 minutes prior to antibiotics or concomitant with their administration, even though the etiology is initially unknown while awaiting culture results. Supportive treatment is needed in all patients, including pain management and fever control with antipyretics such as ibuprofen and acetaminophen/paracetamol. Repeating LP is unnecessary but should be considered in patients whose clinical status does not improve after 48 hours. Once the diagnosis of aseptic meningitis has been established, the patient can often be discharged home except for the elderly, immunocompromised, and children with pleocytosis. Also, if the meningitis is drug-induced, the drug should be stopped or, if essential, be replaced with a drug not associated with meningeal irritation.

(5) Prognosis

Prognosis varies with the age of the patient as well as the etiology of meningitis. Viral meningitis is usually a benign condition, and full recovery generally occurs in 5 ~ 14 days in most patients with only fatigue and light headedness as residual symptoms. It may be complicated by seizures and progress to status epilepticus. This complication requires treatment, but prophylaxis is not recommended. Sensorineural deafness and aqueductal stenosis, causing hydrocephalus, can result from mumps meningoencephalitis. Hydrocephalus, infarcts, epilepsy, mental regression, neurological deficits, and cranial nerve palsies can be caused by tuberculosis meningitis.

7.6 Acute Transverse Myelitis

Acute myelopathies (AM) can be of inflammatory, compressive, neoplastic, vascular, metabolic or biological practice, given the varied underlying pathophysiology. Acute transverse myelitis (ATM), the commonest AM, is defined as an acute inflammatory spinal cord syndrome leading to motor and/or sensory impairment, with or without sphincter dysfunction, secondary to a wide variety of autoimmune or inflammatory diseases.

(1) Epidemiology and etiology

ATM has an incidence of one to four new cases per million people per year, affecting individuals of all ages with bimodal peaks between the ages of 10~19 years and 30~39 years. There is no sex or familial predisposition. Clinical features such as fever, meningismus, rash, concurrent systemic infection, immunocompromised state, recurrent genital infection, radicular burning pain with or without vesicles suggestive of zoster radiculitis, or adenopathy may suggest an infectious etiology for ATM. Other clinical features (oral or genital ulcers, photosensitivity, anemia/leukopenia/thrombocytopenia) may suggest a systemic inflammatory disease, such as Sjögren syndrome, antiphospholipid syndrome, SLE, sarcoidosis, or mixed connective tissue disease.

(2) Clinical feature

1) Clinical manifestation

ATM is characterized clinically by acutely or subacutely developing symptoms and signs of neurologic dysfunction in motor, sensory, and autonomic nerves and nerve tracts of the spinal cord. When the maximal level of deficit is reached, patients have total paraplegia, bladder dysfunction, and numbness commonly, paresthesias, or band-like dysesthesias. Autonomic symptoms consist variably of urinary urgency, bladder incontinence, incomplete evacuation, or bowel constipation.

Brown-Sequard syndrome (Fig. 7.3) is due to a unilateral lesion involving the hemi-cord that presents as motor weakness and vibration and joint position sensory loss (dorsal column dysfunction) on the same side as the lesion and pain and temperature loss on the opposite side of the lesion (spinothalamic dysfunction). This is often due to MS or a compressive etiology.

A complete loss of spinal cord function may be due to an acute compressive lesion, a necrotizing myelitis or trauma. A central cord lesion can present as autonomic dysfunction, spinothalamic deficits, and a pyramidal distribution weakness below the level of the lesion, and may be due to a syrinx or possibly NMO. An anterior spinal cord syndrome with acute flaccid weakness, spinothalamic dysfunction but preserved dorsal column function may be caused by an anterior spinal artery occlusion. Isolated loss of vibration and joint position sense may be due to Vitamin B_{12} deficiency, copper deficiency, or nitrous oxide toxicity.

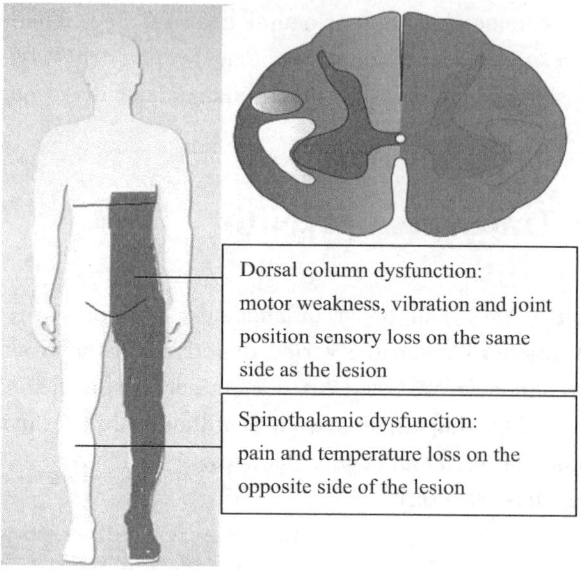

Fig. 7.3 Brown-Sequard syndrome

2) Diagnostic investigation

A sagittal survey of the spine using MRI can be particularly helpful. Inflammatory lesions often produce local enlargement of the spinal cord and increased signal intensity on T_2-weighted sequences of MRI (Fig. 7.4). MRI-T_2WI of a patient with ATM with increased signal intensity at C3 ~ C5. Lumbar puncture is indicated to determine if there are signs of inflammation within the CSF once MRI has excluded a compressive etiology. After measuring the opening pressure, it is critical that routine CSF studies include cell count with differential protein and glucose concentrations. If the CSF shows signs of inflammation (pleocytosis, elevated protein concentration, oligoclonal bands, or elevated IgG index), then the subsequent work-up should focus on demyelinating, infectious, or other inflammatory causes of an acute myelitis. In addition, bacterial, fungal, and AFB cultures should be considered. If the CSF is non-inflammatory, then vascular, toxic/metabolic, neurodegenerative, or neoplastic myelopathies become much more likely and the subsequent work-up should focus on these etiologies.

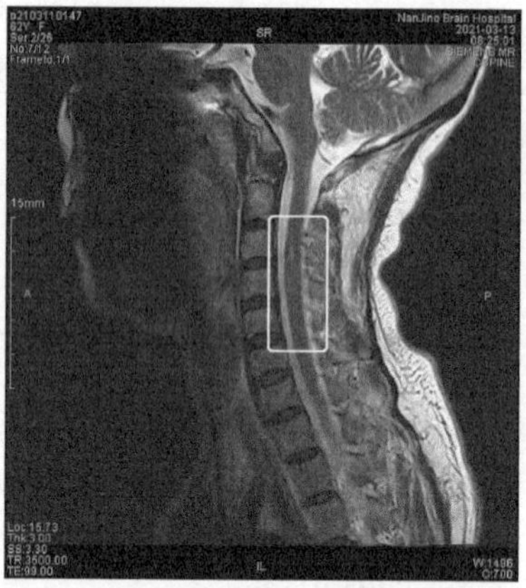

Fig. 7.4 MRI-T_2WI of a patient with ATM showing increased signal intensity at C3~C5

(3) Differential diagnosis

a. Multiple sclerosis: As MS or clinically isolated syndrome (CIS) is the majority of incomplete transverse myelopathy in young persons, they more pronounce on one side, usually slowly spreading from the legs to the upper part of the body. MRI is also quite typical with small demyelinating lesions, involving less than two segments, most often located in the posterior or lateral part of the spinal cord. The oligoclonal bands (OCB) are present in the CSF. But sometimes ATM can be the presenting feature of MS.

b. Neuromyelitis optica spectrum disorders (NMOSD): The symptoms are rarely monophasic, more often aggressively relapsing, limited to the optic nerve and spinal cord, mostly sparing the brain. Visual evoked potentials are recommended to individuals in only spinal forms. Some cases of NMOSD are associated with a highly specific serum autoantibody marker aquaporin-4 antibody (AQP-4), also known as "NMO-IgG".

c. Compressive myelopathies: Spinal cord MRI is very important to exclude compressive lesions of the spinal cord.

d. Spinal tumor: Patients have a lasting history for weeks to months. MRI has an enhancing lesion in the spinal cord like an "inflammation lesion". If significant enhancement with gadolinium persists after a course of steroids, a spinal cord biopsy could be considered.

e. Subacute combined degeneration of spinal cord: The neurological manifestations may be the earliest and frequently the only signs of Vitamin B_{12} deficiency. They may have a relatively sudden onset, including spastic paraparesis, impaired perception of joint position and vibration, commonly involving hands. Contrast enhancement may be present. Vitamin B_{12} (cyanocobalamin), folic acid and Vitamin E deficiencies can be found by serologic test.

(4) Treatment

Once again, there are no clinical controlled trials or specific guidelines to drive therapy. High dose Ⅳ corticosteroids (30 mg/(kg · d) of methylprednisolone to a maximum of 1 g), as first-line treatment, for 3~5 days, either alone or in combination with Ⅳ-Ig is widely accepted. In addition, systemic corticosteroids are used in a variety of systemic infections and shown to be safe when used in tandem with empiric antibiotics. Plasma exchange is sometimes utilized, but only when the first-line therapy fails. Symptomatic treatment of pain, urodynamic evaluation and early involvement of rehabilitation medicine is also extremely important in long-term management.

(5) Prognosis

Most patients have good recovery and show improvement in gait within the first 2 weeks of symptom onset. Rapid progression of symptoms, back pain, and spinal shock predict poor recovery. Abnormal sensory symptoms may also persist as numbness is the most common sensory complaint in up to 75% of patients followed by dysesthesias.

7.7 HIV-co-infection of CNS

7.7.1 Tuberculous Meningitis

In 2017, WHO estimated 10 million incident cases of tuberculosis, which would correlate to 100 000~500 000 cases per year of tuberculous meningitis (TBM). In 2008, nearly one of three TBM-related deaths (29%) worldwide was considered to be related to HIV infection, and TBM contributed to 26% of the estimated deaths due to HIV infection.

(1) Etiology and pathophysiology

a. Macroscopic pathology: Transmission of *M. tuberculosis* is airborne, so the first focus of infection is the lung. It disseminate through the blood either via direct local infection or via lymph nodes. At first, only an initial intracranial lesion of tuberculous meningitis can be found at the meninges or parameninge. Rupture of that focus then lead to further extension of inflammation throughout the meninges, leading to parenchymal tuberculoma formation or to vascular pathology characteristic of the disease. The characteristic feature of TBM is the presence of a thick, gelatinous inflammatory exudate in the basal cisterns and subarachnoid spaces of the brain, which may extend into the spinal canal. The predominantly basal location has important implications: firstly, the major cerebral vessels originating from the base of the brain become encased with exudate; secondly, exudate blocks the circulation of CSF; and thirdly, it envelopes and compresses the local cranial nerves resulting in cranial nerve palsies.

b. Immune and metabolic factors: Bacterial replication must occur in the CNS for TBM pathogenesis to proceed. Once bacilli travers the blood-brain barrier, they are taken up by microglia and can also replicate in these cells, leading to the induction of microglial cytokine and chemokine production. Host immune regulation, pathogen virulence factors and energy related metabolites all act by then. It suggests that the induction of inflammasomes and activation of an innate cytokine response leading to influx of phagocytes are key processes in the pathogenesis of TBM.

c. Bacillary and host genetic factors: *M. tuberculosis* can be divided into seven lineages classified as "ancient" (lineages 1, 5, 6 and 7) or "modern" (lineages 2, 3 and 4). One hypothesis is that some lineages might more frequently cause or affect the severity of meningeal infection. Many immune response genes are under polymorphic genetic (such as TLR9, SIGIRR, SPN, TIRAP, TLR2 and MRC1) influence. A single nucleotide polymorphism in the leukotriene A4 hydrolase (LTA4H) promoter is associated with inflammatory cell recruitment, patient survival and response to adjunctive anti-inflammatory therapy. There are a number of other polymorphisms related to the pathogenesis of TBM, including CD43, G54D, PKP3-SIGIRR-TMEM16J or Taq1 VDR SNP.

(2) Clinical feature

1) Clinical manifestation

TBM has a nonspecific prodrome and has more recognizable symptoms gradually, such as headache, fever, vomiting and neck stiffness. Meningitic symptoms become progressively more dominant, consciousness falls, and focal neurological deficits occur, with cranial nerve palsies (the fifth and third cranial nerves) and limb weakness. Presentation of TBM can be abrupt, and can rapidly progress to severe coma and prostration with high mortality for them.

2) Diagnostic investigation

a. CSF examination is essential for the exact diagnosis of tuberculous meningitis. Typical CSF changes include lymphocytic pleocytosis (150~1 000 leukocytes/μL), decreased glucose levels (CSF: plasma glucose ratios of <0.5) and elevated protein levels (0.8~2.0 g/dL). The "gold standard" for diagnosis confirmation is demonstration of *M. tuberculosis* in the CSF.

b. Microbiological diagnosis: Microscopy and Ziehl-Neelsen staining (50% sensitivity) to detect acid fast bacilli in CSF is the main stay for the rapid diagnosis of tuberculosis. A large volume of CSF (≈10 mL) and examination for 30 minutes by an experienced microscopist, can detect the bacteria in >80% of TBM cases, and also increase the yield of culture. Culture of *M. tuberculosis* is more sensitive than microscopy for diagnosis, but takes 10 days to 8 weeks.

c. Diagnostic imaging: CT and MRI are widely used for detection of basal meningeal exudates, infarcts, tuberculomas and hydrocephalus, and the diffusion-weighted MRI has superior resolution for infarcts and tuberculomas. Neuroimaging characteristics of tuberculous meningitis are leptomeningeal enhancement, hydrocephalus, infarcts and/or tuberculoma (Fig. 7.5). T_1WI shows obvious hydrocephalus from a patient with tuberculous meningitis, male, 58 years, complains of fever and headache for 30 days (Fig. 7.5a); enhanced-T_1WI axial image shows tuberculomas in the lateral fissure cistern, circumferential cistern from another man with tuberculous meningitis (Fig. 7.5b). Spinal cord disease should not be undetected. The basilar exudates manifest as intensely enhancing areas in the regions of basal cisterns and Sylvian fissure. Gadolinium-enhanced MRI is superior to find small leptomeningeal tuberculomas and diffusion-weighted MRI improves the detection of small areas of ischaemia or early infarction. The main limitation of both imaging modalities is that around 30% of individuals at an early stage have normal brain CT scans, and around 15% have normal brain MRI scans. Imaging of organs other than the brain can also yield important diagnostic information. Radiographic evidence of tuberculosis at other sites (chest, abdomen and pelvis) can provide supportive diagnostic information.

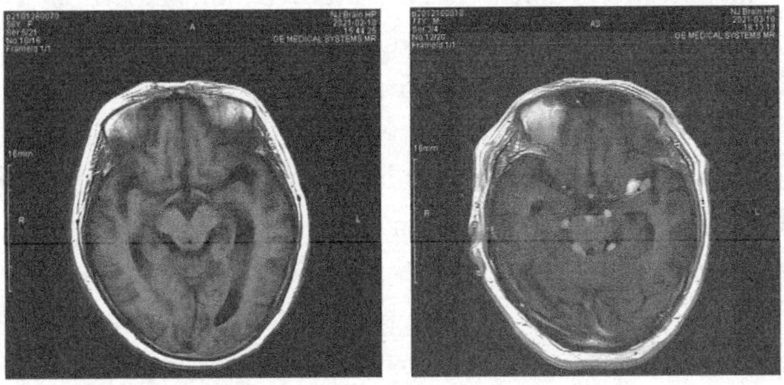

(a) Obvious hydrocephalus (b) Tuberculomas

Fig. 7.5 Different neuroimagings of tuberculous meningitis

Radiographic evidence of tuberculosis at other sites (chest, abdomen and pelvis) can provide supportive diagnostic information.

(3) Treatment

1) Antimicrobial therapy

Anti-tuberculosis therapy is the main stay of treatment for tuberculous meningitis. The antituberculosis treatment needs to be continued for at least 9~12 months. Treatment is started with first-line antituberculous drugs, which include isoniazid, rifampicin, pyrazinamide, streptomycin and ethambutol (Tab. 7.4). The second-line drugs known to have good penetration into the CSF include fluoroquinolones, ethionamide, cycloserine and linezolid; pyrazinamide and high-dose isoniazid also have good penetration into the CSF.

Tab. 7.4 Antituberculosis drugs (first-line) for TBM recommended by WTO

Drug	Daily dose	Duration	Adverse effect
Rifampicin	8~12 mg/kg, max. 600 mg	12 months	Hepatotoxicity, orange urine, many drug interactions
Oniazid	4~6 mg/kg, max. 300 mg	12 months	Hepatotoxicity, peripheral neuropathy, lupus-like syndrome, confusion, seizures
Pyrazinamide	20~30 mg/kg	First 2 months	Hepatotoxicity, arthralgia, gout
Ethambutol	15~20 mg/kg	First 2 months	Dose-related retrobulbar neuritis, more common in renal impairment
Streptomycin	12~18 mg/kg, max. 1 g	First 2 months	Monitor plasma concentrations when possible; causes nephrotoxicity and ototoxicity

2) Adjunctive host-directed therapies

a. Corticosteroids. Corticosteroids increase survival in HIV-1-negative children and adults with TBM, but the benefit of corticosteroids is uncertain in individuals co-infected with HIV-1, and is not found to reduce long-term neurological disability. Inflammatory complications can occur weeks or even months after the start of antituberculosis chemotherapy for TBM, when initial corticosteroid treatment is reduced or stopped, with symptoms of fever, progressively worsening headache, and sometimes seizures or reduced consciousness. In these circumstances, alternative anti-inflammatory agents can be tried. Thalidomide, anti-TNF biological agents (such as infliximab) and IFN-γ treatment have been reported successfully.

b. Aspirin. Brain infarction is the most common cause of long-term neurological disability owing to TBM. So treatment with aspirin might improve outcome from TBM by reducing the incidence of brain infarction.

c. Antiretroviral therapy. Aside from corticosteroids, antiretroviral drugs are the only adjunctive agents with proven benefit for patient with HIV co-infection. But whether this therapy should be started concurrently with antituberculosis drugs or delayed until the tuberculosis is partially or completely treated remains uncertain.

3) Supportive management

Raised intracranial pressure (ICP), cerebral ischaemia, hydrocephalus, hyponatraemia and seizures all contribute to poor outcome in patients with TBM, and should be actively tested and treated. Clinical management should be directed at the careful and continuous monitoring and correction of abnormalities in gas exchange and tissue oxygenation, through mechanical ventilation, meticulous fluid and electrolyte management, control and monitoring of intracranial pressure, and rigorous temperature control.

a. Vascular compromise as a common complication may lead to ischaemia, infarction and raised ICP. TCD performed at the bedside can reliably track TBM-related intracranial vasculopathy in adults patients. Hypertonic saline similar to mannitol might be effective in treating TBM-associated ICP.

b. Hyponatraemia (plasma sodium < 135 mmol/L) due to SIADH (syndrome of inappropriate antidiuretic hormone secretion) or cerebral salt wasting occurs in around 40% ~ 50% of patients with TBM. But it is not reliable that SIADH is managed by fluid restriction, and cerebral salt wasting by fluid administration.

c. Hydrocephalus is the most common cause of raised ICP and should be treated with ventriculo-peritoneal shunting (VPS) or endoscopic third ventriculo-stomy (ETV).

4) Prevention

Childhood disease can also be prevented by giving isoniazid to children exposed to infectious adults. For people with HIV, antiretroviral therapy is the most effective preventive strategy against tuberculosis.

(4) Prognosis

The outcomes of TBM are better if the earlier treatment is started. TBM severity degrade established by the Medical Research Council (MRC) (Tab. 7.5) remains the most widely used tool to define TBM disease severity, and strongly predicts outcome. Disease caused by multidrug-resistant *M. tuberculosis* (resistant to at least rifampicin and isoniazid) confers a major risk of death. Other important risk factors for death from TBM include extremes of age, and interruptions to first-line antitubercular treatment because of drug-induced adverse events.

Tab. 7.5 **TBM severity grade combined to the Glasgow coma scale (GCS) (1974, UK)**

Grade	Defination	Death rate/%
Grade Ⅰ	GCS score 15; no focal neurological signs	15
Grade Ⅱ	GCS score 11~14, or 15 with focal neurological sign	30
Grade Ⅲ	GCS score≤10	50

7.7.2 Cryptococcal Meningitis

Cryptococcal meningitis (CM) is the most common manifestation of systemic fungal infection in HIV-1-infected patients and is the third most frequent neurological complication in patients with AIDS.

(1) Epidemiology and pathophysiology

Although the incidence of HIV-associated cryptococcal infection has reduced significantly in industrialised countries with the widespread implementation of successful anti-retroviral therapy (ART) programs, the incidence of cryptococcal meningitis is still high, especially in sub-Saharan Africa and some parts of Asia. Cryptococcal meningitis one-year mortality in low-income countries would be higher than 70% for those in care and 100% for those not in care. In 2011, the World Health Organization (WHO) and the Centre for Disease Prevention and Control (CDC) recommended cryptococcal antigenaemia screening for people living with HIV with CD4 counts<100 cells/μL and who are not on ART.

Pathologic examination reveals a basilar, nonexudative chronic meningitis and microabscesses, usually in the basal ganglia region, as well as crypto-coccomas, may also develop. It is in association with excreta from certain birds such as pigeons, environmental scavengers such as ameba and sowbugs and in a variety of tree species in their hollows. It occurs primarily by inhalation of the infectious propagules (either poorly encapsulated yeast cells or basidiospores) from environmental reservoirs with deposition into pulmonary alveoli.

It is not established whether CM occurs as a result of dissemination of newly acquired infection or represents reactivation of latent infection. Enhanced immune function secondary to HAART may unmask latent infection and precipitate clinically apparent meningitis. Clearly, cryptococcosis emphasizes the Goldilocks paradigm of immunity. It produces disease when immunity is too little or too much, but when the human host immunity is just right, disease does not appear.

(2) Clinical feature

1) Clinical manifestation

CM usually presents solely with neurologic manifestations, without evidence of systemic infection. The onset and duration of CM are variable. The signs and symptoms of meningitis in immunocompetent patients, such as nuchal rigidity and/or meningismus and photophobia, have not been shown to correlate well with CM in a study of HIV-1-infected patients. Patients often present with nonspecific complaints such as headache, fever, altered mental status, nausea, and vomiting. Focal neurologic signs and seizures occur in about 10% of patients. Elevated ICP occurs in excess of 50% of HIV-1-infected patients with CM, without accompanying hydrocephalus or cerebral edema.

2) Diagnostic investigation

a. The CSF changes are relatively minor, and in some cases the CSF is normal. CSF examination may reveal increased protein and depressed glucose levels. In approximately 70% of the patients, the CSF white cell count is below 20 cells/mL, and the pleocytosis is almost always mononuclear. The opening pressure on lumbar puncture is often elevated. India ink smear of CSF is a valuable supportive test for diagnosis, with a sensitivity ranging 30%~50% (non-AIDS-related cryptococcal meningitis) and up to 80% (AIDS-related disease). Cryptococcus can be visualized as a globular, encapsulated yeast cell with or without budding, ranging 5~20 μm in diameter.

b. CSF Cryptococcal antigen should be tested too, and a titer above 1 : 8 is considered presumptive evidence of the infection.

c. Cryptococcal polysaccharide capsular antigen (CrAg) performed by latex agglutination assays (LA) or enzyme immunoassay (EIA) is positive in more than 99% of cases of AIDS-related CM, usually at titers more than 1 : 2 048. A positive CrAg test is shown to be useful as a predictor of cryptococcal meningitis and mortality after ART initiation.

d. Mycological culture of CSF samples is considered the "gold standard" diagnostic method. A quantitative culture of defined volumes of CSF is of great value in assessing the value and rapidity of fungal killing by different antifungal regimens.

e. Neuroimaging studies are useful to confirm the diagnosis of obstructive hydrocephalus. Actually, there are some important imaging findings of the cryptococcal meningoencephalitis, including dilated Virchow-Robin spaces (VRS), pseudocysts, cryptococcoma, leptomeningeal or parenchymal enhancing lesions and hazy brain base. Lots of mimics can combine with the cryptococcal meningoencephalitis, especially in patients with AIDS. The enhanced lesions in the basal ganglia should be considered toxoplasmosis or primary lymphoma. Subependymal contrast lesions may be primary lymphoma or cytomegalovirus encephalitis.

(3) Treatment

1) Optimal antifungal therapy

Intravenous amphotericin B combined with 5-flucytosine is the initial treatment of choice for 2-week induction therapy. Fluconazole is recommended for consolidation therapy for 8 weeks, or until CSF cultures are negative. Fluconazole plus flucytosine may be an alternative for induction therapy. The induction phase is followed by a consolidation phase and long-term suppressive antifungal therapy using fluconazole monotherapy. Amphotericin B is an alternative for maintenance therapy. The addition of granulocyte-macrophage colony stimulating factor to standard antifungal therapy may provide a useful therapeutic option in HIV-1-infected patients with CM associated with CSF leukopenia.

2) Antiretroviral therapy (ART) after initiation of antifungal therapy

Clinical guideline for the management of cryptococcal meningitis established by the Infectious Diseases Society of America (IDSA) recommends no initiation of ART 2~10 weeks until at least four weeks after induction antifungal therapy, in order to prevent other HIV-related complications without exacerbating immune reconstitution reactions.

3) Management of intracranial pressure

Along with the optimization of antifungal therapy, management of increased intracranial pressure is critically important in cryptococcal meningoencephalitis. Treatment options for managing acutely elevated intracranial pressure include repeated lumbar punctures (daily until pressure and symptoms are stable for >2 days), lumbar drain insertion, ventriculostomy, or ventriculoperitoneal shunt, if obstructive hydrocephalus develops. Early neurosurgical consultation rather than medical treatments (corticosteroids, mannitol, acetazolamide) is recommended in severe cases of meningoencephalitis.

(4) Prognosis

Cryptococcal meningitis is one leading cause of early mortality among HIV-infected adults in sub-Saharan Africa. Poor prognostic factors for CM in HIV-1-infected patients include positive blood cultures, altered mental status, CSF antigen titer above 1 : 1 024, positive CSF India ink smear, CSF white cell count below 20 cells/mL, and elevated CSF pressure. Visual loss is the major complication of sustained high ICP in cryptococcal meningitis. Other complications include hearing loss, strabismus, diplopia in association with reduced acuity, and marked papilledema.

7.7.3 Neurosyphilis

Syphilis is a sexually and vertically transmitted infection caused by the spirochaete *Treponema pallidum* (*T. pallidum*) *subspecies pallidum* (Spirochaetales). Neurosyphilis, the clinical result of infection of CNS, can occur during any stage of syphilis. There has been a resurgence of neurosyphilis in decades, with a rate estimated at 0.47 ~ 2.1 cases per million population. *T. pallidum* is cleared from peripheral sites by opsonization, followed by ingestion and killed by activated macrophages. It can evade the host immune response by antigen-poor surface membrane or produce of antigenically variant surface proteins during the course of infection. An increased risk of neurosyphilis, particularly the early forms, is seen in HIV-infected individuals. Risk factors include lower peripheral blood $CD4^{+}$T cellcounts, detectable plasma HIV-RNA, high serum rapid plasma reagin titer (RPR), and lack of antiretroviral use.

The histologic hallmark of neurosyphilis vary: CNS gummas are composed of a dense perivascular infiltrate of lymphocytes, plasma cells, epithelioid cells, and multinucleated giant cells surrounding a caseous, necrotic core and endarteritis. Diffuse leptomeningitis characterizes asymptomatic neurosyphilis and syphilitic meningitis. The pathologic findings of meningovascular syphilis include diffuse thickening and lymphocytic infiltration of the meninges with superimposed arteritis. Paresis is a late stage when perivascular lymphocytic and plasma cell infiltration in the brain parenchyma is typically observed, with neuronal loss and atrophy, and identification of treponemes in the cerebral cortex. Tabes dorsalis features demyelination, axonal degeneration, and atrophy of the posterior columns in the spinal cord.

(1) Clinical feature

The diagnosis of neurosyphilis depends upon a combination of clinical findings, serological tests for syphilis, and confirmatory testing of CSF.

a. Depending on the time since infection, early neurosyphilis is distinguished from late neurosyphilis. Early neurosyphilis (weeks to months to a few years) primarily includes syphilitic meningitis and meningovascular neurosyphilis (the latter can also occur at late stage). Classical forms of late neurosyphilis (years to decades) are tabes dorsalis and paralytic neurosyphilis.

b. Serologic tests for syphilis are divided into treponemal and nontreponemal. The treponemal tests measure IgG and IgM antibodies to *T. pallidum* or to recombinant *T. pallidum* proteins. These tests include *T. pallidum* particle agglutination (TPPA), fluorescence treponemal antibody absorption test (FTA-ABS), and various *T. pallidum* enzyme immunoassays (TP-EIAs) or chemiluminescence immunoassays. Nontreponemal tests include the RPR, Venereal Disease Research Laboratory (VDRL), and toluidine red unheated serum test (TRUST), of which RPR is the most commonly used. Success of therapy is based on the nontreponemal test decreasing response.

c. The CSF is frequently abnormal in patients with neurosyphilis with both pleocytosis and a raised protein concentration. The VDRL assay performed on CSF is considered the gold standard for specificity but is recognized to have limited sensitivity. Other CSF tests, including serological assays, such as RPR, FTA-ABS and TPHA, and molecular assays including PCR have variable specificity and sensitivity for the diagnosis of neurosyphilis. Clinical features of established neurosyphilis can be summarized in Tab. 7.6.

Tab. 7.6 Clinical features of early and late established neurosyphilis

Stage		Disease duration	Clinical feature	Laboratory test
Early stage	Asymptomatic neurosyphilis	<1 year	Serological evidence of syphilis; lack neurological symptoms	SerumVDRL (+); CSF-VDRL (+), elevated WBC or protein
	Meningitis	0.2~2 years	Headache, meningismus, cranial-nerve palsies, blindness or deafness	Serum VDRL (+); CSF: WBC pleocytosis (50 ~ 2 000/mL) with protein up to 250 mg/dl; Wasser-mannreaction (+)
	Meningovascular neurosyphilis	0.2~8 years	Stroke, meningismus, cranial-nerve palsies, meningomyelitis with progressive myelopathy or sphincter dysfunction	Serum VDRL (+); CSF lymphocytic pleocytosis or normoglycorrhachia; CSF-VDRL (+)
Late stage	Tabes dorsalis	10 years	Ataxic gait, prominent Romberg sign, lightning pains in legs and trunk, greatly impaired deep and proprioceptive sensation, Charcot joint, common Argyll Robertson pupil, paraparesis, sphincter dysfunction.	Serum VDRL (+/-); CSF normal or mild pleocytosis with protein elevation; CSF-VDRL (+)
	General paresis	8~20 years	Progressive dementia, psychiatric syndrome, personality change, manic delusion tremor, dysar-thria, Parkinsonism, Argyll Robertson pupil	Serum VDRL (+) CSF-VDRL (+), WBC pleocytosis or protein

(2) Differential diagnosis

The diagnosis of neurosyphilis is challenging, as it is often referred to as "the great imitator" and it can present in countless ways. Firstly, neurosyphilis should always be considered as a differential diagnosis in any patient with ischaemic stroke of unknown aetiology, particularly in young people. Other potential differential diagnosis of neurosyphilis include meningitis, chronic headache, psychiatric illness cognitive impairment, seizures, mass lesion cranial (poly) neuropathy, optic neuritis/optic atrophy, transverse myelitis, myelopathy (poly) radiculopathy or peripheral neuropathy. All HIV positive patients with neurological symptoms above should be subject to an appropriate diagnostic workup to rule out neurosyphilis.

(3) Treatment

Intramuscular penicillin G is the preferred drug for treating patients in all stages of syphilis. It is the first-line option drug for treating people at any stage of syphilis, and remains as an effective first-line treatment. The preparation used, dosage, and length of treatment depend on the stage and clinical manifestations of the disease. According to international guidelines for treating neurosyphilis, crystalline penicillin should be administered in doses of 24 million units intravenous from 10 ~ 14 days. Procaine penicillin should be administered in doses of 2.4 million units intramuscular once daily plus probenecid 500 mg orally four times a day, both for 10 ~ 14 days. There is a particular reaction in people with syphilis when they receive antibiotic, namely the Jarisch-Herxheimer reaction. Ceftriaxone, is as an alternative antibiotic used for treating people with penicillin allergy. It should be administered in doses of 2 g daily intravenous or intramuscular for 10 ~ 14 days. Doxycycline, a second-generation tetracycline, is also considered an alternative regime for neurosyphilis treatment and can be used at 100 mg orally, twice a day, for 21 ~ 30 days. Another option is tetracycline 500 mg orally, four times daily, for 30 days. The CDC recommends that CSF examination be repeated every 6 months after completion of therapy until abnormalities resolve. A first post therapy lumbar puncture should be performed at 3 months after therapy to minimize loss to follow-up and to identify early treatment failure (increased in CSF-WBCs/fourfold increase in CSF-VDRL).

Q: What is Jarisch-Herxheimer reaction?

A: The Jarisch-Herxheimer reaction is an acute febrile reaction frequently accompanied by headache, myalgia, and fever that can occur within the first 24 hours after the initiation of any syphilis therapy; it is a reaction to treatment and not an allergic reaction to penicillin. Patients should be informed about this possible adverse reaction and how to manage it if it occurs. The Jarisch-Herxheimer reaction occurs most frequently among persons who have early syphilis, presumably because bacterial loads are higher during these stages. Antipyretics can be used to manage symptoms.

7.8 Parasite Infection

7.8.1 Neuroschistosomiasis

Neuroschistosomiasis is an infection of the CNS by schistosome and may manifest it as cerebral and/or spinal schistosomiasis. WHO estimates that at least 236. 6 million people required preventive treatment for schistosomiasis in 2019 in 51 endemic countries, out of which more than 105.4 million people were reported to had been treated. The infection is prevalent in tropical and sub-tropical areas, in poor communities without potable water and adequate sanitation. Schistosomiasis is radiating to new geographical areas owing to demographic, environmental and climatic factors. In endemic countries the infection rate may be increased by co-infection with HIV because schistosomiasis is associated with horizontal transmission of AIDS. Five species are known to infect humans: *Schistosoma mansoni* (*S. mansoni*), *Schistosoma haematobium* (*S. haematobium*), *Schistosoma japonicum* (*S. japonicum*), *Schistosoma intercalatum* (*S. intercalatum*) and *Schistosoma mekongi* (*S. mekongi*). The first three species are the most widely distributed.

(1) Pathophysiology

The immunogenic interaction between schistosome egg deposition and the delayed hypersensitivity reaction of the host are the basis of the pathogenic mechanism in cerebral and spinal schistosomiasis. Host's cellular inflammatory response range from a minimal inflammatory reaction to scattered ova to a severe reaction resulting in space-occupying granulomatous mass and nervous tissue necrosis. The number, size and morphology of ova may also play a role in the pathogenesis of neuroschistosomiasis. The smaller eggs of *S. japonicum* can reach the brain more easily, whereas *S. mansoni* and *S. haematobium* eggs are larger and may be retained much more frequently in the spinal cord. Some adult worms may aberrantly migrate to the CNS via the valveless venous plexus of Batson. Egg embolism have been found in the cerebral cortex, and collections of schistosome ova in the leptomeninges, brain parenchyma, cerebellum, brainstem and choroid plexus.

(2) Clinical feature

Cerebral and/or spinal schistosomiais should be suspected in people presenting with acute encephalopathy or myelopathy who has exposed to freshwater in endemic areas.

1) Clinical manifestation

① Cerebral schistosomiais

The involvement of the CNS in schistosomiasis can occur during all stages, including the early postinfective, the asymptomatic and the chronic stages. The asymptomatic form of CNS is far more frequent than the symptomatic ones. The acute phase occurs a few weeks after exposure to schistosome-infected water. Acute cerebral schistosomiasis may manifest itself as Katayama syndrome or headache, seizures and focal neurological deficit (visual field impairment, speech disturbances, hemiparesis, cerebellar syndrome). As schistosome eggs accumulate, about 3 months or more after infection, they form agranuloma which enters the chronic phase. The severity of symptoms may depend on the location of the granulomas and the severity of the immune response. Large single or multiple schistosome necrotic-exudative granulomatous lesions located in brain hemispheres may provoke a prominent mass effect and deviation of brain structures, resulting to hydrocephalus and increased intracranial pressure. It may also cause cerebrovascular complications (stroke, cerebral haematomas, subarachnoid haemorrhage and cerebellar haematomas), which owe to a chronic hypereosinophilic syndrome.

② Spinal schistosomiasis

Schistosomal myelopathy tends to occur early and is more likely to be symptomatic than cerebral schistosomiasis. The clinical syndrome is usually an acute or subacute myelopathy, with or without polyradiculitis, causing lumbosacral and lower limbs pain, paraparesis or paraplegia, bowel and bladder sphincter dysfunction, and sensory, sexual and reflexic disturbances.

2) Diagnostic investigation

① Cerebral schistosomiais

A definitive diagnosis can only be made by means of histopathological study demonstrating schistosome eggs and granulomas. Neuroimaging studies have revealed the presence of multiple oedematous inflammatory granulomas in the brain cortex that are heterogeneously enhanced after intravenous administration of gadolinium, which are isointense on T_1-weighted images and hyperintense on T_2-weighted images. Cerebral schistosomiasis sometimes presents pseudotumoral form because of an expanding tumor-like lesion surrounded by oedema. *Schistosome* ova in stool, urine and/or rectal mucosa (rectal biopsy) can be detected in approximately 40% of acute neuroschistosomiasis patients. However, the search for ova in the stool is usually unsuccessful in the early post-infective stage. The enzyme linked immunosorbent assay (ELISA) technique for detection of egg antigen is a reliable method. The combination of ELISA and hemagglutination has higher sensitivity and specificity. The antibody occurs commonly several weeks after the onset of neurological symptoms and remains positive for life. CSF findings are unspecific and may be found in other parasite infections of the CNS. The ELISA can be positive in the CSF.

② Spinal schistosomiasis

MRI is a useful technique that provides valuable information to assess the location and extension of spinal granulomas, and the degree of spinal inflammation, necrosis and oedema. In spinal schistosomiasis, swelling of conus medullaris, enlargement of the spinal cord at the thoracic level, usually below T8, thickening of spinal roots and cauda equine, and high-intensity signal on sagittal T_2-weighted images can be observed. Granulomas of conus medullaris can be heterogeneously enhanced by gadolinium contrast medium on T_1-weighted images. Eosinophils, lymphocytic pleocytosis, increased protein concentration and raised IgG index can be found in CSF.

(3) Differential diagnosis

Differential diagnosis of pseudotumoral brain schistosomiasis should include neurocysticercosis, gliomas, cerebral tuberculomas, mycosis of the CNS and even brain abscesses. Differential diagnosis of spinal schistosomiasis should include ependymoma, spinal cord astrocytoma, metastatic tumor, spinal dural arteriovenous fistula and spinal neurocysticercosis. Differential diagnosis can be summarized in Tab. 7.7.

Tab. 7.7 Differential diagnosis of neuroschistosomiasis

Brain schistosomiasis	Spinal schistosomiasis
Brain abscesses	Ependymoma
Neurocysticercosis	Spinal cord astrocytoma
Gliomas	Metastatic tumor
Cerebral tuberculomas	Spinal dural arteriovenous fistula (SDAVF)

(4) Treatment

1) Medical treatment

Schistosomicidal drugs (praziquantel, oxamniquine and artemisinin derivatives) and steroids are used to treat cerebral and spinal schistosomiasis. Praziquantel is safely co-administered with albendazole and ivermectin, in areas where these drugs are used separately for preventive chemotherapy.

a. Praziquantel is a safe and effective chemotherapy against all species of schistosomes. The recommended dose for treatment of neuroschistosomiasis is 50 mg/(kg · d) bid for 5 days. Patients should be followed-up by stools and urine re-examined 1 month after treatment to assess the efficacy of chemotherapy.

b. Artemether, an antimalarial drug, can kill schistosomula during the first 3 weeks of life. It has been used for schistosomiasis chemoprophylaxis in China.

c. Oxamniquine, a tetrahydroquinoline derivative, is effectively used against Caribbean and South American *S. mansoni* strains by a single dose (30~50 mg/kg).

d. Corticosteroids are used to suppress the inflammatory response and granuloma formation, thereby preventing further tissue destruction, and reduce ova deposition. Patients usually receive intravenous methylprednisolone (15 ~ 20 mg/kg; maximum dose 1 g) over 5 ~ 7 days followed by oral prednisone for 2 ~ 6 weeks.

2) Surgical treatment

Surgery and combination of therapies are needed in severe condition. Rehabilitation and multidisciplinary team care are necessary in severely disabled and paraplegic patients.

(5) Prognosis

Cerebral schistosomiasis is associated with a better outcome than the spinal cord disorder. Most treated patients recover quickly and without any residual deficits.

7.8.2 Taeniasis/Cysticercosis

Neurocysticercosis (NCC) is the most common helminthic infection (the larval stage of the pork tapeworm *Taenia solium*) of the nervous system in humans. It is also the most frequent preventable cause of epilepsy worldwide. In 2015, WHO states that the total number of people suffering from neurocysticercosis, including symptomatic and asymptomatic cases, is estimated to be between 2.56 ~ 8.30 million, based on the range of epilepsy prevalence data available. *Taenia solium* (*T. solium*), the pork tapeworm, is endemic in most developing countries where domestic pig coexist with human in poor sanitary conditions. *T. solium* is a two-host zoonotic cestode. The life cycle of *T. solium* involves an intermediate host (pigs) harboring the parasitic larvae or encysted cysticerci in its tissues, and a definitive host (humans) carrying the adult tapeworm in intestines. Humans acquire cysticercosis by fecal-oral contamination, so a tapeworm carrier can originate NCC cases even in a non cysticercosis-endemic region.

(1) Clinical feature

1) Clinical manifestation

The prepatent period between infection and symptoms in NCC is estimated between 3 and 5 years. The most frequent clinical manifestations are seizures, intracranial hypertension, focal deficits, and cognitive alterations. The location of the parasite in the CNS and its expansion toward the inside of the brain parenchyma or toward the subarachnoid and ventricular spaces is a major determinant of its process of evolution and the subsequent clinical manifestations.

① Intraparenchymal cysts

Cysticerci in the brain parenchyma establish initially as viable cysts (Cysticercus cellulosae) usually measuring 0.5 ~ 1.5 cm in diameter, with a clear liquid content. Parenchymal brain cysts primarily manifest with seizures and epilepsy (most characteristic symptom), though headache, focal signs, and cognitive deficits are common. The semiology of seizures frequently correlates with the anatomic location of one of the brain parasites in any stage of the parasite. Focal deficits may occur after repeated partial seizures, from Todd paralysis, and may take a few days to resolve. Depression also seems a common event in NCC. The real prevalence of cognitive alterations and psychiatric symptoms by type of NCC, however, is yet unknown.

② Extraparenchymal cysts

Extraparenchymal NCC frequently presents with intracranial hypertension obstructive hydrocephalus, large cyst masses or cysticercotic encephalitis. The information on the natural evolution of cysts inside the ventricular cavities (ventricular NCC) is limited by their clinical expression. Ventricular cysts frequently block the circulation of cerebrospinal fluid (CSF) causing obstructive hydrocephalus. Cysts in the subarachnoid space tend to grow and expand their membranes forming vesicular clusters which present as space-occupying lesions, called racemose cysticercosis in the classic literature. Subarachnoid NCC can present in different locations, most typically in the sylvian fissure, interhemispheric spaces, or in the basal cisterns. Subarachnoid NCC is progressive and associated with significant mortality, reported to be more than 20% even in well-equipped centers.

2) Diagnostic investigation

A diagnosis of NCC is based on neuroimaging examinations and supported by specific serologic assays.

① Neuroimaging examinations

A patient with suspected NCC should be commended to perform both CT and MRI, because MRI provides better imaging of small lesions or that in the posterior fossa and gives more information on parenchymal inflammation or periventricular effusion in hydrocephalus. CT is much better to detect calcifications, and it is common to miss calcified cysts if MRI is used alone. A 38-year-old otherwise healthy woman presents seizures. Her MRI-enhanced demonstrates multiple cystic lesions with a dot (rings) in both hemisphere. Viable intraparenchymal cysts (Fig. 7.6) are seen as well-defined, rounded cystic structures with liquid contents whose signal is similar to CSF, with minimal or no surrounding inflammation initially noticeable as pericystic edema and contrast enhancement. When the cyst collapse into a granulomatous lesion, the fluid inside the cyst becomes turbid and dense, the cyst shrinks and eventually is replaced with a residual calcification. Intraventricular cysts appear on MRI also as well-defined viable or degenerating cysts but the subarachnoid cysts are less defined just in shape. These lesions may grow and occupy large spaces, particularly in the sylvian fissures and in the basal cisterns.

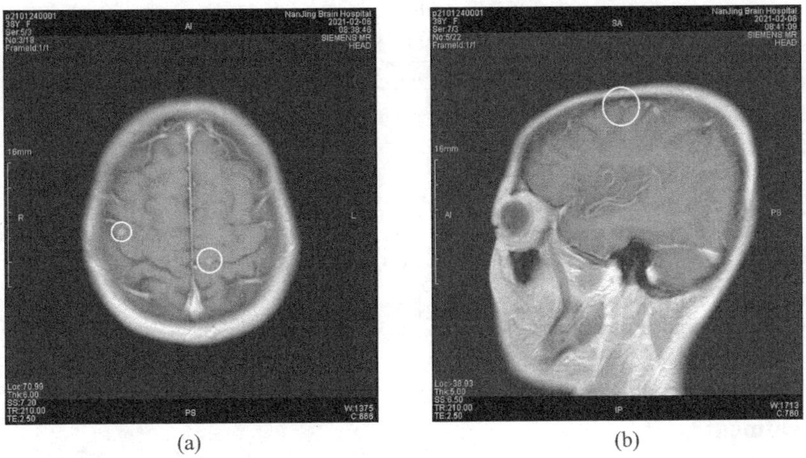

(a) (b)

Fig. 7.6 MRI-enhanced shows NCC (ring) in both hemisphere

② Antibody assays

Serum samples are preferred for antibody diagnosis although CSF examination may complement the serological diagnosis and also add information, such as cell counts and CSF biochemistry. Serology for NCC aims to detect specific antibodies to the parasite or circulating parasite antigens. Antigen detection using a monoclonal antibody-based ELISA can confirm the presence of living parasites. Antibody detection using lentil lectin purified parasite glycoprotein antigen (LLGP-EITB) is the tool of serological diagnosis of cysticercosis. Some individuals with multiple cysts may have persistently detectable antibodies on LLGP-EITB years after successful antiparasitic treatment, while a few patients may become seronegative after 9 months or so.

③ Diagnostic criteria

The diagnosis of neurocysticercosis is difficult because clinical manifestations are nonspecific, most neuroimaging findings are not pathognomonic, and some serologic tests have low sensitivity and specificity. A set of diagnostic criteria was proposed in 1996 and recently revisited (Tab. 7.8), based on objective clinical, imaging, immunological, and epidemiological data; these criteria consist of three parts that are stratified according to their diagnostic strength.

Tab. 7.8 Diagnostic criteria for human neurocysticercosis (2017)

Part 1 Absolute criteria		
A. Histological demonstration of the parasite from biopsy of a brain or spinal cord lesion; B. Direct visualization of sub-retinal cysticercus; C. Conclusive demonstration of a scolex within a cystic lesion on neuroimaging studies		
Part 2 Neuroimaging criteria		
Major	Confirmatory	Minor
A. Cystic lesions without a discernible scolex; B. Enhancing lesions; C. Multilobulated cystic lesions; D. Typical parenchymal brain calcifications	A. Resolution of cystic lesions after cysticidal drug therapy; B. Spontaneous resolution of single small enhanced lesions; C. Migration of ventricular cysts documented on sequential neuroimaging studies	A. Obstructive hydrocephalus (symmetric/asymmetric); B. Abnormal enhancement of basal leptomeninges
Part 3 Clinical/exposure criteria		
Major	Minor	
A. Detection of specific cysticercal antibodies/cysticercal antigens; B. Cysticercosis outside the central nervous system; C. Evidence of a household contact with *T. solium* infection	A. Evidence of a household contact with *T. solium* infection; B. Individuals exposed to cysticercosis endemic area; C. Not included	

(2) Treatment

1) Antiparasitic treatment

a. Praziquantel are effective antiparasitic drugs against *T. solium* cysticerci. A dosage of 50 mg/(kg · d) for 2 weeks is adopted mostly, although a single-day regimen of 75 mg/kg has recently been described with similar rates of cyst disappearance in some groups of patients.

b. Albendazole has better penetration into cerebrospinal fluid. The dose previously used in hydatid disease [15 mg/(kg · d)] is used for cysticercosis for 15 days or 1 week.

2) Supportive therapy

Between the second and fifth days of antiparasitic therapy, there is usually an exacerbation of neurological symptoms, attributed to local inflammation due to the death of the larvae. So steroids are generally given simultaneously in order to control the edema and intracranial hypertension. The most frequent regimen is dexamethasone at doses of 4.5 ~ 12 mg/d. Prednisone at 1 mg/(kg · d) may replace dexamethasone when long-term steroid therapy is required. Analgesics and antiepileptic drugs should be used as indicated in general practice. Control of intracranial hypertension may require steroids, acetazolamide or mannitol.

3) Surgery

The role of surgical therapy in the management of neurocysticercosis has significantly decreased over time and is now mainly restricted to placement of ventricular shunts for hydrocephalus. Less invasive procedures have been described, specifically the use of neuroendoscopic approaches with fenestration of the anterior wall of the third ventricle; rarely, excision of a large lesion or lesion conglomerate.

(3) Prognosis

In general, parenchymal NCC seems to carry a benign prognosis if adequate antiparasitic agents and supportive therapy is provided. Extraparenchymal NCC, on the other hand, is not benign. Subarachnoid NCC still carries significant risks even in the best available management conditions.

7.9 Prion Diseases

Transmissible spongiform encephalopathies (TSE), or prion diseases, are a group of fatal neurodegenerative disorders that affect both humans and animals. Human prion diseases include Kuru disease, the various forms of Creutzfeldt-Jakob disease (CJD), Gerstmann-Sträussler-Scheinker (GSS) syndrome, fatal familial insomnia, sporadic fatal insomnia, and the variably protease-sensitive prionopathy. The classification of human prion diseases recognizes idiopathic (sCJD), inherited and acquired forms of disease. The first verified cases later known as Creutzfeldt-Jakob disease were reported in 1921 by Jakob. The spectrum of inherited human prion diseases now includes different forms of familial CJD, classical and variant forms of Gerstmann-Sträussler-Scheinker syndrome (GSS), and fatal familial insomnia (FFI). These conditions have been linked to an ever-increasing number of pathogenic mutations and insertions in the PRNP gene. Kuru disease is the first identified acquired form of human prion disease. The first iatrogenic acquired case of CJD was reported in 1974 in a corneal transplant recipient. Epidemiologic evidence has linked this disorder to the epidemic of bovine spongiform encephalopathy in the United Kingdom since 1986, drawing considerable public attention to prion diseases. The most common human prion disease, however, is still idiopathic sCJD (with an incidence of approximately 1 case per million population per year), which is not associated with any known mutations in the PRNP gene or environmental risk factors.

(1) Pathophysiology

Prion is defined as a "proteinaceous infectious particle" consisting a single protein without the involvement of nucleic acids that causes spongiform encephalopathies in mammals by triggering normally healthy proteins in the brain to fold abnormally. It is caused by the conversion of cellular prion protein C (PrP C) into a misfolded pathological isoform (PrPSc or prion-proteinaceous infectious particle) that self-propagates by conformational conversion of PrP C. Once a misfolded prion enters a healthy person, it converts correctly-folded proteins into the disease-associated form. The spongiform changes, neuronal loss, gliosis and accumulation of PrPSc are the characteristic neuropathological lesions. "Spongiform change" refers to vacuolation of the neuropil of the cerebral cortex, the subcortical gray matter, and the cerebellar molecular layer. It is almost always present in the head of the caudate nucleus in cases of sporadic disease but usually is minimal to absent in brain stem and spinal cord. Vacuolation of nerve cell bodies in human prion diseases has been described but is unusual, in contrast to transmissible spongiform encephalopathies of animals, such as scrapie.

The most common molecular strain (Codon 129) is MM1/MV1. Between 60% and 70% of all CJD cases are grouped here, with 95% of these being MM1. MV2 is present in 9% of the patient population and is distinguished from all other subtypes because of the significantly longer disease course. MM2 also has a longer disease course (14 months), and is seen in 2%~8% of cases. The final group, the VV1, is the most uncommon, being seen in just 1% of cases. This is an early-onset subtype. In cases of sporadic, iatrogenic, and familial CJD, the gross appearance of the brain may vary from normal to showing variable degrees of cerebral cortical, striatal, and/or cerebellar atrophy. In general, loss of brain substance is confined to gray matter with relative sparing of white matter. Significant cerebral and cerebellar atrophy also may become apparent only with long disease duration (in excess of 30 months) in patients who have familial and sporadic forms of fatal insomnia.

(2) Clinical feature

1) Clinical manifestation

The hallmark of CJD is rapidly progressive dementia of unknown origin. Also, numerous atypical neurological examination findings are commonly seen: myoclonus, visual changes leading to cortical blindness, ataxia, and usually an akinetic mutism in the last stages of the disease. Myoclonus is the most common sign, but there are atypical findings such as sleep disturbances, chorea, psychiatric symptoms, and peripheral neuropathy. The clinical examination can highlight the heterogeneity of CJD phenotypes, but the common factor is progressive decline in neurological status. The most common physical examination findings stratified by phenotypic strain are listed in Tab. 7.9.

2) Diagnostic investigation

Only a brain biopsy or an exam of brain tissue after death (autopsy) can confirm the presence of CJD. But doctors often can make an accurate diagnosis based on your medical and personal history, a neurological exam, and certain diagnostic tests.

① Diagnostic criteria

In 2015, the WHO published the updated diagnostic criteria for CJD (Tab. 7.10) relying on clinical examination, EEG, and CSF findings, MRI findings, genetic testing, or modern laboratory tests for confirmation of the diagnosis. Criteria for a diagnosis of CJD that includes newer confirmatory tests and incorporates phenotypic strain provide a less invasive means of definitive diagnosis and include the atypical patient.

Tab. 7.9 Clinical and genetic features of human prion diseases

	Idiopathic CJD		Inherited CJD			Acquired Creutzfeldt-Jakob disease		
Subtype	Sporadic CJD	sFI	Familial CJD	GSS	FFI	Variant CJD	Iatrogenic CJD	Kuru
Age of onset	Mean 65 (14~92)	Mean 60.3	50~60 (26~81)	50~60 (2nd~8th decade)	50 (20~63)	26 (12~74)	50~75	5~60
Disease duration	2 weeks~35 months	14 months	6 months (2~41 months)	5~6 years (3 months~13 years)	13~15 months (6~42 months)	14 months (6~39 months)	Similar to sCJD	12 months
Main clinical features	Progressive dementia, myoclonus, visual cerebellar disturbances, pyramidal-extrapyramidal signs, akinetic mutism	Autonomic dysfunction bulbar and gait motor signs	Almost similar to sCJD MM1, but haplotype-related variability	Progressive ataxia, incoordination, dysarthria, pyramidal/extrapyramidal signs, late dementia	Insomnia, autonomic dy-sfunction, bulbar and gait motor symptoms	Early psychiatric symptoms (depression, anxiety, delusions, withdrawn), persistent painful sensory symptoms, ataxia, myoclonus/chorea/dystonia, later dementia	Clinical symptoms similar to sCJD, but usually cerebellar onset with peripheral infections and usually dementing onset with intracerebral infections	Progressive ataxia, tremors, emotional liability, choreoathetotic involuntary movements, dementia not a dominant feature
Cerebrospinal fluid 14-3-3 protein	Positive in 93%	Negative	Positive in more than 90%	Usually negative	Negative	50%	77%	
EEG	PSWC (66%~90%)	Nonspecific alterations	PSWC 70%	Nonspecific alterations	Nonspecific alterations	Nonspecific alterations, no PSWC	Similar to sCJD	
Codon 129	MM 70%, MV 14%, VV 16%	MM		M	M	MM 99%	MM 57%, MV 20%, VV 23%	MM genotype preferentially affected but MV and VV genotypes also present
PRNP mutation	Not demonstrable	Not demonstrable	More than 25 disease-associated mutations	P102L	D1789	Not demonstrable	Not demonstrable	Not demonstrable

Note: M, methionine; PSWC, period short wave complexes; sFI, sporadic fatal insomnia; V, valine.

Tab. 7.10 2015 proposed updated diagnostic criteria for CJD

A	Rapidly progressive dementia
B	1) Myoclonus; 2) Visual or cerebellar signs; 3) Pyramidal/extrapyramidal; 4) Akinetic mutism; 5) VV2 genotype w/predominant ataxia w/o myoclonus in early stage; 6) MV2 genotype w/long disease course (>12 months old) and predominant ataxia in early stage; 7) MM2 genotype and temporal lobe changes on MRI w/o basal ganglia involvement; 8) VV1 genotype and young age at onset (< 50 years old), slowly progressive disease w/ frontotemporal dementia
C	1) PSWCs on EEG routine investigations that do not indicate an alternative diagnosis; 2) Positive 14-3-3 CSF assay; 3) MRI high-intensity signal abnormalities in caudate nucleus and/or putamen on DW or FLAIR imaging
D	Routine investigations that do not indicate an alternative diagnosis

Probable CJD = (A) + at least 2 of [B(criteria 1~4)] + positive result on at least 1 of (C) + (D).

Possible CJD = (A) + at least 2 of (B) + absent (C) + absent (D).

Definite CJD = diagnosed by standard neuropathological techniques/immunocytochemically/CDI-confirmed PrP/positive RT-QuIC of CSF/nasal brushings.

② EEG findings

Periodic sharp wave complexes (PSWCs) are found in the EEG recordings of approximately two-thirds of patients with sCJD, and have therefore been incorporated into probable sCJD diagnostic criteria by the WHO. The typical appearance for sCJD is that of a periodic triphasic sharp wave complex. Historically, PSWCs for CJD were described as typically presenting in a bilateral frontal midline. However, there is growing evidence to support a more temporal EEG diagnostic template among patients diagnosed with sCJD. The PSWCs are likely to present while patients are awake and to be exacerbated with sleep deprivation. Benzodiazepines mask PSWC findings on EEG for patients with sCJD.

③ MRI findings

The term pulvinar sign, or bilateral FLAIR hyperintensity of the pulvinar area, is coined with patients of vCJD. DWI is considered superior to any other MRI sequence in the early stages of CJD. In patients with hyperintensity of basal ganglia on DWI, there is a shorter disease duration and higher incidence of myoclonus. Shorter time between symptom onset and akinetic mutism is strongly correlated with the patients having hyperintense lesions in the occipital cortex on DWI. Hyperintensity decreases in the later stages of the disease, and the only findings may be cortical atrophy. In all sCJD cases with basal ganglia or thalamic DWI hyperintensities, there is associated restricted diffusion in the ADC map. The pattern of FLAIR/DWI hyperintensity and restricted diffusion can differentiate sCJD from other forms of progressive dementia.

④ CSF biomarkers

Both 14-3-3 protein and tau protein are biomarkers for rapid neuronal destruction, and so the total concentrations increase as CJD progresses. 14-3-3 protein is a surrogate marker for CJD with the sensitivity of 92% ~ 96% in CSF for classic sCJD. Tau protein in classic sCJD has a sensitivity of 81% and a specificity of 85%. They should only be used to give confidence in the diagnosis with the right clinical picture, and should not be used to rule out the disease, as they are also found in many other diseases of the brain in which the pathology is neuronal loss. Real-time quaking-induced conversion (RT-QuIC) is a recently described laboratory technique that provides definitive diagnosis of CJD from CSF samples by detecting PrPSc. RT-QuIC with nasal brushings shows a sensitivity of 97% and specificity of 100%, with positive results seen within 30 hours.

⑤ Utility of biopsy

The gold standard for diagnosis is pathological confirmation from a brain biopsy, but the frequency of a positively diagnostic biopsy is surprisingly low. The CDI is a newer method that can detect the disease with a better diagnostic success rate than the current tests. Brain biopsy should only be done after all noninvasive diagnostic avenues are exhausted, and still do not point to a cause.

(3) Treatment

Despite all the advances in the understanding of this disease, the prognosis remains grim—CJD is a terminal disease. The mainstay of treatment is symptomatic and supportive, for example, using clonazepam for the treatment of myoclonus. Future targets of therapy involve preventing the conversion of PrP C to PrPSc.

References

[1] RAJNIK M, OTTOLINI M G. Serious infections of the central nervous system: encephalitis, meningitis, and brain abscess[J]. Adolescent Medicine, 2000,11(2):401-425.

[2] SOETERS H M, DIALLO A O, BICABA B W, et al. Bacterial meningitis epidemiology in five countries in the meningitis belt of sub-Saharan Africa, 2015—2017[J]. The Journal of Infectious Diseases, 2019,220(9):S165-S174.

[3] KAMEI S. Current clinical management of bacterial meningitis[J]. Brain and Nerve, 2015,67(7):787-798.

[4] ROPPER A H, SAMUELS M A, KLEIN J, et al. Adams and Victor's principles of Neurology[M]. New York: McGraw-Hill Education, 2019.

[5] BROUWER M C, TUNKEL A R, MCKHANN G M, et al. Brainabscess[J]. The New England Journal of Medicine, 2014,371(5):447-456.

[6] WIDDRINGTON J D, BOND H, SCHWAB U, et al. Pyogenic brain abscess and subdural empyema: presentation, management, and factors predicting outcome[J]. Infection, 2018,46(6):785-792.

[7] BRADSHAW M J, VENKATESAN A. Herpes simplex virus-1 encephalitis in adults: pathophysiology, diagnosis, and management[J]. Neurotherapeutics, 2016,13(3):493-508.

[8] GRAUS F, TITULAER M J, BALU R, et al. A clinical approach to diagnosis of autoimmuneencephalitis[J]. Lancet Neurology, 2016,15(4):391-404.

[9] DALMAU J, ARMANGUÉ T, PLANAGUMÀ J, et al. An update on anti-NMDA receptor encephalitis for neurologists and psychiatrists: mechanisms and models[J]. Lancet Neurology, 2019,18(11):1045-1057.

[10] SHUKLA B, AGUILERA E A, SALAZAR L S, et al. Aseptic meningitis in adults and children: diagnostic and management challenges[J]. Journal of Clinical Virology, 2017, 94:110-114.

[11] ROMAN G C. Proposed diagnostic criteria and nosology of acute transverse myelitis [J]. Neurology, 2003,60(4):730-731.

[12] GROSSO A, RYAN O, TRAM K H, et al. Financing the response to HIV among gay men and other men who have sex with men: Case studies from eight diverse countries[J]. Global Public Health, 2015,10(10):1172-1184.

[13] MEINTJES G, BRUST J C M, NUTTALL J, et al. Management of active tuberculosis in adults with HIV[J]. Lancet HIV, 2019,6(7):e463-e474.

[14] GRAYBILL J R, SOBEL J D, SAAG M, et al. Diagnosis and management of increased intracranial pressure in patients with AIDS and cryptococcal meningitis. The NIAID mycoses study group and AIDS cooperative treatment groups[J]. Clinical Infections Diseases, 2000,30(1):47-54.

[15] MAKADZANGE A T, MCHUGH G. New approaches to the diagnosis and treatment of cryptococcal meningitis[J]. Seminars in Neurology, 2014,34(1):47-60.

[16] O'BYRNE P, PHERSON P M. Syphilis[J]. BMJ, 2019,365:l4159.

[17] FERRARI T C A, MOREIRA P R R. Neuroschistosomiasis: clinical symptoms and pathogenesis[J]. Lancet Neurology, 2011,10(9):853-864.

[18] GELLIDO C L, ONESTI S, LLENA J, et al. Spinal schistosomiasis[J]. Neurology, 2000,54(2):527.

[19] WHITE A C, COYLE C M, RAJSHEKHAR V, et al. Diagnosis and treatment of neurocysticercosis: 2017 clinical practice guidelines by the Infectious Diseases Society of America (IDSA) and the American Society of Tropical Medicine and Hygiene (ASTMH)[J]. Clinical Infections Diseases, 2018,66(8):1159-1163.

[20] PUOTI G, BIZZI A, FORLONI G, et al. Sporadic human prion diseases: molecular insights and diagnosis[J]. Lancet Neurology, 2012,11(7):618-628.

[21] MANIX M, KALAKOTI P, HENRY M, et al. Creutzfeldt-Jakob disease: updated diagnostic criteria, treatment algorithm, and the utility of brain biopsy[J]. Neurosurgical Focus, 2015,39(5):E2.

(Zhu Ying, Jiang Ping)

Chapter 8
Demyelinating Diseases

Nerve fibers are classified into unmyelinated and myelinated nerve fibers. Myelinated nerve fibers such as plant preganglionic fibers and larger somatic nerve fibers have an outer sheath on their axons, called myelin sheath. Myelin is made up of the membrane of myelin cells. Myelin cells of central nerve are oligodendrocytes and myelin cells of peripheral nerve fibers are cell membranes of Schwann cells. Myelin sheaths are composed of lipids and proteins. They can protect axon and have insulating effect on nerve impulse, and can accelerate conduction of nerve impulse. Fibers with thick myelin sheath transmit impulses quickly. When myelin is damaged, the conduction velocity is slowed. Nerve conduction is also affected by temperature, and an increase in body temperature during myelination can cause conduction block. Demyelinating disease is a disease of the nervous system in which myelination is the main or primary lesion and the damage of axons, cell bodies and glia is relatively minor. It can occur in the central or peripheral nervous system. Demyelinating diseases of the central nervous system (CNS) can be classified according to their pathogenesis into several categories: demyelination due to inflammatory processes, viral demyelination, demyelination caused by acquired metabolic derangements, hypoxic-ischaemic forms of demyelination and demyelination caused by focal compression.

8.1 Multiple Sclerosis

Multiple sclerosis (MS) is a chronic inflammatory disorder of the central nervous system (CNS) which predominantly affects patients aged 20 to 40 years. It is characterized by demyelination and subsequent degeneration leading to neuronal damage and axonal loss. The incidence and prevalence rates continue to rise worldwide, with highest reports originating from North America and Europe. Although the exact etiology remains unknown, our current understanding of the natural history of MS and its immunopathogenesis points toward an immune dysregulation resulting from an interaction between genetic predispositions and environmental factors.

(1) Pathophysiology

The etiology of MS is unknown. There is some geographical and racial variation in disease prevalence: lower rates are found in tropical countries and migrants from low prevalence areas remain at low risk if they move over the age of 15 years; if younger, they take on the risk of their new home. There is a minor genetic component and there is a tendency for an association with HLA antigens DR2 and DW2. The pathological hallmark of MS is the area of demyelination, with loss of myelin and relative preservation of axons (Fig. 8.1). Active lesions may have an associated inflammatory response and oedema. In more chronic lesions, the oedema and inflammation have resolved and there is a demarcated area of gliotic scarring, with atrophy and axonal loss. Plaques can be found in any part of the white matter of the brain and spinal cord. There is a predilection for the periventricular white matter, the corpus callosum and optic nerves. The area of demyelination disrupts the conduction of a nerve impulse. This initially blocks conduction, but recovery conduction is slow and the refractory period is prolonged.

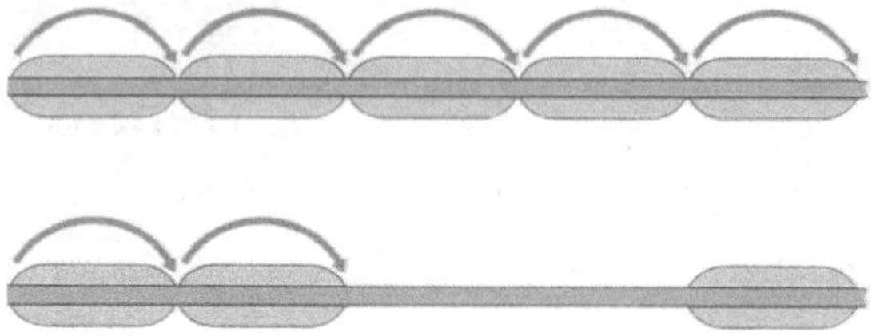

Fig. 8.1 Effects of demyelination on an axon: saltatory conduction is blocked

(2) Clinical feature

1) Clinical manifestation

The peak age of onset of MS is 25~35. It is rare below 15 years old and over 60 years old. It is more frequent in women than men (about 1.5 : 1).

Sensory symptoms are the most common presentation, occurring as the first symptom in up to 40% of patients. The feelings are described as numbness, coldness, pins and needles, swelling or tightness. They may be radicular, especially in the limbs and over the lower trunk. The onset is usually over a few days with resolution in weeks to months. Signs may be absent or relatively subtle, usually affecting vibration sense and proprioception more than superficial modalities. Sometimes signs can be more prominent than the symptoms with a sensory level or occasionally a marked loss of proprioception in a hand. Optic neuritis is a common initial manifestation of MS. A visual disturbance evolves over a few days with distortion of the central vision and impairment of colour perception. There may be pain on eye movement. Visual loss can be mild to severe. Patients have a relative afferent pupillary defect and a central scotoma. The optic disc usually appears normal (retrobulbar optic neuritis) though it may be swollen with papillitis. Vision improves over months, though may be incomplete, particularly if visual loss is severe initially. Optic atrophy may develop following an episode of optic neuritis. Uhtoff's phenomenon is the decrease in visual acuity following a rise in temperature, due to exercise, a hot bath or a fever. Double vision is a common early symptom. This can be associated with a range of eye movement abnormalities (3rd, 6th or occasionally 4th nerve palsies), skew deviation and lateral gaze palsies and, most characteristic, an internuclear ophthalmoplegia (INO). Dizziness, usually with other brain stem symptoms (diplopia, facial numbness or dysarthria), may occur. Nystagmus is a common finding, and ataxic nystagmus is found with an INO. Gait and truncal ataxia are commonly found later in the disease. There may be marked limb incoordination with associated cerebellar tremor. Weakness usually affects the legs. It can be an early symptom. Later in the disease it produces a paraplegia, which may have marked spasticity, increased reflexes and extensor plantars. An evolving paraparesis is the usual pattern of primary progressive MS. The development of urgency and frequency of micturition, and to a lesser extent defecation, usually parallels the motor weakness in the legs. Urinary symptoms can arise with detrusor sphincter dyssynergia leading to retention and a bladder that empties incompletely, which reflect unstable upper motor neurone type bladder. This can result in repeated infections and overflow incontinence. Impotence is a common problem in men.

Motor and sensory problems can be clearly localized to a single lesion in the spinal cord:

myelitis. In MS, this is usually incomplete, for example, producing a hemicord lesion (Brown-Séquard syndrome), though it can be complete-transverse myelitis. Some patients have a progressive spinal cord involvement. Lhermitte's phenomenon is an electric shock feeling going down the back and into the arms and legs after bending the neck. It occurs in MS and to a lesser extent in patients with other cervical cord disease. Epilepsy is slightly more common (3%) than in the general population. Fatigue is often a very prominent syndrome in MS. This is often very debilitating and can occur in patients with relatively mild disease.

There are essentially three patterns of disease (Fig. 8.2): a. Relapsing remitting form, with clear relapses followed by recovery. The frequency of relapses and duration of remission vary considerably. This may go on to produce a secondary progressive form, where there is a progressive increase in disability. Relapses occur more commonly after infections. There is a slight increase after trauma, though evidence is less clear-cut. There is a relative reduction during pregnancy with a slight increase afterward—over the whole period, the rate is stable. b. Secondary progressive form. Approximately 50% of patients with relapsing remitting MS have no relapses after 10 ~ 15 years of disease, with a slow progressive progression. c. Primary progressive form that deteriorates from onset. This accounts for about 10% of patients. The diagnosis of primary progressive MS (PPMS) relies on demonstrating retrospectively or prospectively, steady disability progression without relapses over a period of at least one year and at least two of the three following criteria: one or more T_2 lesions in at least one of the three brain areas (periventricular, cortical/juxtacortical, or infratentorial region); at least two or more spinal cord lesions; positive oligoclonal bands by isoelectric focusing immunoassay.

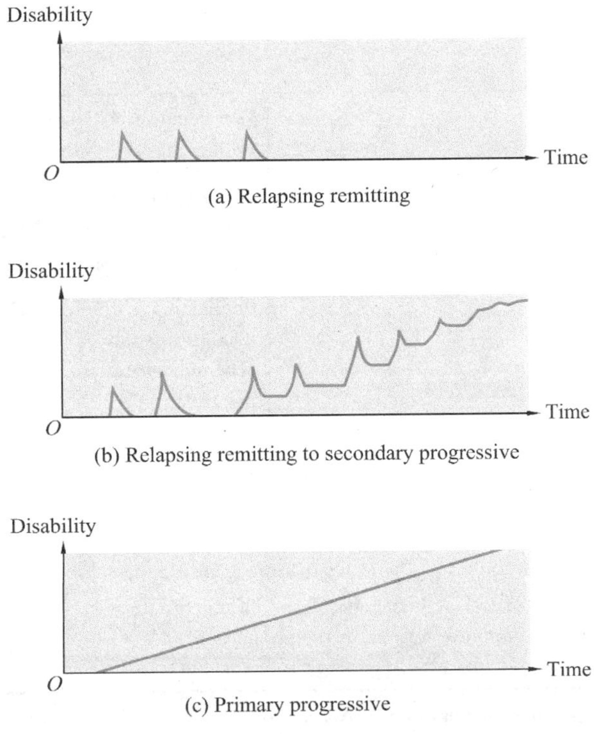

Fig. 8.2 Various patterns of progression in multiple sclerosis over time

2) Diagnostic investigation

The diagnosis of MS remains clinical despite recent advances in diagnostics and the availability of several radiological and neuro-immunological surrogate markers. The diagnosis relies on comprehensive history-taking and neurological examination to determine dissemination in time and space and signs of certain clinical symptoms while excluding mimickers. Supportive diagnostic evidence may be provided by paraclinical tests such as MRI, evoked potential studies (identifying clinically silent lesions in the visual, brainstem, and spinal cord pathways) and cerebrospinal fluid (CSF) analysis [looking for inflammatory markers such as oligoclonal bands (OCB) and/or elevated IgG index]. These CSF inflammatory markers are present in up to 90% of patients with MS.

In the latest revised criteria (Tab. 8.1), diagnosis of MS still requires evidence of dissemination in space (DIS) and time (DIT). DIS can now be fulfilled by demonstrating ≥1 T_2 lesions in at least 2 out of the 4 following regions of the CNS: periventricular, cortical-juxtacortical, infratentorial and spinal cord. It is important to note that symptomatic lesions in the spinal cord and brainstem are now included in the revised criteria. DIT can be fulfilled by the presence of a new T_2 and/or gadolinium-enhancing lesion(s) on follow-up MRI, or the simultaneous presence of gadolinium-enhancing and non-enhancing lesions at any point in time. Again, unlike the 2010 McDonald criteria, no distinction between symptomatic and asymptomatic MRI lesions is required. If criteria for DIS are fulfilled, the presence of CSF-specific oligoclonal bands allows a diagnosis of multiple sclerosis in the absence of DIT.

Tab. 8.1 2017 McDonald criteria for diagnosis of MS[a]

	Number of clinical attacks	Number of MRI lesions with objective clinical evidence	Additional data needed for diagnosis
Relapsing-remitting multiple	≥2	≥2	None[b]
	≥2	1[c]	None
	≥2	1	DIS demonstrated by an additional clinical attack implicating a different CNS site or by MRI
	1	≥2	DIT demonstrated by additional clinical attack, MRI, or CSF-specific oligoclonal bands
	1	1	DIS demonstrated by additional clinical attack implicating a different CNS site/by MRI and DIT demonstrated by an additional clinical attack/by MRI/demonstration of CSF-specific oligoclonal bands
Primary progressive multiple sclerosis	• Required: 1 year of disability progression (retrospectively or prospectively determined) independent of clinical relapse • Plus 2 of the following: A. 1 or more T_2-hyperintense lesions characteristic of MS in any of the following brain regions: periventricular, cortical or juxtacortical, or infratentorial; B. 2 or more T_2-hyperintense lesions in the spinal cord; C. presence of CSF-specific oligoclonal bands.		

Note: [a] Adapted with permission from *Lancet Neurology*.

[b] Although no MRI is required for the diagnosis, an MRI scan of the brain should be obtained in all patients with a suspected diagnosis of MS unless impossible.

[c] One lesion as well as clear-cut historical evidence of a previous attack involving a lesion in a distinct anatomical location.

(3) Differential diagnosis

The diagnosis of MS depends on identification of multiple episodes of demyelination separated in space and time. The occurrence of a single episode does not lead to a diagnosis of MS. The differential diagnosis for the most characteristic episodes will be considered individually. The differential diagnosis of multiple episodes will then be considered.

1) Optic neuritis

The most important differential is with optic nerve compression. This is usually more insidious in onset and is progressive. This can be ruled out by MRI scan. Patients of 25% to 60% first present with optic neuritis, and then develop MS.

2) Spinal cord syndromes

The most important differential diagnosis is spinal cord compression. In more insidious spinal cord syndromes, the differential diagnosis includes rarer spinal cord disease, such as Vitamin B_{12} deficiency, HTLV-1 myelopathy and familial spastic paraparesis. For patients lacking sensory signs, amyotrophic lateral sclerosis should be considered; associated lower motor neurone signs allow a distinction. After first presentation with complete transverse myelitis, patients later develop MS; those with partial spinal cord syndromes more often progress (70%).

3) Brain stem syndromes

The differential diagnosis is wide, including tumours, brain stem encephalitis, cranial polyneuritis, an Arnold-Chiari malformation or vascular disease, the last being the most common alternative in older patients. MRI may clarify this differential; CSF examination and other investigations may be needed.

4) Multifocal CNS disease

The relapsing remitting form of MS can be mimicked by other inflammatory diseases, such as systemic lupus erythematosus, sarcoid, Behçet's disease and polyarteritis nodosa, and infectious diseases such as Lyme disease and syphilis. These are all rare. A monophasic illness characterized by widespread multifocal demyelination can occur either in isolation (acute disseminated encephalomyelitis) or after an infection (post-infectious encephalomyelitis). In these conditions, there are multiple areas of demyelination separated in space but not in time.

(4) Management and treatment

1) Management

It is important that a newly diagnosed patient and their family appreciate that many patients can follow a more benign course. They need help to come to terms with the condition, particularly with the uncertainty of the future. The range of problems that may accompany the patients means that a range of help is required from the family doctor, physiotherapists and occupational therapists, making it important for a team approach supporting the patients and carers.

2) Treatment

There is as yet no cure for MS. Treatment is aimed at alleviating symptoms. Some newer therapies may prove useful in reducing the frequency of relapses and slow progression of disability.

① Symptomatic treatment

Steroids accelerate the recovery following a relapse. They are usually given intravenously (as methylprednisolone) over 3 days. Steroids can be used in patients with progressive MS, but the response is usually more disappointing than in relapsing remitting disease. Pain may occur and usually responds to pain modulating drugs, such as amitriptyline or gabapentin. Carbamazepine may also help some paroxysmal symptoms such as Lhermitte's or trigeminal neuralgia. Tremor is usually difficult to treat; occasionally stereotactic thalamotomy may be helpful. Depression is common and needs to be treated with appropriate support and antidepressants. Physiotherapy is helpful at optimizing the level of function of the patient and occupational therapy optimizes the patient's environment to minimize the impact of disabilities. Speech therapy may be helpful in some patients.

② Disease-modifying treatment

Some immune-modulating drugs such as cyclophosphamide and azathioprine have been shown to have minor beneficial effects. Beta-interferon is given either subcutaneously or intramuscularly; side-effects include local irritation at the site of injection and flu-like symptoms. Some patients develop antibodies to beta-interferon though the significance is not clear. Natalizumab, a monoclonal antibody affecting permeability of the blood-brain barrier, has a greater effect on relapse rate than beta-interferon, but a small risk of developing fatal progressive multifocal leucoencephalopathy means it is licensed in the UK for only a small proportion of patients with aggressive disease.

(5) Prognosis

The prognosis is variable and any comments about long-term prognosis are complicated by the improved diagnostic methods that allow milder disease to be recognized. On the basis of currently available studies, life expectancy is reduced by 10 ~ 20 years. Half of the patients move into the progressive phase of the disease by 10 years and half require aids to walk by 17 years. About 15% have a very benign form of the disease with only a few relapses and minor, if any, disability. The disease is mild after 5 years, severe disease develops infrequently. Several factors influence prognosis. Relapsing remitting disease has a better prognosis than primary progressive. Men tend to do worse than women. Sensory symptoms or optic neuritis at onset tend to indicate a better prognosis.

8.2 Neuromyelitis Optica

In recent years, the definition of neuromyelitis optica (NMO), or Devic disease has been expanded as a specific antibody discovered in the serum of affected patients. Because of this, the term neuromyelitis optica spectrum disorder (NMOSD) is now used to include optic neuritis with spinal cord manifestations and include other neurologic disorders associated with the serum aquaporin-4 immunoglobulin G (AQP4-IgG) antibodies. Beside MS, recent discoveries have highlighted rarer, more sinister manifestations of optic neuritis such as NMOSD and myelin oligodendrocyte glycoprotein (MOG), which necessitate additional evaluation and treatment. The etiology of NMOSD is still unclear. In the past, NMOSD was characterized as a variant of MS, but recent studies have elucidated the differences in the disease process, manifestations, and management. Whole-genome sequencing has identified some at-risk genotypes for NMOSD, and two major histocompatibility complexes have been identified. The prevalence of NMOSD is approximately 0.3 ~ 4.4 per million. NMOSD characteristically occurs in females (80%) and younger patients (aged 30 ~ 40). Worldwide, NMOSD has a variable prevalence among demyelinating diseases. Among all demyelinating diseases, NMOSD comprises only 1% ~ 2% in the United States and Italy but comprises 13.7% in India and over 30% in Thailand. Ethnicity appears to play a role in the phenotype of the disease. NMOSD can correlate with other auto-immune diseases, such as systemic lupus erythematosus, celiac disease, Sjögren syndrome, and sarcoidosis. NMOSD attacks have been shown to occur in 20% ~ 30% of cases after an environmental trigger, such as post-vaccination or post-infection.

(1) Pathophysiology

NMOSD is an inflammatory disease that primarily affects the optic nerve and spinal cord. It has been recognized more broadly as a distinct entity with a unique mechanism and pathogenesis based on the IgG antibodies against aquaporin-4 (AQP4) rather than a variant of MS. AQP4 is a membrane-bound protein with a high concentration in certain parts of the central nervous system, such as the optic nerve, the spinal cord, and the area postrema. In essence, NMOSD is an autoimmune demyelinating astrocytopathy where AQP4-IgG mediates perivascular lymphocytic infiltration leading to axonal loss with a preference for the aforementioned at-risk areas.

(2) Clinical feature

1) Clinical manifestation

Classically, optic neuritis occurs in a younger, caucasian patient and present with an episode of acute onset, painful, monocular vision loss, with a relative afferent pupillary defect in the affected eye. The clinical exam of a patient with acute optic neuritis should always have the visual acuity, pupils, and intraocular pressure tested, followed by a thorough neuro-ophthalmic exam. A fundus exam will typically reveal optic nerve head elevation on the affected side. If the patient suffers from intractable hiccups, unexplained nausea or vomiting, or symptomatic narcolepsy, these could be clues that the optic neuritis may be caused by NMOSD. NMOSD may alternatively present less classically, and AQP4-IgG can be presented in other disorders. These disorders can present as isolated longitudinal extensive transverse myelitis, brainstem clinical manifestations, brainstem encephalitis, monophasic optic neuritis, or recurrent optic neuritis.

2) Diagnostic investigation

NMOSD is evaluated by clinical examination and serologic testing for AQP4-IgG as well as MRI with and without gadolinium. Diagnosis is based on core clinical characteristics and supplemented by additional testing, and several criteria exist. Because of this, the international consensus diagnostic criteria was established in 2015, which separated NMOSD into AQP4-IgG status (with testing, without testing, or unknown) and defined clinical and MRI characteristics of NMOSD. Color vision testing may show a decrease in color vision, and visual field evaluation may show a central scotoma. Ancillary testing with optical coherence tomography can aid in the diagnosis and may reveal a thinner nerve fiber layer than in MS cases. Characteristic findings in optic neuritis include white matter lesions and optic nerve enhancement (T_2-hyperintense lesions or T_1-weighted contrast-enhancing images). Other MRI manifestations of NMOSD include acute myelitis, which shows longitudinal intramedullary lesions or focal spinal cord atrophic segments. Those patients with area postrema syndrome will demonstrate lesions at the dorsal medulla region or area postrema. Those with acute brainstem syndrome will show lesions at the peri-ependymal brainstem. When MRI lesions show enhancement in the optic nerves and spinal cord, the main differential diagnosis of NMOSD is MS. It is important to distinguish these clinical entities as the prognosis and management differ considerably, and some MS drugs can worsen NMOSD. In contrast with MS, NMOSD has some distinct radiologic features that differentiate it as a clinical entity. NMOSD shows longitudinal spinal cord lesions extending over three or more segments, while MS typically has short, multiple lesions.

(3) Differential diagnosis

The differential diagnosis of a patient with optic neuritis typically includes MS, NMOSD, and MOG. MS is the most common of these entities and should therefore be ruled out first (Tab. 8.2). Still, the clinician should be especially aware of the other two as they typically portend a less favorable prognosis and different treatments. Because NMOSD can also present without ocular symptoms, the presentation and differential of NMOSD broaden significantly when the patient does not have ocular involvement. Still, the primary clinical entity on the differential is MS, but theoretically, any lesion causing MS-like symptoms could be on the differential of NMOSD. The CSF findings in NMO include moderate pleocytosis, elevated protein, and absence of OCBs. A serum marker for NMO is available commercially, NMO-IgG antibody. This NMO-IgG binds selectively to aquaporin-4 water channel, which is found in high amounts in astrocytic foot processes at the blood-brain barrier. The NMO-IgG antibody test is useful in identifying NMO from MS, with sensitivity of 73% and specificity of 91%. Specific radiologic and laboratory criteria have been proposed to differentiate NMO from MS: a. a spinal cord MRI lesion extending contiguously three or more vertebral segments; b. a brain MRI that fails to meet diagnostic criteria for MS; c. a positive NMO-IgG antibody titer. Two of these three supporting criteria need to be met for the diagnosis of NMO. Other mimics to exclude based on imaging are Schilder disease and tumefactive MS, which are seen as large tumor-like lesions associated with edema and mass effect; Marburg virus variant of MS, which also presents with encephalopathy and multiple, large lesions on MRI; brain abscess, which is usually a solitary, complete ring-enhancing lesion with hypointense center on MRI. Symmetric bithalamic lesions can be seen in cerebral venous thrombosis, hypernatremia, acute necrotizing encephalopathy, and extrapontine myelinolysis. Basal ganglia lesions can be seen in organic aciduria and infantile bilateral striatal necrosis.

Tab. 8.2 Differences between NMOSD and MS

Character	MS	NMOSD
Frequency of disease	Common	Rare
Latitude gradient	Present	Not proven
Incidence in females/%	70	90
Ethnic variation	Common in Caucasians	Common in Africans and Asians
Age at onset/years old	20~40	40~60
Progressive course	Common	Rare
Coexistent autoimmune disease	Rare	Common: MG, SLE, Sjogren's syndrome, APL
Tissue involvement	White matter	White and gray matter
Necrosis/cavitation	Rare	Common
Leukocyte infiltrate	T and B lymphocytes	Neutrophils, eosinophils
Perivascular IgG and complement	Common	Common
Attack severity	Often mild	Often severe
Spinal cord	Short-segment peripheral cord lesions, asymptomatic	Usually symptomatic LETM, extending into medulla, central cord involvement

(4) Treatment

1) Drug treatment

Treatment of the acute phase of NMOSD flare usually involves the use of intravenous steroids such as methylprednisolone, often used in high doses (500 ~ 100 mg/d) for 5 ~ 10 days. Others studies advocate for plasmapheresis treatment (55 mL/kg) as well as intravenous immunoglobulin. Chronic immunosuppressive therapy can be accomplished with azathioprine or rituximab as first-line agents. Second-line agents may include mycophenolate or methotrexate. These second-line agents may be advantageous due to their less frequent dosing. Newer biologic agents are directed against specific immune mediators, such as anti-IL-6, anti-complement, or anti-AQP4-IgG. A retrospective multicenter analysis showed reductions in relapse rate with rituximab, mycophenolate, and azathioprine (with prednisone) of 88.2%, 87.4%, and 72.1%, respectively.

2) Deterrence and patient education

Patients diagnosed with NMOSD should be aware of the potential complications of the disorder, the comorbid associated autoimmune conditions, and the importance of medication compliance and follow-up. Currently, there are no known preventive strategies for NMOSD.

3) Enhancing healthcare team outcomes

The neuro-ophthalmologist is often initially involved in diagnosing patients with NMOSD, but patients may also initially present to a primary care provider or neurologist. It is essential to consult with an interprofessional team that includes the ophthalmologist, neurologist, and primary care provider to provide adequate care for these patients. The nurse's role is vital as these patients often require hospital admission with rapid induction of intravenous steroids. The pharmacist will be critical in adjusting the appropriate steroid dose for the patient, which will need to be done considering the other medical issue of the patient. The radiologist is also key in making the appropriate diagnosis based on the MRI results. To date, there are no large randomized clinical trials on the diagnosis and treatment of NMOSD; therefore, we rely primarily on consensus based on expert opinion. Diagnostic criteria are based on historical and case-control studies for diagnosis.

(5) Prognosis

Complications of NMOSD include visual field defects and motor impairment, with potential blindness and irreversible motor deficits. In severe cases, myogenic respiratory failure is the cause of increased mortality. NMOSD has a variable course and prognosis. It is either relapsing (80% ~ 90%) or monophasic. Some patients suffer chronic disability as a result of relapsing episodes.

8.3 Acute Disseminated Encephalomyelitis

Acute disseminated encephalomyelitis (ADEM) is an acute multifocal demyelinating disease of the central nervous system (CNS) that typically follows an infectious illness. ADEM can occur at any age, with higher frequency in children than adults. Predominant age of occurrence in children is 5 ~ 8 and adults between 19 and 61. The diagnosis of ADEM is usually made in the setting of a viral illness or vaccination. Hence, the incidence of disease varies with the triggering infectious agent. Worldwide distribution of ADEM is unknown in part because regional cases of ADEM are often linked to specific vaccinations. Several different viruses, mainly exanthematous, could produce febrile encephalopathy shortly after the infection. Hence, the illnesses are named after the disease-causing viruses, such as varicella encephalomyelitis, rubella encephalomyelitis, and rabies encephalomyelitis, also known as neuroparalytic accident. Although there is a temporal relationship between the febrile illness and onset of neurologic symptoms, the neurologic illness is probably not due to direct invasion of the infectious agent into the CNS. It is likely that the infectious agents trigger an autoimmune response against the CNS antigens, which in turn produces the CNS pathology. The pathogenesis of ADEM has most resemblance to the animal model experimental autoimmune encephalomyelitis (EAE), which is an acute demyelinating disease induced by immunization of animals with myelin protein products. Histologic analysis shows inflammatory demyelinating lesions typically in the spinal cord and in some animal strains in the brain. Since EAE is a T-cell-mediated disease, it is likely that ADEM is also a T-cell-mediated disease by its close resemblance to the EAE model. Several theories have been postulated to explain how infections or vaccinations prime T-cell responses against myelin antigens in the CNS. It is likely that more than one immune mechanism is involved in triggering ADEM in susceptible patients.

Although ADEM typically has a monophasic course, recurrences after a delay are common. The incidence of these relapses has been variably reported from 5.5% to as high as 21%. Several terms have been used to describe relapsing forms of ADEM: a. If a subsequent neurologic event takes place within 4 weeks of tapering steroid therapy or within 3 months from the initial event, then this event is not considered a "true" relapse but still temporally related to the initial event. Such a relapse has also been dubbed "pseudorelapsing ADEM" or "steroid-dependent ADEM". b. A true recurrent ADEM is defined as a new clinical event occurring at least 3 months after the initial ADEM presentation and at least 4 weeks after the completion of steroid treatment. Importantly, the clinical presentation and distribution of demyelinating lesions on MRI should be very similar to the initial ADEM event. c. Multiphasic ADEM is defined as future ADEM episodes, but involving new clinical deficits and MRI lesions different from the initial ADEM event. Recrudescences occur at least 3 months after the initial ADEM episode and greater than 4 weeks after the completion of steroid treatment.

(1) Clinical feature

1) Clinical manifestation

Clinical manifestations of ADEM can be pleotropic. Symptoms can range from non-specific, such as malaise and fatigue, to fulminant, progressing rapidly to obtundation and coma. The clinical course of ADEM is classically monophasic, with most patients reporting an antecedent infection or vaccination. In children, a prodromal phase precedes the neurologic symptoms and consists of malaise, fever, headache, nausea, and vomiting, progressing within days to maximal neurologic symptoms. The presenting neurologic manifestation varies according to the initial CNS site affected by the inflammation. As the disease progresses, multiple CNS sites become involved, with resulting deficits including hemiplegia, ataxia, cranial nerve deficits, optic neuritis, myelitis, speech impairment, hemiparesthesias, and seizures. A hyperacute variant of ADEM is known as acute hemorrhagic leukoencephalopathy (AHL), also variably called AHEM or acute necrotizing hemorrhagic leukoencephalitis (ANHLE). AHL occurs within days to a few weeks after an infection, usually upper respiratory, or vaccination. Clinical presentation includes fever, headache, confusion, seizures, and weakness, progressing rapidly to stupor and coma. CT or MRI scans show large lesions associated with edema and mass effect, tissue displacement, and petechial or frank hemorrhages. Death can occur within days from the onset of encephalopathy due to herniation caused by cerebral edema and hemorrhage. Most patients do not survive this illness and few who endure are left with permanent deficits. Besides ADEM and AHL, there are certain isolated syndromes, such as optic neuritis, acute cerebellar ataxia (Bickerstaff's encephalitis), and transverse myelitis, that may also follow an infection or vaccination. In contrast to the typical ADEM, prodromal symptoms in these restricted syndromes usually do not occur and the clinical presentation is only limited to the relevant CNS site of injury. Imaging studies confirm CNS involvement relevant to the clinical manifestation and diffusely distributed lesions are not seen, as in ADEM. These restricted syndromes are more frequently seen in adults than in children. It is uncertain whether these isolated syndromes represent a restricted form of ADEM or entirely different forms of inflammatory demyelinating diseases. But, if an antecedent infection is not observed and these syndromes have a relapsing course, then other diseases need to be considered, such as MS, neuromyelitis optica (NMO), and neurologic complication of connective tissue diseases.

2) Diagnostic investigation

MRI is the imaging for evaluating patients for possible ADEM. The initial MRI may be normal if done at the onset of prodromal symptoms. During the progressive course of the disease, T_2 MRI sequences show several lesions scattered throughout the brain involving both the white-matter and gray-matter structures, such as cerebral cortices, thalamus, basal ganglia, brainstem, and cerebellum. In ADEM, contrast-enhancing lesions have been observed in 30%~100% of patients. The pattern of enhancement can be variable, from complete enhancement of smaller lesions to incomplete enhancement of larger lesions, such as ring-shaped, open ring, gyral, and nodular patterns. Rarely, large solitary lesions can be seen in the brain, often resembling neoplasm. In addition to the brain, spinal cord can also be affected in ADEM. Spinal cord lesions are typically large and appear edematous on MRI. Often there is a predilection for the thoracic cord, but lesions can occur at any level. Serial MRI after the initial episode plays a vital role in establishing the diagnosis of ADEM. In monophasic ADEM, MRI can be obtained at least 6 months after the initial episode shows lesion resolution and, more importantly, no evidence of any new lesions. Further specificity for the diagnosis of ADEM can be obtained by continual MRI follow-up over 2~3 years.

(2) Differential diagnosis

ADEM usually presents with subacute encephalopathy, which has a broad differential diagnosis, such as strokes, cerebral autosomal dominant arteriopathy with subcortical infarcts and leukoencephalopathy (CADASIL), multiple sclerosis, neurosarcoidosis, etc. No specific criteria exist for diagnosing ADEM, but the antecedent history, temporal course of the illness, neuroimaging, CSF analysis, and probably repeat imaging during remission are most important in arriving at the diagnosis and excluding other causes of encephalopathy. In the differential diagnosis, conditions to consider and rule out relevant treatment and prognosis are MS and NMO. Tab. 8.3 provides key clinical, radiologic, and laboratory features distinguishing ADEM from MS and NMO. The diagnosis can be further reassured if follow-up MRI after 6 months or more continues to show lesion resolution and absence of new lesions. If there is accrual of additional T_2 lesions over time, then patients need to be evaluated for possible MS.

Tab. 8.3 **Features of major central nervous system demyelinating diseases**

	Character	NMO	MS	ADEM
Demographics	Age of onset (median)	40	30	6.5 (pediatric); 33 (adults)
	Female : Male	8 : 1(relapsing)	2 : 1(relapsing)	1 : 1
	Ethnicity	↑ Incidence in non-white	Usually white	All populations at risk
Clinical course	Monophasic	20%	NA	>95%
	Relapsing	80%	85% initially	<5%
	Primary progressive	NA	15%	NA
MRI features	Brain white-matter lesions	Typically absent at onset	Oval, usually perpendicular to ventricles	Large, disseminated; rarely periventricular
	Spinal cord lesions	Longitudinally extensive	Punctate	Punctate to rarely large longitudinal
	Optic nerve lesions	Unilateral or bilateral, with poor recovery	Usually unilateral, with good recovery	Unilateral or bilateral with good recovery
CSF findings	WBC count	↑↑↑ Lymphocytes, neutrophils	↑ Lymphocytes	↑↑ Lymphocytes, occasionally neutrophils
	Total protein	Elevated	Typically normal	Normal to elevated
	Oligoclonal bands (OCBs)	Typically absent *	>90% present	Variable (0~29%)
Pathology	Gray matter	Demyelination with necrosis	Demyelination	Demyelination (AHL: hemorrhage)
	White matter	Demyelination with necrosis	Demyelination	Demyelination (AHL: hemorrhage)
Lesion immuno-pathology	Macrophages	+++	+++	+++
	T cells	+/-	+++	+++
	Eosinophils	++	None	Rare
	Neutrophils	+++	None	Occasional
	Antibodies	+++	Variable	Variable
	Complement	++	Variable	Variable
	Coexisting autoimmune diseases	30%~50%	Infrequent	Not seen
	Disability progression	Relapse-related	Independent of relapses	Relapse-related in recurrent/multifocal

Note: NMO, neuromyelitis optica; ADEM, acute disseminated encephalomyelitis; WBC, white blood cell; AHL, acute hemorrhagic leukoencephalopathy.

* OCBs may be seen during active disease, but disappear during remission. In ADEM, persistence of OCBs during disease remission raises suspicion for later risk of developing MS.

(3) Treatment

Symptomatic and supportive care involves admission of patients usually to a step-down unit or intensive care unit due to moderate to severe encephalopathy and the presence of cerebral edema. Choice of treatment is high-dose glucocorticoid administered systemically for several days (3~5), followed by an extended oral steroid taper over 6~8 weeks. Recrudescences are fewer when this regimen is employed compared to a short steroid taper, strongly suggesting a benefit from glucocorticoid treatment, as might be expected for a T-cell-mediated process. There are cases of ADEM or even fulminant presentation such as AHL where steroids alone are not sufficient for suppressing inflammation and improving clinical findings. PLEX, intravenous immunoglobulin (IVIG), and immunosuppressive drugs have been used with some success. Plasma exchange or IVIG is usually the second step in recalcitrant cases. PLEX is administered every other day for a total of five sessions, with removal of 1 ~ 1.5 L plasma volume. Maintenance doses at 4-week intervals may be needed for the next 3~4 months. IVIG is given at a dose of 400 mg/(kg · d) for 5 consecutive days. Also, maintenance doses at 4-week intervals may be needed for the next 3~4 months. Of the immunosuppressive agents, cyclophosphamide is more often used in ADEM after steroid failure. Its use is rather reserved, often as a third-line agent after inadequate response from PLEX or IVIG.

(4) Prognosis

The prognosis of ADEM has significantly improved from former times. Full recovery occurs in many patients and improvement with minor residual symptoms is up to 70%~90%. In the case of AHL, the mortality can be as high as 50%. A greater percentage of pediatric patients recover completely from ADEM compared to adults (60%~80% versus 46%), implying greater recovery potential of the developing CNS in children. It is generally agreed that ADEM needs to be promptly treated upon diagnosis because of the beneficial effects of limiting clinical symptoms and possibly preventing recurrences. In addition to the physical disability, long-term cognitive deficits have been reported in ADEM. Patients with onset of ADEM at an older age also had slower verbal processing when assessed after a mean of 2.2 years. Perhaps the neuroanatomic basis for these cognitive deficits is subtle damage in the cortical regions of the brain, an area that is difficult to visualize on routine MRI scans. Non-conventional MRI techniques such as diffusion tensor, magnetization transfer ratio, MR spectroscopy, and high-resolution cortical imaging may be more sensitive in assessing damage in the cortical gray matter than the conventional MRI measures.

8.4 Guillain-Barré Syndrome

Guillain-Barré syndrome (GBS) is an immune-mediated polyradiculoneuropathy that accounts for an estimated 100 000 new cases annually worldwide. Guillain-Barré syndrome has been reported in many countries and has a wide range of reported incidences. There is a 20% increase in incidence for every 10-year increase in age, and unlike other autoimmune diseases, the risk of Guillain-Barré syndrome is higher in men than in women. In comparison to North America and Europe, population-based studies in east Asia report lower incidences of Guillain-Barré syndrome with 0.44 cases per 100 000 person-years in Japan, and 0.67 in China. Seasonal variation of incidence has close association with infections. Studies in western countries suggest a peak in winter, whereas northern China, India, Bangladesh, and Latin America witness a summer peak. In most patients, the acute onset of neurological symptoms is preceded by an infective illness, followed by progressive limb weakness, which can last up to 4 weeks before reaching plateau. Several infections are associated with Guillain-Barré syndrome, but *Campylobacter jejuni* is the most common and extensively reported.

(1) Pathophysiology

Up to the late 1980s, Guillain-Barré syndrome was considered to be a single disease entity with immune-mediated attack on myelin components, resulting in demyelination and secondary axonal damage. It subsequently became clear that GBS could be broadly classified into acute inflammatory demyelinating polyradiculoneuropathy (AIDP), acute motor axonal neuropathy (AMAN)/acute motor-sensory axonal neuropathy (AMSAN) and Miller-Fisher syndrome (MFS), depending on the site of target antigen. This classification, together with the discovery of antiglycolipid antibodies, expanded the understanding of Guillain-Barré syndrome pathogenesis. Deposition of activated complement products can be detected on Schwann cells, suggesting nerve injury that is antibody-mediated. By contrast with AIDP, patients with AMAN show primary axonal injury without substantial T-cell inflammation or demyelination. IgG and activated complement are deposited on nodal and internodal axolemma. Macrophages appear to invade the periaxonal space, and there is nodal lengthening following paranodal myelin detachment, leading to slowing of conduction due to an increase in nodal membrane capacitance. Immunisation of rabbits with GM1 ganglioside can produce disease that resembles AMAN, with circulating anti-GM1 antibodies, motor neuropathy, and pathological findings of IgG deposition on motor axons and periaxonal macrophages.

(2) Clinical feature

1) Clinical manifestation

Most patients with Guillain-Barré syndrome have an antecedent event up to 4 weeks before developing neurological symptoms, mainly upper respiratory tract infections (35%) in Europe, North America, and east and southeast Asia, whereas gastroenteritis (27%) is more common in Bangladesh. Guillain-Barré syndrome is also associated with particular vaccinations and inimmune check point inhibitor therapy. Other less common triggers include ganglioside administration and surgery. GBS is clinically heterogeneous, and the classic presentation of Guillain-Barré syndrome features progressive (ascending) limb weakness associated with reduced or absent reflexes. However, patients can present with localised weakness and these variants include a pharyngeal-cervical-brachial variant and facial diplegia with paraesthesia. Patients can also present with completely different sets of clinical features to classic Guillain-Barré syndrome but can share similar serological biomarkers. These disorders include Miller-Fisher syndrome and Bickerstaff brainstem encephalitis.

2) Diagnostic investigation

① Electrodiagnostic classification

At the early stages of disease, nerve conduction can be normal, but in most patients there is evidence of a neuropathy. Some early studies on nerve conduction changes in Guillain-Barré syndrome include absent Hoffmann reflexes and F waves, and abundant A waves. Guillain-Barré syndrome electrophysiology is a dynamic process, and a single nerve conduction study might not reflect the true underlying pathophysiology. Antibodies against target antigens at these sites lead to myelin detachment, which is reflected on nerve conduction studies as slowing and block of conduction. Serial nerve conduction studies can show reduction in distal compound muscle action potential amplitude with relatively preserved velocities. By contrast, repeated nerve conduction studies of AIDP show progressively slower parameters with prolongation of distal latencies and slower conduction velocities, even in the recovery stages, reflecting the remyelinating process.

② Neuroimaging

Peripheral nerve imaging is an emerging area of disease biomarkers. On nerve ultrasound, cervical root enlargement can be seen in early Guillain-Barré syndrome, especially when weakness is substantial. In differentiating from chronic inflammatory demyelinating polyradiculoneuropathy (CIDP), one study found the application of ultrasound features of sensory sparing pattern, enlarged cervical roots or the vagus nerve had sensitivity, specificity, and positive predictive value of over 85%. Another feature that supports Guillain-Barré syndrome is an improvement in nerve enlargement with clinical recovery.

③ Diagnostic criteria

Both the NINDS and the Brighton criteria continue to be widely used. At minimum, a diagnosis of GBS requires the presence of symmetrical flaccid weakness and decreased reflexes in the absence of alternative causes. The Brighton collaboration criteria (Tab. 8.4) also considers a separate case definition for Miller-Fisher syndrome, which requires the presence of the clinical triad of bilateral ophthalmoplegia, decreased reflexes, and ataxia, together with the absence of limb weakness and CNS involvement to fulfil a Level 3 diagnostic certainty. Reaching higher diagnostic certainties in both GBS and Miller-Fisher syndrome requires the presence of a monophasic illness reaching nadir within 28 days, cerebrospinal fluid albumincytological dissociation, and electrodiagnostic evidence of neuropathy. Cerebrospinal fluid albumincytological dissociation is one of the characteristics of GBS, that is, increased protein level and normal cell number; the CSF protein level is normal at the beginning of the disease, and usually increases at the first weekend. The protein level could still continue to increase after the clinical symptoms are stabilized, and reach the peak at 3~6 weeks after the onset. The CSF protein could be as high as 20 g/L in patients with persistent and unhealed disease. Oligoclonal bands could be detected in CSF and peripheral blood, but they are not identical, suggesting that part of Ig is intrathecal, suggesting that the disease is related to immunity.

Tab. 8.4 Brighton collaboration criteria of GBS (level of diagnostic certainty)

Classic GBS (AIDP/AMAN/AMSAN)	Miller-Fisher syndrome
① Clinical features A. Bilateral and flaccid weakness of limbs; B. Decreased or absent deep tendon reflexes; C. Absence of alternative diagnosis; D. Monophasic course, time between onset to plateau 12 h~28 days ② CSF analysis A. CSF white cell count<50/μL (usually<10); B. CSF protein raised (after 1 week) ③ Nerve conduction studies consistent with conduction slowing and block	① Clinical features A. Bilateral opthalmoparesis; B. Ataxia; C. Absent limb weakness; D. No altered consciousness or corticospinal tract signs ② CSF analysis A. CSF cell count<50/μL (usually<10) B. CSF protein raised (after 1 week) ③ Nerve conduction studies normal or only sensory abnormalities
Level 1 ①+②+③ Level 3 ①	Level 2 ①+②/③ Level 4 only①−D verified

(3) Treatment

The management of patients with Guillain-Barré syndrome can be stratified according to different stages of the disease.

a. In the acute phase, typically within the first 2 weeks of disease onset, patients are at risk of developing complications and extensive nerve damage. In patients with potential respiratory and autonomic failure, admission to a high-dependency unit is advisable for close monitoring of disease progression. Immunotherapy should be initiated as soon as patients show features of disability.

b. Currently, intravenous immunoglobulin and plasma exchange have been shown to be equally effective in improving symptom by accelerating recovery, but do not halt disease progression or alter the extent of nerve damage. Both treatments are associated with few adverse events. Rarely, liver dysfunction and thromboembolic events can occur with intravenous immunoglobulin, whereas plasma exchange should be avoided in patients with autonomic instability because the large shifts in fluids lead to a hypotensive state. Steroids are not effective when used on their own but could be beneficial in combination with intravenous immunoglobulin. In patients with autonomic dysfunction and in children, intravenous immunoglobulin is preferred. A dose of 2 g/kg administered over 5 days has shown efficacy in accelerating recovery. A shorter 2-day course was effective in children, but associated with more frequent treatment-related fluctuations. For plasma exchange, four sessions (50 mL/kg plasma per session) have been shown to be effective, but in most clinical practice, five sessions are chosen.

c. During the progressive phase, patients are at risk of indirect complications including aspiration, pneumonia, and deep vein thrombosis. These complications can be prevented with supportive measures, such as enteral tube feeding, regular respiratory physiotherapy, and deep vein thrombosis prophylaxis. Physiotherapy should commence as early as possible. Symptoms of pain, fatigue, and low mood require appropriate management. Close monitoring should continue as Guillain-Barré syndrome mortality is highest during the recovery phase. The causes of death are typically from respiratory, cardiovascular, or autonomic complications.

References

[1] LASSMANN H. Multiple sclerosis pathology and its reflection by imaging technologies: introduction[J]. Brain Pathology, 2018,28(5):721-722.

[2] KAMIŃSKA J, KOPER O M, PIECHAL K, et al. Multiple sclerosis-etiology and diagnostic potential[J]. Postępy Higieny i Medycyny Do Świadczalnej, 2017,71(0):551-563.

[3] YAMOUT B, SAHRAIAN M, BOHLEGA S, et al. Consensus recommendations for the diagnosis and treatment of multiple sclerosis: 2019 revisions to the MENACTRIMS guidelines[J]. Multiple Sclerosis and Related Disorders, 2020,37:101459.

[4] HUDA S, WHITTAM D, BHOJAK M, et al. Neuromyelitis optica spectrum disorders [J]. Nature Reviews Cancer, 2019,19(2):169-176.

[5] WU Y, ZHONG L M, GENG J. Neuromyelitis optica spectrum disorder: pathogenesis, treatment, and experimental models[J]. Multiple Sclerosis and Related Disorders, 2019, 27(1):412-418.

[6] JARIUS S, PAUL F, WEINSHENKER B G, et al. Neuromyelitis optica[J]. Nature Reviews Disease Primers, 2020,6(1):85.

[7] RAMAKRISHNAN P, NAGARAJAN D. Neuromyelitis optica spectrum disorder: an overview[J]. Acta Neurobiologiae Experimentalis, 2020,80(3):256-272.

[8] JAVED A, KHAN O. Acute disseminated encephalomyelitis[J]. Handbook of

Clinical Neurology, 2014,123:705-717.

[9] GHEUENS S, SMITH D R, WANG X, et al. Simultaneous PML-IRIS after discontinuation of natalizumab in a patient with MS[J]. Neurology, 2012,78(18):1390-1393.

[10] TAN I L, MCARTHUR J C, CLIFFORD D B, et al. Immune reconstitution inflammatory syndrome in natalizumab-associated PML[J].Neurology, 2011,77(11):1061-1067.

(Zhu Ying, Zhang Tingting)

Chapter 9
Neurodegenerative Diseases

Neurodegenerative diseases (NDs) are common and growing causes of mortality and morbidity worldwide, particularly in the elderly, characterized by progressive degeneration of the nervous system. NDs can be broadly classified according to primary clinical features (e.g., dementia, parkinsonism, or motor neuron disease), anatomic distribution of neurodegeneration (e.g., frontotemporal degenerations, extrapyramidal disorders, or spinocerebellar degenerations), or principal molecular abnormality. Although the diagnosis of NDs mainly depends on clinical manifestations, the diagnostic gold standards are neuropathological evaluation at autopsy. Most NDs are characterized by abnormal folding of potentially cytotoxic protein species associated with degeneration and death of specific neuronal populations. Here, we aim to describe the common NDs, focusing on dementia (e.g., Alzheimer's disease, Dementia with Lewy bodies, Frontotemporal lobar degeneration), movement disorders (e.g., Parkinson's disease, Wilson's disease, Huntington's disease, Essential tremor), and motor neuron disease (MND).

9.1 Dementia

Dementia is an acquired, generalized, and usually progressive impairment of cognitive function that affects the content, but not the level, of consciousness. Although its incidence increases with advancing age, dementia is not an invariable accompaniment of aging. The most common feature of dementia is impairment in short-term and long-term memory, with additional impairment in at least one of the following: abstract thinking, impaired judgment, other disturbances of higher cognitive function, or personality change. The disturbance causes disability in usual social occupational, or personal function. Although a wide variety of diseases can produce dementia, it is generally agreed that Alzheimer's disease (AD) is the most common cause. Dementia with Lewy bodies, which is recognized as a distinct entity rather than simply AD and Parkinson's disease (PD), may be second in frequency. Vascular dementia (VD), sometimes referred to as multinfarct dementia, is the next most common. Other causes of dementia, including reversible dementias, are comparatively rare. Additionally, many neurodegenerative dementias develop without producing symptoms for many years, so-called "preclinical" disease. Consequently, many patients move through an early phase of illness that does not meet standard diagnostic criteria for dementia. This intermediate clinical phase is called mild cognitive impairment (MCI), reflecting the presence of significant cognitive decline minus the expected loss of function typical of dementia. Many of the diseases underlying dementia are definitively diagnosed only at autopsy, including AD. Today, diagnosis of dementia, therefore, remains largely clinical. Although there is no good treatment for dementia, it is imperative to recognize and treat dementia as early as possible, with a goal to maximize and preserve quality of life for both patients and caregivers.

9.1.1 Alzheimer's Disease

AD is the most common cause of dementia. It is a disorder of cognitive and behavioral impairment that markedly interferes with social and occupational function. An estimated 40 million people, mostly older than 60 years, have dementia worldwide. Reliable estimates of the prevalence of early-onset dementia and AD (before the age of 65) are scarce. The prevalence of dementia before age 50 is less than 1 per 4 000, with roughly 30% of cases being attributed to AD. The etiology of AD is unclear. About 5% of AD is familial autosomal dominant, which is named early-onset familial AD. Three genes are directly involved in the abnormal production, clearance or aggregation of Aβ peptide, including Alzheimer precursor protein (APP) gene, presenilin (PSEN) 1 gene and PSEN 2 gene. In late-onset familial AD, the risk of being affected and the age at onset are related to the number of apolipoprotein E-4 (ApoE4) alleles on chromosome 19. Epidemiologic studies identify several potential risk factors for AD. The most consistent risk factors include advanced age, family history (especially in first-degree relatives), and ApoE genotype. Other risk factors include hypertension, stroke, and fasting homocysteine levels. Cholinergic neurons are lost and the acetylcholine-synthesizing enzyme choline acetyltransferase is markedly depleted in the cerebral cortex and hippocampus of patients with AD. The disease is defined by characteristic histopathologic features, especially ncurofibillary tangles and neuritic (senile) plaques (Fig. 9.1). Neurofibrillary tangles are intracellular deposits containing hyperphosphorylated tau and ubiquitin, which has a vital role in the maintenance of neuronal cytoskeleton structure and function. Neuritic plaques are extracellular

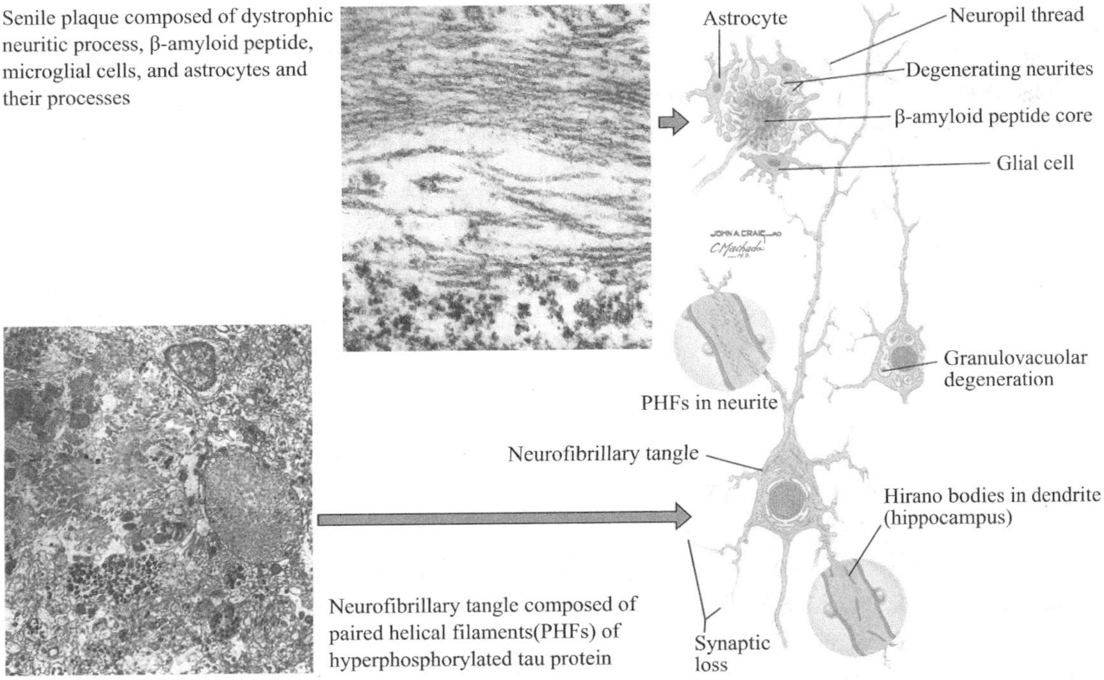

Fig. 9.1 Microscopic pathology in AD

deposits that contain the proteins β-amyloid, PSEN 1, PSEN 2, α_1-antichymotrypsin, apolipoprotein E, α_2-macroglobulin, and ubiquitin. The abnormal accumulation of β-amyloid in AD is responsible for the death of selectively vulnerable neurons.

(1) Clinical feature

1) Clinical manifestation

Commonly, AD begins with short-term memory loss. Often, patients have increasing forgetfulness of words and names, relying more on lists, calendars, and family members for reminders. Family members often notice increasing repetitiveness, patients asking the same question or repeating the same conversation minutes after it was completed. Patients may forget to convey telephone messages or turn off the stove, or lose track of where they place things. Moreover, their ability to recall these incidents is impaired. They "forget that they forget." Affected individuals may become suspicious of others, for example, thinking that misplaced items were stolen. Language function gradually declines. Word-finding and name-finding difficulties are common even in very early stages. Naming impairment and gradual loss of comprehension, expression, or both are universal. The perception of the temporal sequence of events is affected and disorientation eventually becomes pervasive. Geographic orientation declines, first affecting patients' ability to navigate in unfamiliar environments and later within their homes. Visuospatial skills decline and construction deficits may occur early. Behavior and personality in patients with AD are often affected. Psychotic features may become prominent, such as combativeness, irritability, frustration, and anxiety. Some patients also develop delusional thoughts and hallucinations, most commonly visual or auditory in nature. These may be benign, understated, hidden, or frightening and may lead to severe agitation.

As cognitive and behavioral changes appear, the patients' ability to maintain personal independence declines. Altered activities that may occur early include medication mismanagement, financial disorganization, burnt pots on the stove, and driving errors. Eventually patients require assistance with daily activities: personal hygiene/bathing, eating, dressing, and toileting. Often, by this stage, patients exhibit signs of Parkinsonism characterized by midline rigidity, symmetric bradykinesia and hypokinesia, stooped posture, and shuffling stride. The risk of falling increases. Seizures occur in up to 20% of cases. Myoclonic jerks are increasingly noted in advanced stages.

Later stages of AD are characterized by loss of bladder and then bowel control, failure to recognize family members, and eventually severe akinesia, requiring total nursing care. The most common cause of death is aspiration pneumonia. On average, AD has a duration of approximately 8 years. However, this varies substantially. Some patients live 20 years or more. Nursing care marks an important end point for many patients and their caregivers. The most common causes for nursing home placement include behavioral problems, immobility, and incontinence.

2) Diagnostic investigation

① Mental status exam

The mental status examination should assess all major cognitive domains, including memory, attention, language, construction, orientation, and executive function. Standardized global measures of cognitive function such as the MMSE are of limited diagnostic value. The widely used MMSE is relatively insensitive to the milder stages of AD. Other tests, such as the MoCA test, include test items more suited to detecting earlier stages of cognitive impairment allowing improved sensitivity for detecting MCI. Another measure, the Alzheimer's Disease

8 (AD8) is an informant-based tool that may shorten screening considerably. It must be emphasized that such instruments are not diagnostic tests, and interpretation of results must take into consideration level of education, native language, and physical or sensory impairment that might affect performance.

② Blood tests

There is no standard test panel to diagnose AD. Traditionally, levels of Vitamin B_{12}, folate, TSH, and often serum RPR are measured. These tests may reveal a reversible cause of cognitive impairment that may contribute to overall dementia severity.

③ Brain imaging

The CT scan or MRI often shows cortical atrophy and enlarged ventricles (Fig. 9.2), but such changes may also be seen in elderly nondemented patients. Functional imaging, such as FDG-PET and single photon emission computed tomography (SPECT) scans, may also be considered. FDG-PET scanning may be useful in differentiating AD from frontotemporal dementia (FTD) and could be considered in selecting cases as a diagnostic tool (Fig. 9.3).

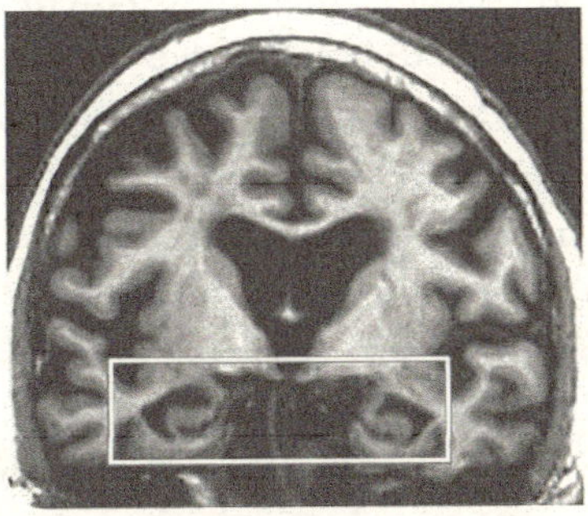

Fig. 9.2 Atrophy of temporal lobe in AD

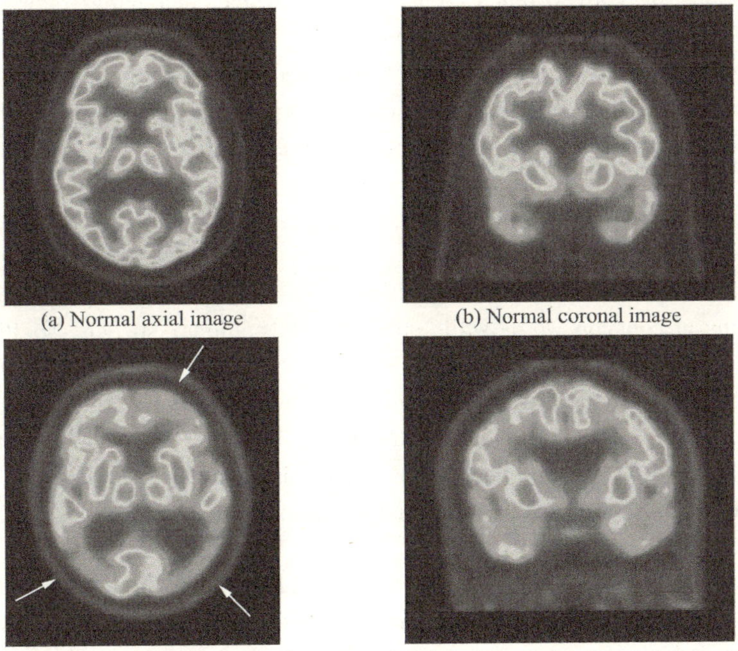

(a) Normal axial image

(b) Normal coronal image

(c) Reduced activity within temporal and parietal lobes (arrows)

(d) Early decreased activity in left frontal lobe consistent with advancing disease

Fig. 9.3 FDG-PET typical pattern for AD

④ CSF tests

Core CSF biomarkers for AD are Aβ42, which shows cortical amyloid deposition; total tau (t-tau), which reflects the intensity of neurodegeneration; and phosphorylated tau (p-tau), which correlates with neurofibrillary pathological changes. These core CSF biomarkers have high diagnostic accuracy, with sensitivity and specificity of 85%~90%, to identify prodromal AD in the mild cognitive impairment stage.

⑤ Genetic tests

APP, PS1, PS2 can be performed in patients with family history. ApoE genotyping is not diagnostic of AD. Moreover, ApoE genotyping should not be used routinely in family members because there is no specific genetic counseling to offer. The presence of an ApoE e4 genotype may only heighten anxiety unnecessarily.

(2) **Diagnosis**

The clinical diagnostic criteria of the National Institute on Aging Alzheimer's Association (NIA-AA, 2011) are listed below.

1) Criteria for all-cause dementia

Dementia is diagnosed when there are cognitive or behavioral (neuropsychiatric) symptoms that interfere with the ability to function at work or at usual activities, and represent a decline from previous levels of functioning and performing; and cannot be explained by delirium or major psychiatric disorder. Cognitive impairment is detected and diagnosed through a combination of history-taking from the patient and a knowledgeable informant and an objective neuropsychological testing. The cognitive or behavioral impairment involves a minimum of two of the following domains.

a. Impaired ability to acquire and remember new information. The symptoms include: repetitive questions or conversations, misplacing personal belongings, forgetting events or appointments, getting lost on a familiar route.

b. Impaired reasoning and handling of complex tasks, poor judgment. The symptoms include: poor understanding of safety risks, inability to manage finances, poor decision-making ability, inability to plan complex or sequential activities.

c. Impaired visuospatial abilities. The symptoms include: inability to recognize faces or common objects or to find objects in direct view despite good acuity, inability to operate simple implements, or orient clothing to the body.

d. Impaired language functions (speaking, reading, writing). The symptoms include: difficulty thinking of common words while speaking, hesitations; speech, spelling, and writing errors.

e. Changes in personality, behavior, or comportment. The symptoms include: uncharacteristic mood fluctuations such as agitation, impaired motivation, initiative, apathy, loss of drive, social withdrawal, decreased interest in previous activities, loss of empathy, compulsive or obsessive behaviors, socially unacceptable behaviors.

2) Probable AD dementia

It meets criteria for dementia described above and the following characteristics. Symptoms have a gradual onset over months to years, not sudden over hours or days. Clear-cut history of worsening of cognition by report or observation. The initial and most prominent cognitive deficits are evident on history and examination, including amnestic presentation and nonamnestic presentations (e.g, language presentation, visuospatial presentation, executive dysfunction). However, the diagnosis of probable AD dementia should not be applied when there is the following evidence: a. substantial concomitant cerebrovascular disease; b. core features of Dementia with Lewy bodies other than dementia itself; c. prominent features of behavioral variant frontotemporal dementia; d. prominent features of semantic variant primary progressive aphasia or nonfluent/agrammatic variant primary progressive aphasia; e. evidence for another concurrent, active neurological disease, or a non-neurological medical comorbidity or use of medication that could have a substantial effect on cognition.

(3) Differential diagnosis

The absence of motor deficits early in AD differentiates it from most other dementias. Other dementias lacking motor signs include amnestic syndrome (Korsakoff encephalopathy), Pick disease, vascular dementia, and HIV dementia complex. Depression can also produce dementia-like symptoms without motor deficits. Poor concentration and short-term memory impairment result from lack of effort, disinterest, or distractibility.

Reversible causes of dementia without motor signs include toxic and metabolic causes of chronic delirium. Chronic use of medication with anticholinergic side effects (e. g., antihistamines and tricyclic antidepressants) is a possible cause of chronic delirium that may mimic AD. β-blockers, digoxin, H_2-blockers, and various antibiotics may also contribute to chronic delirium.

Dementia with motor deficits includes a longer list of possibilities. Thyroid disease, Vitamin B_{12} deficiency, and tertiary neurosyphilis are often considered; however, these conditions rarely cause dementia and usually present with characteristic metabolic or sensorimotor symptoms.

(4) Treatment

The current pharmacologic treatment of AD is purely symptomatic. Long-term benefits of these medications may include a delay in need for nursing home placement. The various agents available include donepezil, rivastigmine, and galantamine. These medications are primarily effective at maximal doses. Rivastigmine is most effective at 4.5 or 6 mg twice a day. Donepezil is only mildly effective at 5 mg/d, but greater benefit occurs with 10 mg/d doses. Similarly, galantamine should always be titrated to 12 mg twice a day to maximize benefit. Galantamine is available in an extended-release formulation to allow for once a day dosing. Typical adverse effects that may cause discontinuation include cholinergic effects, especially vomiting and persistent loose stools. Memantine is an *N*-methyl-D-aspartate (NMDA) receptor antagonist that is approved for patients with moderate to severe AD. Memantine is most effective at 5 or 10 mg twice a day. Furthermore, memantine shows promise when used in combination with cholinesterase inhibitors.

There are currently no therapies approved by Food and Drug Administration for MCI. Much of the management of the patient with AD revolves around family interactions. Caregivers should provide patients with a comforting and respectful living environment. As their cognitive abilities slip away, it is important to provide a setting that preserves patient dignity. AD patients particularly benefit from a structured simple approach to daily life, maintaining a routine of social and physical activities.

(5) Prognosis

In the early days of AD, patients can usually remain at home and continue social activities, and limited professional activities. Patients in advanced stages of the disease may require care in a nursing facility and the use of psychoactive medications. These patients must be protected and prevented from injuring themselves and their families by injudicious actions or decisions. Death from inanition or infection generally occurs 5 ~ 10 years after the first symptoms.

9.1.2 Dementia with Lewy Bodies

Dementia with Lewy bodies (DLB) is probably the second most common cause of dementia. DLB is age-related disease, onset of which is usually after age 65 and is more common in men than in women. Lewy bodies, α-synuclein neuronal inclusions, are the hallmarks of DLB, with neuronal loss. Lewy bodies in Nigro-striatal are related with Parkinson's disease. In autonomic ganglia, Lewy bodies cause postural hypotension, and if in the limbic cortex and neocortex, Lewy bodies produce cognitive dysfunction and psychosis.

(1) Clinical feature

1) Clinical manifestation

DLB is characterized clinically by cognitive decline without prominent early memory impairment. The core clinical features include fluctuating cognitive ability, well-formed visual hallucinations, and signs of Parkinsonism, especially rigidity and bradykinesia.

① Fluctuation

DLB fluctuations are typically delirium-like, occurring as spontaneous alterations in cognition, attention, and arousal. They include waxing and waning episodes of behavioral inconsistency, incoherent speech, variable attention, or altered consciousness that involves staring or zoning out. Direct questioning of an informant about fluctuations may not reliably discriminate DLB from AD, but questions about daytime drowsiness, lethargy, staring into space, or episodes of disorganized speech do.

② Visual hallucinations

Recurrent, complex visual hallucinations occur in up to 80% of patients with DLB and are a frequent clinical signpost to diagnosis. They are typically well-formed, featuring people, children, or animals, sometimes accompanied by related phenomena including passage hallucinations, sense of presence, and visual illusions.

③ Parkinsonism

Spontaneous Parkinsonian features, not due to antidopaminergic medications or stroke, are common in DLB, eventually occurring in over 85%. Parkinsonism in PD is defined as bradykinesia in combination with rest tremor, rigidity, or both. Many DLB patients' Parkinsonism falls short of this, so documentation of only one of these cardinal features is required.

④ REM sleep behavior disorder (RBD)

RBD is now included as a core clinical feature which often begins many years before other symptoms and becomes less vigorous or even quiescent over time, and it should be screened using a scale that allows for patient or bed partner report. Conditions mimicking RBD are common in people with dementia (e.g., awakenings, severe obstructive sleep apnea, and periodic limb movements), all of which must be excluded by careful supplementary questioning to avoid a false-positive diagnosis.

2) Diagnostic investigation

The clinical evaluation for DLB is similar to that for AD. Formal neuropsychological tests can be useful early in the course to differentiate DLB from other dementing illnesses. There are no specific findings on blood or spinal fluid analysis. Brain MRI do not reveal any specific abnormalities. EEG shows nonspecific abnormalities, including focal or diffuse brain wave slowing. PET imaging may be helpful in the future, particularly in highlighting affected dopaminergic systems. The utility of DAT imaging in distinguishing DLB from AD is well-established, with sensitivity (78%) and specificity (90%). PSG demonstration of REM sleep without atonia is desirable whenever feasible, since it is a highly specific predictor of Lewy-related pathology. If the PSG shows REM sleep without atonia in a person with dementia and a history of RBD, there is a ≥90% likelihood of a synucleinopathy, sufficient to justify a probable DLB diagnosis even in the absence of any other core feature or biomarker.

(2) Diagnosis

In 2017, the diagnostic criteria of DLB was revised for the fourth time.

1) Core clinical features

a. Fluctuating cognition with pronounced variations in attention and alertness.

b. Recurrent visual hallucinations that are typically well formed and detailed.

c. REM sleep behavior disorder, which may precede cognitive decline.

d. One or more spontaneous cardinal features of Parkinsonism: these are bradykinesia (defined as slowness of movement and decrement in amplitude or speed), rest tremor, or rigidity.

The first 3 typically occur early and may persist throughout the course.

2) Supportive clinical features

Severe sensitivity to antipsychotic agents: postural instability, repeated falls, syncope or other transient episodes of unresponsiveness; severe autonomic dysfunction, e.g., constipation, orthostatic hypotension, urinary incontinence, hypersomnia, hyposmia, hallucinations in other modalities, systematized delusions, apathy, anxiety, and depression, etc.

(3) Differential diagnosis

1) AD

The cognitive impairment in DLB may be similar to that in AD, although there are some important differences. The memory loss in DLB tends to be less severe than in AD; however, retrieval deficits are more pronounced than encoding deficits. Therefore, patients with DLB have a greater problem retrieving previously learned information and show a greater benefit with cueing than patients with AD. In DLB, visuospatial and construction skills may be impaired earlier than in AD. Patients with DLB may present with geographic disorientation in familiar neighborhoods or even in their own homes while their memory is mildly impaired. Executive function is also impaired significantly earlier in DLB than in AD, manifested as impaired problem solving, inability to complete tasks, and marked disorganization of daily activities. Formal neuropsychological tests help to differentiate AD from DLB, particularly in early disease stages.

2) PD

Motor signs of DLB include all the typical features of PD; however, here the bradykinesia and rigidity are more characteristic, whereas tremor is relatively uncommon. Signs tend to be distributed more symmetrically and axially than they are in PD. Unexplained falls occur early and often in patients with DLB, unlike postural instability in PD, which tends to mark more advanced disease. Response to dopaminergic medications is limited or absent with DLB, although they may exacerbate hallucinations. Parkinsonism is also seen in advanced AD and in frontotemporal dementia. When Parkinsonism occurs within 1 ~ 2 years of dementia, either before or after the onset of cognitive decline, DLB is a prime consideration in the differential diagnosis.

(4) **Treatment**

DLB patients may respond well to anticholinesterase drug. Patients with DLB often exhibit sensitivity to various centrally acting drugs, most prominently to neuroleptic medications, and may become completely incapacitated by severe akinesia, dystonia, or delirium. The incidence of neuroleptic malignant syndrome in DLB is unknown. Good clinical judgment and conservative dosing strategies should be used in every case. The treatment of psychotic features in DLB is one of the most challenging management issues. If at all possible, neuroleptic medication should be avoided.

9.1.3 Frontotemporal Dementia

Frontotemporal dementia (FTD) is the third most common type of dementia in population ≥65, and the second most common type of dementia in population < 65, accounting for approximately 15% ~ 20% of all degenerative dementias. Men and women are equally affected. Up to 40% FTD are familial, four genes for FTD are identified: the microtubule-associated protein tau gene (MAPT) associated with tau aggregates, the progranulin gene (PGRN) associated with transactive response DNA-binding protein-43 (TDP-43) aggregates, the charged multivesicular body protein 2B gene (CHMP2B), and the valosin containing protein gene (VCP). The molecular pathology involves several proteins (tau and TDP-43) distributed in different cortical and subcortical distributions, and corresponds to specific clinical manifestations of various FTD syndromes. The term Pick complex has been suggested to provide a more inclusive diagnostic entity to encompass the pathologic and clinical features of these dementias inclusively. A positive labeling for pathologic tau protein within Pick bodies, astrocytes, and oligodendrocytes is common thread in the pathogenesis of these disorders, termed tauopathies. Associated dementias of the tauopathy group (FTLD-tau), besides Pick disease, include progressive supranuclear palsy (PSP), corticobasal degeneration (CBD), and amyotrophic lateral sclerosis-Parkinsonism dementia complex of Guam (ALS-PDC). Tau is involved in the pathogenesis of AD. However, the mechanism by which tau is affected in AD and Pick disease differs. Other FTD cases demonstrate no significant tau labeling. These forms of FTLD (FTLD-U) occur in the behavioral subtype of FTD (bvFTD), FTD in motor neuron disease (FTD-MND), semantic dementia (SD), and progressive nonfluent aphasia (PNFA).

(1) **Clinical feature**

bvFTD and primary progressive aphasia (PPA) are the two clinical types of FTD. The latter one includes three subtypes, including semantic variant PPA (svPPA), nonfluent/agrammatic variant PPA (nfvPPA) and logopenic variant PPA (lvPPA).

1) Clinical manifestation

a. Patients with bvFTD have focal atrophy of the orbital and mesial frontal lobes and anterior temporal lobes. They have changed personality, such as apathy, social withdraw, and loss of empathy. They lack wills to speak, move and communicate and have delayed response to inquiries. They can hardly maintain attention, switch thought, follow social conventions and inhibit their impulses. Changed eating patterns are common. Impairment of problem solving, judgment, organization and planning occur as disease progresses, but these executive function impairments can also occur early and patients may partially recognize their deficits. Frontal release signs such as snout, grasp and sucking reflexes and incontinence may be observed at early stage.

b. svPPA, also known as semantic dementia (SD), have characteristic bilateral asymmetric atrophy of temporal lobes, usually severer on the left side. svPPA patients have difficulties in retrieving and understanding words and nonverbal information, while their speech remains fluent. Behavioral abnormalities, especially disinhibited outbursts, changed eating pattern, obsessions and compulsions are common. svPPA patients have difficulty in differentiating faces and voices, understanding inner nature and links of things.

c. nfvPPA, also known as progressive nonfluent aphasia (PNFA), have atrophy in left frontal lobe and around lateral fissures. The patients have slow, nonfluent and sometimes telegraphic speech with difficulty in following grammars (agrammatism) and pronouncing words correctly. They can hardly understand complex sentences. Ultimately, the patients become mute. At early stage, patients only have language problems, other problems in cognition occur in several years.

d. lvPPA, also known as logopenic PPA, is the most recently described variant of PPA. Word retrieval and sentence repetition deficits are the core features of lvPPA. Spontaneous speech is characterized by slow rate, with frequent pauses due to significant word-finding problems, but there is no frank agrammatism.

2) Diagnostic investigation

Formal neuropsychological tests are helpful in localizing deficits in cortical function. Brain MRI, important for excluding other mechanisms for frontal lobe syndromes such as tumor or infection, may demonstrate atrophy predominating within frontal and temporal lobes in neurodegenerative disease (Fig. 9.4). Grey matter atrophy and hypometabolism are validated diagnostic biomarkers that are clinically applied at an individual level for the differentiation between FTD, AD and control individuals.

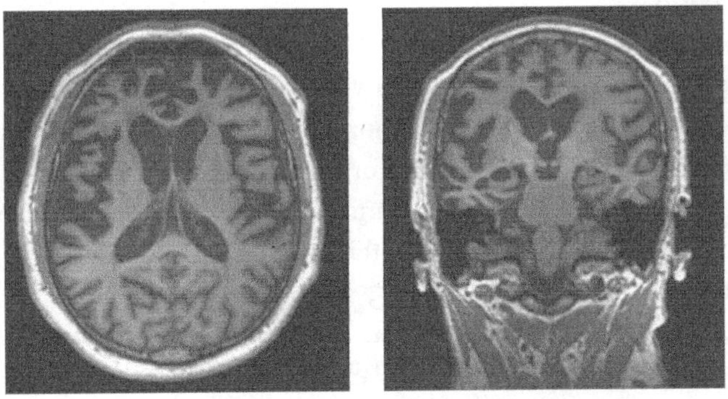

(a) Bilateral frontotemporal lobes (b) Temporal lobe and hippocampus

Fig. 9.4 Symmetrical atrophy in FTD and AD

(2) Diagnosis

There is no unified standard for the diagnosis of FTD. According to the behavior, personality change or progressive language disorder of patients with concealed onset and progressive exacerbation, the diagnosis of FTD can be considered, while the symptoms of memory are relatively not obvious, combined with the special manifestations of limited atrophy of frontotemporal lobe in imaging, excluding other factors that may cause cognitive impairment of frontotemporal lobe.

(3) Treatment

Treatment of FTD is supportive. Caregiver education and reduction of caregiver stress are essential in successful management of agitation and other behavioral problems. When patients become aggressive and combative, distraction and redirection are more effective than verbal instruction in these instances. There is no proven benefit to use cholinesterase inhibitors, commonly used in AD. Limited use of sedatives is recommended to avoid overmedication. Paradoxically, benzodiazepines may exacerbate agitation in some patients. SSRIs may reduce anxiety and restlessness. Other drugs, including mood stabilizers, and atypical anxiolytics (e.g., trazodone, buspirone), sometimes help with problematic behavior when used as monotherapy or in combination.

9.1.4 Vascular Cognitive Impairment

Vascular Cognitive Impairment (VCI) is thought to be the third most common cause of dementia, after AD and DLB. Most patients with this diagnosis have either multiple large cortical infarcts from occlusion of major cerebral arteries or several smaller infarcts (lacunar state) affecting subcortical white matter, basal ganglia, or thalamus. The risk of VCI increases with age just as the risk of stroke increases with age. There is often a prevalence of patients with mixed dementia, including the effects of both vascular and neurodegenerative disorders; this in fact may be much higher than current estimates. In general, diagnostic criteria for VCI lack sufficient sensitivity and specificity to recognize cases of VCI reliably. Many patients may also have other dementia types, like AD, DLB, or normal pressure hydrocephalus. Interestingly, cerebrovascular disease is extremely common and shares several risk factors for AD. These include hypertension, diabetes, and hyperlipidemia. Recent investigations also suggest a link between AD and metabolic syndrome.

(1) Clinical feature

Clinical presentation is arbitrarily divided into large-vessel and small-vessel disease, which are not mutually exclusive clinically. Large-vessel disease tends to affect large vascular territories, producing well-known clinical syndromes. For example, frontal lobe involvement may produce aphasia, apraxia, disinhibition, or apathy. Mesial temporal involvement produces amnesia, angular gyrus lesions lead to constructional apraxia, and parietal lesions produce alexia or apraxia. Small-vessel disease typically eventuates in subcortical infarcts. These are sometimes localized within strategic locations, such as the thalamus or basal ganglia, and involve white matter tracts such as frontosubcortical and thalamocortical tracts. The clinical correlates of small-vessel disease may include executive dysfunction, apathy, inattentiveness, and personality changes typical of frontal lobe syndromes as occur with hydrocephalus and frontotemporal dementia.

There is no specific characteristic appearance on imaging studies that provide a diagnosis of VCI per se. The absence of specific cerebrovascular lesions of course mitigates this diagnosis. MRI is more sensitive than CT in showing subcortical and periventricular white matter changes consistent with small-vessel disease, and smaller infarcts. Therefore, a VCI diagnosis requires recognition of various syndromic features to correlate with findings on imaging studies.

(2) Diagnosis

In order to differentiate from AD, the diagnostic criteria of probable VaD are listed in AHA/ASA: cognitive impairment and imaging evidence of cerebrovascular disease; a clear temporal relationship between a vascular event (e.g., clinical stroke) and onset of cognitive deficits; a clear relationship in the severity and pattern of cognitive impairment and the presence of diffuse, subcortical cerebrovascular disease pathology (e.g., as in CADASIL); no history of gradually progressive cognitive deficits before or after the stroke that suggests the presence of a nonvascular neurodegenerative disorder.

(3) Treatment

Primary prevention must be pursued aggressively. When at-risk patients are identified, treatment of arterial hypertension, cardiac disease, lipid abnormality, and diabetes are important in reducing dementia risk. Secondary prevention, that is, treatment when cerebrovascular disease is initially recognized, begins with appropriate acute management of stroke and its complications. Prevention of stroke recurrence by appropriate antiplatelet or anticoagulant therapy and addressing primary risk factors are also very important. Use of calcium channel blockers in the treatment of hypertension may be more effective in dementia prevention than other antihypertensive medications. Dietary supplementation with folic acid and Vitamins B_6 and B_{12} may help to reduce the levels of homocysteine, a possible contributory precursor to VCI. The role of "neuroprotective agents" in prevention of poststroke dementia is unknown.

9.2 Movement Disorders

Movement disorders (sometimes called extrapyramidal disorders) impair the regulation of voluntary motor activity without directly affecting strength, sensation, or cerebellar function. They include hyperkinetic disorders associated with abnormal, involuntary movements and hypokinetic disorders characterized by poverty of movement. Movement disorders result from dysfunction of deep subcortical gray matter structures termed basal ganglia.

9.2.1 Parkinson's Disease

Parkinson's disease (PD) is one of the most common neurologic disorders worldwide. It affects at least 1 500 000 persons within the United States. Its incidence typically peaks in the sixth decade; however, one can see classic clinical cases with onset as early as the fourth decade. In contrast, PD sometimes presents well into the late eighth or even the ninth decade. Usually the patient's clinical status progresses from a relatively modest limitation at diagnosis to an ever-increasing disability over 10 to 20 years in many but not all patients. Gender is an established risk factor, with the male-to-female ratio being approximately 3 : 2. Ethnicity is also a risk factor for the disease. Age is the greatest risk factor for the development of PD. The prevalence and incidence increase nearly exponentially with age and peak after 80 years of age. This trend has important public health implications; with an aging population and rising life expectancy worldwide, the number of people with PD is expected to increase by more than 50% by 2030. Other risk factors for PD includes environmental exposures. The factors that increase risk are pesticide exposure, prior head injury, rural living, β-blocker use, agricultural occupation, and well-water drinking. Environmental factors found to be associated with a decreased risk are tobacco smoking, coffee drinking, non-steroidal anti-inflammatory drug use, calcium channel blocker use, and alcohol consumption. The contribution of genetics to PD is suggested by the increased risk of disease associated with a family history of PD or tremor. PARK1 (SNCA), which encodes the protein α-synuclein, is the first gene to be associated with inherited PD. Mutations in LRRK2 and parkin are the most common causes of dominantly and recessively inherited PD, respectively.

(1) Pathology and pathogenesis

The characteristic pathological feature of PD is the loss of the pigmented dopaminergic cells of the zona compacta of the substantia nigra (Fig. 9.5). In some of the remaining neurons, there are eosinophilic cytoplasmic inclusions called Lewy bodies which are made up of α-synuclein (Fig. 9.6). Overexpression of α-synuclein in animal models leads to dose-dependent neurodegeneration, with dopaminergic cells in the substantia nigra being particularly susceptible. Lewy bodies are proteinaceous cytoplasmic inclusions specifically found in the brains of PD patients, however, even today, the exact role of Lewy bodies is still unknown. The confirmation that triplication of the alpha-synuclein gene (PARK4) and the subsequent elevated protein levels (in the CSF) could cause PD has greatly strengthened the hypothesis that accumulation of protein is a fundamental event in the pathogenesis of PD. Both dopamine and acetylcholine are present in the corpus striatum, where they act as neurotransmitters. In PD patients, it is generally believed that the normal balance between these two antagonistic neurotransmitters is disturbed because of dopamine depletion in the dopaminergic nigrostriatal system. Disorder of the balance of inhibition and excitation within the basal ganglia and its connections via direct and indirect pathways has been proposed to explain the impaired motor function in PD.

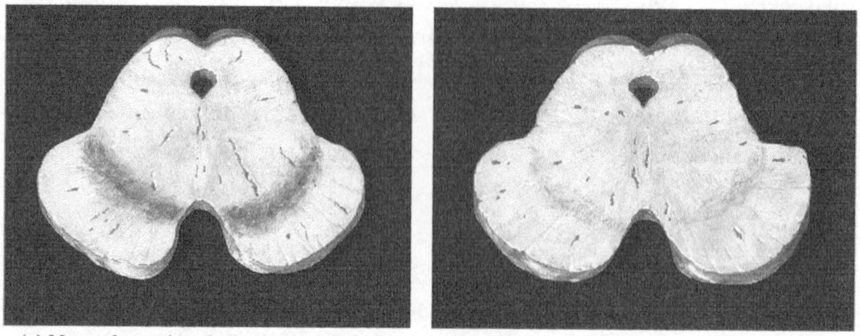

(a) Normal: section through cerebral peduncles and substantianigra

(b) PD: substantia nigra depigmented

Fig. 9.5 Neuropathology of PD

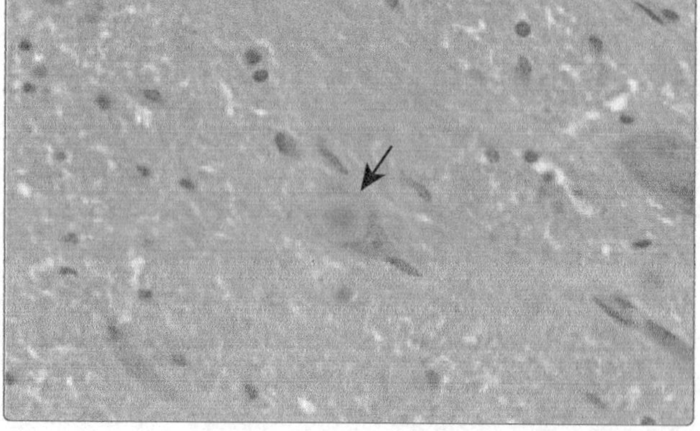

Fig. 9.6 Lewy bodies (head) in substantia nigra

(2) Clinical feature

1) Clinical manifestation

① Motor signs

There are four primary motor signs including tremor, rigidity, bradykinesia, and gait disturbance.

a. Tremor. The 4~6 Hz and pill rolling tremor of PD is characterisically most conspicuous at rest, it increases at times of emotional stress and often improves during voluntary activity.

b. Rigidity. Rigidity is a characteristic clinical feature of PD. The disturbance in tone is responsible for the flexed posture of many patients with PD. There is an initial marked resistance to passive movement and then a sudden release, for example, clasp-knife phenomena. The classic cogwheel rigidity is from a tremor superimposed on the altered muscle tone.

c. Bradykinesia. Bradykinesia is the most disabling PD symptom, which manifests a slowness of voluntary movement and a reduction in automatic movement, such as swinging the arms while walking. The patient's face is relatively immobile (masklike face), with widened palpebral fissures, infrequent blinking, a certain fixity of facial expression, and a smile that develops and fades slowly. The voice is of low volume and tends to be poorly modulated. Fine or rapidly alternating movements are impaired, but power is not diminished if time is allowed for it to develop. The handwriting is small, tremulous, and hard to read.

d. Gait disturbance. The patient generally finds it difficult to get up from bed or an chair and tends to adopt a flexed posture on standing. It is often difficult to start walking, so that the patient may lean farther and farther forward while walking before being able to advance. The gait itself is characterized by small, shuffling steps and absence of the arm swing that normally accompanies locomotion; there is generally some unsteadiness on turning, and there may be difficulty in stopping. In advanced cases, the patient tends to walk with increasing speed to prevent a fall (festinating gait) because of the altered center of gravity that results from the abnormal posture.

② Non-motor symptoms

Autonomic dysfunction is seen commonly in PD. It is manifested as orthostatic hypotension, impaired gastrointestinal motility, urinary bladder dysfunction, disorders in thermoregulation, and sexual dysfunction. Hyposmia is also common symptoms. PD patients may experience difficulties with sleep initiation and maintenance. This sleep disturbance can occur to the presence of an early morning dystonia or tremor, restless legs syndrome, or rapid eye movement (REM) behavior disorder. Psychiatric and cognitive symptomatology also frequently accompany or even precede the diagnosis of PD in some patients. Later on in PD, hallucinations, psychosis, and vivid nocturnal dreams are common.

2) Diagnostic investigation

There are no specific diagnostic investigations for PD, which is a clinical diagnosis. Examination is aimed at eliminating alternative diagnoses, for example, CT or MRI scanning is used to look for normal pressure hydrocephalus or small vessel disease. Candidate imaging markers include positron emission tomography (PET) or single photon emission computed tomography (SPECT) methods to measure reduction in SNpc dopaminergic nerve terminals projecting to the striatum. For people whose family members have known monogenic forms of PD, genetic testing can assist in diagnosis.

(3) Diagnosis

Having established that the patient has Parkinsonism, the MDS-PD criteria (Tab. 9.1) will be applied to determine whether the patient meets criteria for PD as the cause of this Parkinsonism.

Diagnosis of clinically established PD requires: a. Absence of absolute exclusion criteria. b. At least two supportive criteria. c. No red flags.

Diagnosis of clinically probable PD can be made in: a. Absence of absolute exclusion criteria. b. Presence of red flags counterbalanced by supportive criteria. If there are more than two red flags, clinically probable PD cannot be diagnosed.

Tab. 9.1 Diagnosis criteria for MDS-PD

<table>
<tr><th colspan="2">Supportive criteria</th></tr>
<tr><td colspan="2">1. Clear and dramatic beneficial response to dopaminergic therapy. To meet this criterion, during initial treatment, patients should have returned to normal or near-normal level of function. In the absence of clear documentation of initial response, a dramatic response also can be classified as: A. Marked improvement with dose increases or marked worsening with dose decreases; B. Unequivocal and marked on/off fluctuations, which must have at some point included predictable end-of-dose wearing off.
2. Presence of levodopa-induced dyskinesia.
3. Rest tremor of a limb, documented on clinical examination. Positive results from at least one ancillary diagnostic test. Currently available tests that meet this criterion include olfactory loss and Metaiodobenzylguanidine scintigraphy clearly documenting cardiac sympathetic denervation</td></tr>
<tr><th colspan="2">Absolute exclusion criteria</th></tr>
<tr><td>1. Unequivocal cerebellar abnormalities on examination, such as cerebellar gait, limb ataxia, or cerebellar oculomotor abnormalities;
2. Downward vertical supranuclear gaze palsy, or selective slowing of downward vertical saccades;
3. Diagnosis of probable behavioral variant frontotemporal dementia or primary progressive aphasia within the first 5 years of disease;
4. Parkinsonian features restricted to the lower limbs for more than 3 years;
5. Treatment with a dopamine-depleting agent in consistent with drug-induced Parkinsonism;</td><td>6. Absence of observable response to high-dose levodopa despite at least moderate severity of disease;
7. Unequivocal cortical sensory loss (i. e., graphesthesia, stereognosis with intact primary sensory modalities), clear limb ideomotor apraxia, or progressive aphasia;
8. Normal functional neuroimaging of the presynaptic dopaminergic system;
9. Expert evaluating physician, based on the full diagnostic assessment, believes that an alternative syndrome is more likely than PD</td></tr>
<tr><th colspan="2">Red flag</th></tr>
<tr><td>1. Rapid progression of gait impairment requiring regular use of wheelchair within 5 years of onset;
2. A complete absence of progression of motor symptoms or signs over 5 years unless stability is related to treatment;
3. Early bulbar dysfunction, defined as one of severe dysphonia, dysarthria, or severe dysphagia within the first 5 years of disease;
4. Inspiratory respiratory dysfunction defined as either diurnal or nocturnal inspiratory stridor or frequent inspiratory sighs;</td><td>5. Severe autonomic failure in the first 5 years of disease. This can include orthostatic hypotension and severe urinary incontinence/urinary retention in the first 5 years of disease;
6. Recurrent (> 1/year) falls because of impaired balance within 3 years of onset;
7. The presence of disproportionate anterocollis or contractures of hand or feet within the first 10 years;
8. Absence of any of the common nonmotor features of disease despite 5 years disease duration of 5 years</td></tr>
</table>

(4) Differential diagnosis

1) Secondary causes of Parkinsonism

These causes include medications, stroke, head injury, hydrocephalus, encephalitis, depression and brain tumor. Dopamine receptor-blocking agents used in psychiatry and for gastrointestinal symptoms are the most common drugs causing Parkinsonism.

2) Atypical Parkinsonism

The most common syndromes are as follows. a. Diffuse Lewy body disease (DLB): DLB occurs especially in patients aged between 60 and 80 and is marked clinically by the combination of a rapidly progressing neurobehavioral syndrome of dementia and hallucinations and extrapyramidal motor features characteristic of PD. Myoclonus may also be seen. There is only an incomplete response to levodopa, but patients are extremely sensitive to Parkinsonian complications of neuroleptics as well as to the side effects of antiparkinsonian drugs. b. Multiple-system atrophy (MSA): MSA is a degenerative disorder characterized by Parkinsonian features, autonomic insufficiency and signs of more widespread neurologic involvement. Antiparkinsonian drugs are typically ineffective. c. Progressive supranuclear palsy (PSP): PSP is a disorder in which there may be bradykinesia and rigidity, but its characteristic features are early postural instability and fall, loss of voluntary control of eye movements (especially vertical gaze), frontotemporal dementia, pseudobulbar palsy, dysarthria, and axial dystonia. The disorder responds poorly, if at all, to antiparkinsonian drugs.

(5) Treatment

PD treatment remains symptomatic, there is no neuroprotective therapy available to prevent ongoing evolution of this neurodegenerative disorder. Treatment can be divided into nonpharmacologic therapy, pharmacologic therapy, and surgical treatment.

1) Nonpharmacologic therapy

Physical therapy and speech therapy are beneficial to many patients with PD, and the quality of life can often be improved by providing simple aids to daily living. Such aids may include extra rails or banisters placed strategically for additional support, table cutlery with large handles, nonslip rubber table mats, devices to amplify the voice, and chairs that will gently eject the occupant at the push of a button.

2) Pharmacologic therapy

Pharmacologic therapy for PD consists of five types of medication. There is no simple approach to treating PD, guidelines depend on functional impairment and response to therapy.

a. Levodopa: Levodopa with carbidopa is used most commonly, and it is the most potent antiparkinsonian medication which is equally beneficial for all symptoms. Levodopa is the immediate natural precursor of dopamine and is converted to dopamine by enzyme aromatic amino acid decarboxylase. Carbidopa-levodopa is available in immediate-release form as tablets (Sinemet) and controlled-release formulations (Sinemet CR). Early side effects, including nausea and orthostatic hypotension, are more easily managed than the late motor complications. Late side effects include involuntary movements, motor fluctuations, vivid dreams, nightmares, confusion, psychosis and typically hallucinations. With increasing duration of usage, there is a slower or delayed response to levodopa's therapeutic effect. Levodopa also appears to have a shorter duration of action, a "wearing off" between doses. The patient's classic PD symptoms that have disappeared early in the course of treatment become prominent once again. Two of the most disabling long-term levodopa therapeutic side effects are the appearance of a variety of dyskinesias and motor fluctuations developing in a modest number of PD individuals. The treatment of these complications is most difficult.

b. Dopaminergic agonists (DAs): DAs directly stimulate dopaminergic receptors. They are particularly indicated for monotherapy in younger patients, who are more prone to the early development of levodopa-related clinical fluctuations and require long-term treatment. DAs are used mainly early in the illness because they reduce the need for levodopa. Commonly utilized preparations include pramipexole, ropinirole. Impulse control disorders or dysfunctional behaviors are problems that are increasingly recognized with dopaminergic agonists but that occur much less commonly with levodopa.

c. Anticholinergic: Anticholinergics are most effective for tremor, but these medications must be used with significant caution in the elderly because of their innate side effects. They are usually used as monotherapy or an adjunct to dopaminergic therapy, and the most commonly used anticholinergic agents include benztropine, procyclidine, and trihexyphenidyl. Side effects, resulting from both peripheral and central cholinergic blockade, include dry mouth, narrow-angle glaucoma, constipation, urinary retention, memory impairment, and confusion with hallucinations.

d. COMT inhibitors: Inhibition of the enzyme catechol-*O*-methyltransferase (COMT) blocks dopamine metabolism. COMT inhibitors prolong levodopa's benefits by extending the life span of the dopamine to which it is converted. There are two major COMT inhibitors. Entacapone is generally used adjunctively to levodopa.

e. Monoamine oxidase B inhibitors (MAO-B): Selegiline is a selective inhibitor of monoamine oxidase B. Its primary mechanism of action is blockade of central dopamine metabolism. It may improve response to levodopa, especially in patients with mild dose-related fluctuations. Selegiline has been studied as a neuroprotective agent because it can block free radical formation from the oxidative metabolism of dopamine. Rasagiline is a newer MAO-B inhibitor which is as available as Azilect. It received Food and Drug Administration approval for the treatment of signs and symptoms of PD as initial monotherapy and as adjunct therapy to levodopa. As monotherapy, it may reduce parkinsonian disability. As adjunctive therapy, it may reduce over time and increase dyskinesia-free on time. Side effects include insomnia, hallucinations, and orthostatic hypotension.

f. Amantadine: Amantadine has a mild beneficial effect on tremor, bradykinesia, and rigidity. Its mechanism of action, thought to include blocking an *N*-methyl-D-aspartate receptor, is controversial. It is the only antiparkinsonian medication that can decrease the severity of levodopa-induced dyskinesias. Common side effects include livedo reticularis and lower extremity edema.

3) Surgical treatment

Deep brain stimulation (DBS) is a well established treatment for the motor symptoms of PD. Thalamic deep brain stimulation is also an option for treatment of tremor. Surgical treatment is an option when the parkinsonian motor features continue to respond to levodopa but motor fluctuations and dyskinesia become disabling. Specific non-motor features, including non-motor fluctuations, sleep-related symptoms, and behavioural abnormalities, can improve with deep brain stimulation, although further study is needed to establish the contributions of the stimulation versus the effect of improvement in motor function and reduction in dopaminergic drugs that accompany deep brain stimulation.

4) Non motor symptoms treatments

Hallucinations can occur, both from drug therapy or an underlying cognitive disturbance. An alteration in dopaminergic therapy or a small dose of quetiapine may help. Anticholinesterase inhibitors (such as rivastigmine) may also help but their use is currently controversial. A significant number of patients with PD are depressed and may benefit from antidepressants.

(6) Prognosis

After 5 years, 75% of patients will develop a complication of treatment by a reduction in responsiveness to levodopa and a narrowing of the therapeutic window. These complications include motor fluctuations (wearing off and on-off phenomenon) and dyskinesias (abnormal involuntary movements). As the therapeutic window narrows, patients notice a more dramatic change in their symptoms when the drug levels are above or below a critical threshold. Initially this occurs at the end of the dose when the drug effect wears off. This can be helped by increasing the frequency of doses, adding selegiline or a COMT inhibitor, adding a dopamine agonist or using a controlled-release form of levodopa. In some patients, the transitions seem to be more marked and random and the patient can swing violently from the rigid immobile "off" state to an "on" state where the patient has severe dyskinesias without any period of useful mobility. This is the "on-off effect" which is difficult to treat, but may be improved by using strategies to smooth levodopa levels (e.g., by adding a dopamine agonist that has a longer halflife or by using apomorphine given subcutaneously by pump). Most patients can continue to work in the early stage, but gradually lose the ability to work after a few years. To the late stage of the disease, due to systemic stiffness, leading to bedridden, PD patients often died of pneumonia and other complications.

9.2.2 Atypical Parkinsonian Syndromes

Atypical parkinsonian syndromes previously called Parkinson-plus syndromes, are chronic, progressive neurodegenerative disorders, characterized by rapidly evolving parkinsonism in association with other signs of neurologic dysfunction beyond the spectrum of idiopathic PD. These include early postural instability, supranuclear gaze palsy, early autonomic failure, and pyramidal, cerebellar, or cortical signs. The most common disorders are progressive supranuclear palsy (PSP), corticobasal degeneration (CBD), and multiple-system atrophy (MSA). Unlike idiopathic PD, these uncommon syndromes have poor or transient responses to dopaminergic therapy and consequently a worse prognosis. These disorders are classified as tauopathies and synucleinopathies based on the accumulation of the abnormal protein tau or α-synuclein within neurons and glial cells having various anatomic distribution within certain brain areas. There are no effective therapies for these syndromes.

9.2.2.1 Progressive Supranuclear Palsy (PSP)

PSP is a sporadic tauopathy that has a progressive clinical course characterized by parkinsonism with supranuclear gaze palsy, early postural instability, falls, bradykinesia, and dysarthria. Its etiology is unknown. It is primarily a subcortical neurodegenerative tauopathy. Macroscopically, depigmentation is observable within the substantia nigra (SN) and locus coeruleus (LC), as well as atrophy of the pons, midbrain, and globus pallidum. Microscopically, the most affected regions are brainstem nuclei Ⅲ, Ⅳ, Ⅸ, and Ⅹ, the red nucleus, LC, SN, globus pallidus, and cerebellar dentate nucleus. Tau protein accumulates within neurons as neurofibrillary tangle (NFT) and in glia as spherical neuropil threads.

(1) Clinical feature

1) Clinical manifestation

PSP typically occurs between the sixth and seventh decades. Patients usually present with gait instability and tendency to unexpectedly fall backwards; in contrast, neither of these symptoms occurs early on in PD. The parkinsonism of PSP is typically axial and symmetric, unlike the asymmetric often single limb presentation of PD. Most patients with PSP carry an erect posture in contrast to the flexed PD stance. Often they lack the typical PD tremor. Dystonia is a common finding particularly early on affecting limbs, neck dystonia, or even as blepharospasm. The hallmark of PSP is the classic and characteristic finding of limited vertical eye movements; eventually a horizontal supranuclear gaze palsy may also become evident. In this clinical setting, the patient usually does not recognize the loss of eye movement per se but rather perceives these limitations as blurry vision particularly manifested by difficulties with routine activities, such as reading or walking down the stairs. Dysarthria and dysphagia are also commonly experienced early in the disease course. Cognitive dysfunction is a later development for most PSP patients.

2) Diagnostic investigation

The most important diagnostic clues are the results of a careful clinical evaluation and a poor response to dopaminergic therapy. CT and MRI often demonstrate generalized or brainstem (dorsal midbrain) atrophy. The combination of atrophy of the midbrain tegmentum with relative sparing of the basis pontis resembles "a lateral view of a standing penguin (especially, the king penguin), with a small head and big body" on a midsagittal MRI scan (Fig. 9.7). Sagittal T_1-weighted MRI shows atrophy of the midbrain, with preservation of the volume of the pons. There is also atrophy of the tectum, particularly the superior colluculi. This appearance is called the "penguin sign". Previously, appearance of the midbrain tegmentum was stated to resemble the head of a hummingbird. Whether the penguin or hummingbird sign will take flight remains to be seen, but the implication of both studies is the same: the midbrain in PSP is atrophic and MRI can be helpful to verify the clinical diagnosis. There are no more specific diagnostic studies available. Metabolic PET studies have demonstrated global reduction in cerebral metabolism; ^{18}F-fluorodopa PET uptake studies revealed reduced caudate and putamen uptake. SPECT revealed bifrontal hypometabolism.

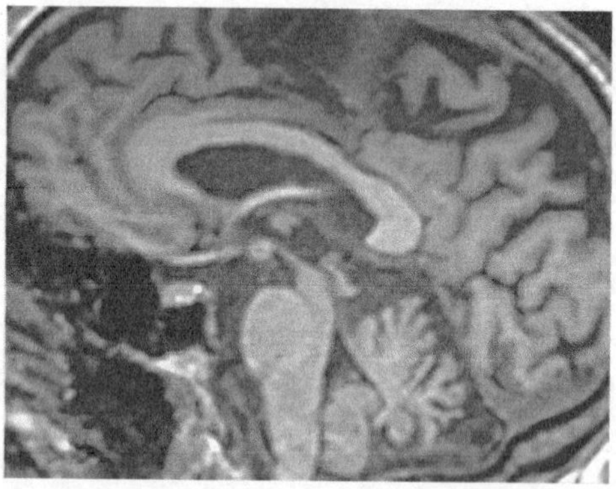

Fig. 9.7 MRI in PSP

(2) Treatment and prognosis

There are no effective specific therapies available for the PSP patient. Although some of these individuals with slowness, stiffness, and balance problems initially may respond to antiparkinsonian therapies, such as levodopa, or levodopa combined with anticholinergic agents, this effect is usually limited and at best a temporary one. Visual limitations, dysarthria, and dysphagia are usually unresponsive to any pharmacologic intervention. Antidepressant drugs have had modest success in PSP; fluoxetine, amitriptyline, and imipramine are the most commonly used, although their benefit seems to be unrelated to their ability to relieve depression. Botulinum toxin injections are used when blepharospasm is an issue. Physical and occupational therapy are the most important patient management aspects. PSP has an inexorably progressive course. The average PSP patient has a survival of 5~6 years from symptom onset to death. Head injury and fractures from falls are common. Because of dysphagia, PSP patients are predisposed to other serious complications such as choking and pneumonia, which are the most common causes of death.

9.2.2.2 Corticobasal Degeneration (CBD)

CBD is a rare sporadic neurodegenerative tauopathy. It occurs mainly after age 60 and shows no population clusters; its incidence, prevalence, and etiology are unknown. The patient's clinical presentation correlates well with the later finding of an asymmetric cortical atrophy contralateral to the involved limb. The frontoparietal cortex is the most involved with most prominent changes of cortical atrophy demonstrated within the perirolandic area. A reduction in amount of cerebral white matter is also apparent in the cerebral peduncles and corpus callosum. Additionally, neuronal loss is present within the SN and LC. Typical microscopic features include neuronal loss (cortex, subcortical regions, SN), astrocytic gliosis, ballooned (achromatic) neurons, NFT, and tau-positive glial inclusions. The microscopic hallmarks of CBD are the ballooned, swollen, or achromatic neurons lacking Nissl substance.

(1) Clinical feature and diagnosis

An asymmetric akinetic-rigid parkinsonism, primarily affecting the arm and hand, is often the major feature. Patients usually present with limb clumsiness, awkward, slow voluntary movements of one arm, with dystonic posturing and tremor. Cortical signs include apraxia, cortical sensory disturbance, and finger myoclonus. The alien limb phenomenon, a failure to recognize ownership of a limb without visual cues, is also a common clinically appreciable sign. Gradually a gait disorder develops, characterized by limb rigidity and impaired position sense. Dementia usually develops late in the course of CBD; however, relatively early on, a declining cognitive function is sometimes a predominant feature. Less commonly, there is an overlap with some similar atypical parkinsonism syndromes. Slowed speech production, dysarthria, swallowing difficulties, and cognitive deficits occur later in this disease. Imaging studies are not diagnostic. MRI and CT can show asymmetric cortical atrophy in the frontoparietal region, maximal on the side contralateral to the involved limb (Fig. 9.8). MRI shows left enlarged lateral ventricle and thin white matter. The asymmetrically reduced pattern in frontoparietal cerebral cortical metabolism, CBF, or both, coupled with bilateral reduction of fluorodopa uptake in the caudate and putamen on PET scanning, provides strong evidence for CBD.

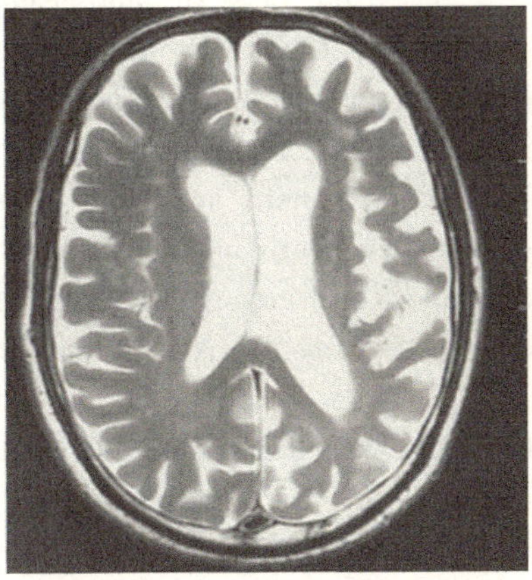

Fig. 9.8 Asymmetric cortical atrophy in MRI

CBD is relatively easy to diagnose because of its stereotypic clinical presentation, particularly the alien hand phenomenon. Some conditions clinically mimic CBD, including PSP, Pick's disease, Alzheimer's disease, some vascular lesions, and rarely adult-onset leukodystrophies. Neuropathologic evaluation is necessary to confirm the diagnosis.

(2) Treatment

There is no definitive treatment. Dopaminergic therapy is of limited benefit, clonazepam can be used for finger myoclonus, and botulinum toxin improves dystonia. Occupational, physical, and speech therapy may also help. There is a significant average survival of usually 5~6 years from symptom onset to death.

9.2.2.3 Multiple-System Atrophy (MSA)

MSA, once called Shy-Drager syndrome, is a sporadic, degenerative CNS disease classified as a synucleinopathy. It presents with a combination of extrapyramidal, pyramidal, cerebellar, and autonomic symptoms and signs. The typical age of onset ranges from late 50s to early 60s, and occasionally between the age of 30 and 40 (i. e. young-onset), and approximately 55% of MSA cases occur in men. MSA is generally considered a sporadic disease. Nevertheless, MSA pedigrees with both autosomal dominant and autosomal recessive inheritance pattern have been reported in Europe and Asia. A loss-of-function mutation in the COQ2 gene, coding for the coenzyme Q10 synthesizing enzyme, was reported in Japanese familial and sporadic MSA cases and is to date the only identified cause of monogenic MSA. Macroscopically, neuronal loss and gliosis are primarily seen in many subcortical areas, such as the SN, LC, putamen, globus pallidus, inferior olive nucleus, pons, cerebellar cortex, autonomic nuclei of the brainstem, and intermediolateral columns of the spinal cord. Glial cytoplasmic inclusions (GCIs) are major microscopic findings that are characteristic of, but not specific for, MSA. These GCIs represent the accumulation of the protein alpha-synuclein within previously normal oligodendrocytes. These inclusions are distributed selectively within the basal ganglia, motor cortex, reticular formation, middle cerebellar peduncle, and the cerebellar white matter.

(1) Clinical feature

1) Clinical manifestation

Based on the signs and symptoms, MSA is classified into two types: Parkinsonian type (MSA-P), the signs and symptoms of which include rigidity, bradykinesia, tremors and impaired posture and balance. Cerebellar type (MSA-C), the signs and symptoms of which include ataxia, unsteady gait and loss of balance, dysarthria, visual disturbances, dysphagia. In addition, there are other general signs and symptoms, including postural hypotension, constipation, urinary retention, incontinence, reduced production in perspiration, sleep disorders, and impotence. The distinction into MSA-P and MSA-C is based on the predominant clinical features. MSA-P is more common in most countries, with an exception of Japan where MSA-C is the predominant phenotype. While approximately half of the patients with MSA-P develop cerebellar signs, even a higher proportion of patients with MSA-C have parkinsonian features. Some authors refer to the combined motor phenotype as "mixed" MSA or MSA P+C. However, these terms are not officially accepted, because it is difficult to delineate the degree of parkinsonian and cerebellar affection in mixed clinical presentations, which include motor and autonomic dysfunction.

a. Motor dysfunction: Ataxia of gait, trunk and limbs, intention tremor and cerebellar oculomotor abnormalities, such as sustained spontaneous or gaze-evoked nystagmus are common in MSA. Parkinsonism is rapidly progressive, poorly responsive to L-dopa and often associated with one or more atypical features. Rapid progression to the wheelchair confinement within 5 years from symptom onset (termed also "wheelchair sign") is present in more than a half of MSA patients. Unilateral symptoms of parkinsonism occur in 40% of MSA patients and a similar proportion of patients retain such asymmetry over the disease course. Early postural instability and gait difficulties coupled with falls are suggestive of atypical parkinsonism rather than PD. Latency to onset of recurrent falls in MSA is significantly shorter compared to PD and longer compared to PSP.

b. Autonomic failure: Early onset, generalized and rapidly progressive autonomic failure is typical of MSA. Rates of autonomic failure of up to 60% are reported at the disease onset. Erectile dysfunction is often the earliest symptom, followed by lower urinary tract symptoms and symptoms of cardiovascular autonomic failure. Isolated autonomic failure in the absence of parkinsonian or cerebellar signs allows the diagnosis of pure autonomic failure. Conversion rates from pure autonomic failure to MSA are reported up to 28% within few years from disease onset. In general, the latency to onset of symptomatic orthostatic hypotension (OH) and urinary incontinence/retention is significantly shorter in MSA compared to PD and very late onset autonomic failure is reported in a minority of MSA patients only.

c. Distinguishing MSA from idiopathic PD and PSP is often challenging early in the illness. Some features such as autonomic dysfunction, poor or marginal response to levodopa with early clinical fluctuations, and dyskinesia can help to differentiate MSA from early PD. Autonomic failure is common in MSA and rare in early PD, whereas dementia and psychiatric features are more common in PD.

2) Diagnostic investigation

Characteristic MRI abnormalities include hypointensity on T_1 or hyperintensities on T_2 in the lateral border of the putamen atrophy. Cerebellar and pontine atrophy with the "hot cross bun" sign in the pons are seen (Fig. 9.9). Typical brain MRI in MSA patient shows "hot cross bun" sign in the pons (arrow in Fig. 9.9a) and putaminal hyperintensity (arrows in Fig. 9.9b). However, MRI is not specific and is often normal. The "hot cross bun" sign is only a surrogate of ponto-cerebellar atrophy and is reported in patients with secondary parkinsonism due to vasculitis as well as in patients with genetically confirmed spinocerebellar ataxia type 2 and 3. Other tests used in diagnosis of MSA include autonomic testing, external anal or urethral sphincter electromyography (EMG), and dopamine transporter scan.

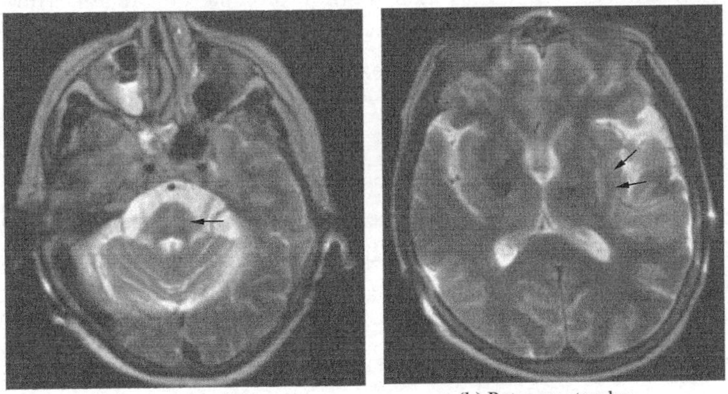

(a) "Hot cross bun" sign (b) Putamen atrophy

Fig. 9.9 MRI findings of MSA

(2) Treatment and prognosis

Only symptomatic therapy is available. Parkinsonism is treated with levodopa despite its inconsistent efficacy. Orthostatic hypotension may respond to conservative measures, such as raising the head of the bed, binding stockings, and liberal salt intake. Medications such as fludrocortisone or midodrine are commonly required. Urinary dysfunction can be treated with antispasmodics, such as oxybutynin and self-catheterization. Typical disease duration is 3 ~ 10 years. Roughly 80% of patients are disabled within five years after motor symptoms occur. Breathing problems such as aspiration and cardiopulmonary arrest are common causes of death.

9.2.3 Other Extrapyramidal Disorders

9.2.3.1 Huntington's Disease

Huntington's disease (HD) is an autosomal dominant disorder of the nervous system characterized by the gradual onset and subsequent progression of chorea and dementia. It is due to a mutation in the Huntingtin gene on chromosome 4p16.3. The disease shows complete penetrance, so that offspring of an affected individual have a 50% chance of developing it. Additional features of the inheritance of HD include anticipation, meaning that there is a trend toward earlier onset in successive generations, and paternal descent, which refers to the tendency for anticipation to be most pronounced in individuals who inherit the disease from their father. Both of these phenomena are related to the unstable nature of the mutation responsible for HD—expansion of a CAG trinucleotide repeat that codes for a polyglutamine tract. The repeat can expand during gametogenesis, especially in the male germline. This leads to an abnormal protein with longer and longer polyglutamine tracts. Normal subjects have between 11 ~ 34 CAG repeats whereas nearly all patients with HD have more than 40. HD occurs throughout the world and in all ethnic groups. Its prevalence rate is about 5 per 10 000 population. Symptoms usually do not appear until adulthood, by which time these patients have often started families of their own; thus, the disease continues from one generation to the next.

(1) Pathophysiology

How an expanded CAG repeat in Huntingtin leads to HD is unknown, but at least two factors may contribute. First, mutant huntingtin is cleaved by proteases and conjugated with ubiquitin, then transported in a complex called the proteasome to the cell nucleus, where it may disrupt the gene transcription machinery and thereby promote cell death. However, loss of the normal function of Huntingtin, which may have an inhibitory effect on programmed cell death, may also contribute to disease pathogenesis. Postmortem examination of patients with the disease reveals cell loss, particularly in the cerebral cortex and corpus striatum. In the latter region, mediumsized spiny neurons that contain γ-aminobutyric acid (GABA) and enkephalin and project to the external segment of the globus pallidus are affected earliest, but other classes of neurons are eventually involved as well. Biochemical studies have shown that the concentrations of the inhibitory neurotransmitter GABA, its biosynthetic enzyme glutamic acid decarboxylase (GAD), and acetylcholine and its biosynthetic enzyme choline acetyltransferase are all reduced in the basal ganglia of patients with HD. The concentration of dopamine is normal or slightly increased. Changes in the concentrations of neuropeptides in the basal ganglia are also found, including decreased substance P, methionine enkephalin, and dynorphin, and increased somatostatin and neuropeptide Y. Neurons containing NADPH diaphorase activity are spared.

(2) Clinical feature and diagnosis

The classic signs of HD include the development of chorea, neurobehavioral changes, and gradual dementia. Symptoms typically become evident during the fourth or fifth decade of life although onset varies from early childhood to late adulthood. The initial clinical presentation may be either neurologic or psychiatric. Characteristic early presentations include the gradual onset of subtle personality changes, forgetfulness, clumsiness, and development of choreiform. Neurobehavioral changes include both emotional and behavioral disturbance. Patients present with increased irritability, suspiciousness, impulsiveness, lack of self-control, and anhedonia. Cognitive decline is characterized by progressive dementia or gradual impairment of the mental processes involved incomprehension reasoning, judgment, and memory. Motor disturbances are characterized by the gradual onset of clumsiness, balance difficulties, and fidgeting movements. Early chorea may be limited to the fingers and toes, later extending to the arms, legs, face, and trunk. Eventually, chorea tends to become widespread or generalized. Parkinsonism and dystonia are sometimes seen later in the disease. Later disease stages are characterized by severe dementia and progressive motor dysfunction, patients usually become unable to walk, have poor dietary intake, become unable to care for themselves, and eventually cease to talk, leading to a persistent vegetative state.

CT scanning or MRI often demonstrates atrophy of the cerebral cortex and caudate nucleus in established cases. PET typically demonstrates glucose hypometabolism within the striatum. Genetic testing now provides an accurate and definitive means of establishing the diagnosis and also permits the presymptomatic detection of the disease. The evaluation of patients with HD includes detailed family history and tests to exclude other possible pathophysiology.

(3) Differential diagnosis

a. Sydenham chorea: This is the other well-recognized form of chorea. It is related to an autoimmune response to infection with group A beta hemolytic streptococci leading to acute rheumatic fever (ARF). The initial illness is usually characterized by pharyngitis, followed within approximately 1 ~ 5 weeks by the sudden onset of ARF. The distribution of chorea is usually generalized, and these movements consist of relatively fast or rapid, irregular, uncontrollable, jerky motions that disappear with sleep and may increase with stress, fatigue, and excitement. Some children are also proved to have emotional and behavioral disturbances. Typically, in a significant majority of children, Sydenham chorea is a self-limited condition, resolving spontaneously within an average duration of 9 months to 2 years.

b. Paroxysmal choreoathetosis: This disease may occur on a familial basis, but the intermittent nature of the symptoms and their relationship to movement or emotional stress usually distinguish this disorder from HD.

c. Neuroacanthocytosis: Neuroacanthocytosis is another hereditary movement disorder also manifested by mild chorea, tics, parkinsonism, and dystonia. Laboratory findings include increased serum creatine phosphokinase and red cell acanthocytes.

(4) Treatment and prognosis

There is no cure for HD, which, as a rule, terminates fatally 10 ~ 20 years after clinical onset. There is no treatment for the dementia, but the movement disorder may respond to drugs that interfere with dopaminergic inhibition of striatal output neurons. Patients should be advised of the risk of transmitting the disease, and living offspring should receive genetic counseling.

Adult-onset HD typically lasts approximately 15 ~ 20 years, whereas the course of juvenile HD tends to last approximately 8 ~ 10 years. Life-threatening complications may result from serious falls, sometimes even leading to subdural hematomas, poor nutrition, infection, choking, aspiration pneumonia, or heart failure.

9.2.3.2 Wilson's Disease

Wilson's disease (WD), sometimes called hepatolenticular degeneration (HLD), is an autosomal recessive disorder of copper metabolism that produces neurologic and hepatic dysfunction. Symptoms vary widely and present most commonly between 5 and 35 years of age. In 1984, the global prevalence of WD was estimated as 1 case per 30 000 individuals in non-isolated populations, with a mutation carrier frequency (individuals with one disease-associated allele) of 1 in 90 individuals (which corresponds to almost 1% of the general population);

these epidemiological data are still widely cited today. The prevalence of WD is higher in Asian countries than in Western countries.

(1) Etiology and pathogenesis

The genetic defect of WD is the ATP7B gene located on the long arm of chromosome 13. ATP7B binds copper and transports it across cellular membranes using ATP as an energy source. In WD, this defect leads to reduced copper binding to apoceruloplasmin, which normally forms ceruloplasmin. The absence or decreased function of ATP7B also results in dysfunction of biliary copper excretion and consequently leads to copper accumulation within the liver. The most frequently observed point mutation, H1069Q, results from the substitution of a histidine to a glutamine. This is present in nearly 30% of WD patients of European descent. Excess copper accumulation results in generation of free radicals, lipid peroxidation of membranes and DNA, and inhibition of protein synthesis leading to hepatocellular injury and necrosis. Release of free copper, from injured hepatocytes, into circulation is thought to be responsible for causing extrahepatic deposition of copper in the brain, kidneys, eyes, and joints.

(2) Clinical feature

1) Clinical manifestation

WD usually presents in childhood or young adult life. The average age at onset is about 11 for patients presenting with hepatic dysfunction and 19 for those with initial neurologic manifestations, but the disease may begin as late as the sixth decade. Hepatic and neurologic presentations are about equally common. Pathological copper accumulation in the eyes can cause ophthalmological manifestations of WD, which include the Kayser-Fleischer ring and sunflower cataract. Kayser-Fleischer rings occur in almost 100% of patients with neurological WD, 40% ~ 50% of patients with hepatic WD and 20% ~ 30% of presymptomatic patients with WD and as such are an important diagnostic feature.

Liver disease is the first clinical manifestation in 40% ~ 60% of patients with WD but may be accompanied by other symptoms. The clinical presentation of WD with liver involvement includes a wide spectrum of signs and symptoms, ranging from asymptomatic subtle morphological changes to the liver and simple acute self-limited hepatitis-like illness to severe hepatitis, recurrent jaundice, cirrhosis with or without portal hypertension and even acute liver failure. Similar to many other hepatic diseases that may involve cirrhosis, the model for end-stage liver disease and Child-Pugh scores are commonly used to assess the severity of chronic liver disease.

After hepatic manifestations, neurological symptoms are the most frequent clinical symptoms of WD. The main clinical spectrum of neurological symptoms includes different movement disorders with a wide variety of involuntary movements, which often overlap. Summarizing the most common neurological features of WD, different clinical forms are distinguished where there is a predominance of tremor, dystonia or parkinsonism; all of these movement disorders are often associated with dysarthria, gait and posture disturbances, drooling and dysphagia. These disturbances may severely affect the activities of daily living.

Dystonia is reported as the first WD symptom in 11% ~ 65% of patients. It can be focal, segmental, multisegmental or may even be generalized. The most characteristic dystonic presentation of WD is an abnormal facial expression or risus sardonicus, which presents as a fixed smile due to dystonia of the risorius muscle. If WD remains untreated, symptoms usually progress to generalized dystonia, contractures and full immobilization.

In addition to the classical movement disorders of WD, it is notable that other neurological syndromes such as dysarthria, dysphagia, epilepsy may occur. Psychologic disorders in WD include dementia, characterized by mental slowness, poor concentration, and memory impairment; disorders of affect, behavior or personality; and psychosis with hallucinations.

2) Diagnostic investigation

Serum levels of ceruloplasmin can be tested if WD is suspected. But the predictive value of ceruloplasmin for diagnosis of WD in patients with liver disease is poor. Total serum copper is usually decreased in proportion to reduced levels of ceruloplasmin (holoceruloplasmin and apoceruloplasmin) in the circulation. Normal or elevated serum copper levels with decreased levels of ceruloplasmin indicate an increase in the concentration of non-ceruloplasmin-bound copper, which is suggestive of WD. 24-hour urinary copper excretion is a useful measure, which is helpful to diagnose WD and to monitor treatment. The conventional level taken as diagnostic of WD is >100 μg excreted over 24 h (>1.6 μmol per 24 h) in patients with signs and symptoms of WD. If WD is suspected, a liver biopsy with measurement of hepatic parenchymal copper concentration is required, if the clinical signs and non-invasive tests do not allow a final diagnosis or if there is suspicion of additional liver pathology from other causes. A hepatic copper content of >250 μg (4 μmol) per gram of dry liver weight is considered robust biochemical evidence for WD.

MRI is abnormal in most WD patients, mirroring the underlying basal ganglia pathology of both gliosis and neuronal loss with a concomitant significant increase in copper concentration. There are a wide variety of relatively symmetric MRI abnormalities resulting from combinations of edema, necrosis, cystic changes, and gliosis. These typically involve the striatum (caudate and putamen), globus pallidus, thalamus, and midbrain.

(3) Diagnosis

A diagnostic score based on all available tests was proposed by the European Association for the Study of the Liver (EASL) at the 8th International Meeting on WD, Leipzig 2001 (Tab. 9.2). The WD scoring system provides a good diagnostic accuracy.

Tab. 9.2 Scoring system developed at the 8th International Meeting on Wilson's disease

Typical clinical symptoms and signs			Other tests		
KF rings	Present	2	Liver copper (in the absence of cholestasis)	>5x ULN (>4 μmol/g)	2
	Absent	0		0.8~4 μmol/g	1
Neurologic symptoms	Severe	2		Rhodanine-positive granules	−1
	Mild	1	Normal (<0.8 μmol/g)	Urinary copper (in the absence of acute hepatitis)	1
	Absent	0		Normal	0
Serum ceruloplasmin	Normal (>0.2 g/L)	0		>2x ULN	1
	0.1~0.2 g/L	1	1~2x ULN	Normal, but>5x ULN after D-penicillamine	2
	<0.1 g/L	2		Mutation analysis	2

Continued

Typical clinical symptoms and signs			Other tests		
Coombs-negative hemolytic anemia	Present	1	On both chromosomes detected	On 1 chromosome detected	1
	Absent	0		No mutations detected	0
Total score	4 or more		Evaluation	Diagnosis established	
	3			Diagnosis possible, more tests needed	
	2 or less			Diagnosis very unlikely	

(4) Differential diagnosis

Acute hepatitis with WD presents similarly to any other acute cases of hepatitis. Similarly, WD should enter into the diagnosis of all patients with chronic hepatitis and cirrhosis, as routine histologic changes are nonspecific. WD should be considered when acute hepatitis is accompanied by rapid onset of jaundice and hemolytic anemia. During adolescence, WD presenting with neurologic symptoms may be misdiagnosed as a behavioural problem because initial symptoms may be subtle. More advanced movement disorders in a young person should provoke consideration of WD, but the diagnosis may be overlooked where the presentation suggests a primarily psychological or psychiatric disorder.

(5) Treatment

Penicillamine, a copper-chelating agent that promotes extraction of copper from tissue deposition sites, should be started as early as possible and customarily employs 1.5~2 g/d of orally administered penicillamine. The response to treatment may take several months and can be monitored by serial slit lamp examinations and blood chemistries. Side effects of penicillamine include nausea, nephrotic syndrome, myasthenia gravis, arthropathy, pemphigus and diverse blood dyscrasias. Zinc salts are also used as an alternative to penicillamine for trientine-intolerant WD patients, as well as for safe and effective maintenance therapy. Zinc salts block intestinal absorption of dietary copper and also stimulate endogenous production of chelators in the liver. These often have a delayed onset of action, therefore, chelation therapy is preferred.

Orthotopic liver transplantation now provides another important treatment option for WD patients, particularly when they are compromised by significant cirrhosis or fulminant liver failure. After liver transplantation, there is no need to continue long-term therapy because the diseased liver is removed and replaced with a healthy liver. Transplantation may reduce neurologic symptoms in some patients.

(6) Prognosis

Untreated WD is universally fatal, with most patients dying from liver disease and a minority from complications of progressive neurologic disease. Prognosis is excellent for compliant patients with WD, even if cirrhosis is present at time of initiating therapy. Rapid progressive liver failure due to WD carries a poor prognosis, unless liver transplantation is performed.

9.2.3.3 Dystonia

Dystonia is a hyperkinetic movement disorder characterized by involuntary, sustained muscle contractions that frequently cause twisting and repetitive movements or abnormal postures. There is simultaneous contraction of agonist and antagonist muscles. One of the characteristic features of dystonia is that it is often temporarily diminished by tactile sensory tricks (gestes antagonists). For example, a patient with cervical dystonia may be able to reduce dystonic movements by placing a hand on the chin or the side of the face. The initial presentation of dystonia is usually focal. In the majority of patients, the dystonia remains focal without spreading to other parts of the body. If dystonia spreads, it tends to involve contiguous body parts and becomes a segmental dystonia. Dystonia is frequently worsened by fatigue and stress and diminishes with relaxation and sleep.

Although the genetics of a number of primary dystonias have been elucidated, the pathophysiology of dystonia remains unclear. Lesions in the basal ganglia, particularly the thalamus and putamen, point to these structures as having key roles in the development of dystonia. A more complex pathophysiological model of dystonia is emerging that incorporates not only rate but pattern, synchronization, and somatosensory responsiveness of neuronal activity.

(1) Clinical feature

There are several recognized classification schemes for dystonia: age at onset, anatomic distribution, and etiology.

1) Age at onset

Early-onset dystonia is defined as dystonia developing at or before the age of 26 and late onset is defined as dystonia developing after the age of 26. Age at onset is an important factor determining prognosis in patients with dystonia, with earlier age at onset correlating with increased likelihood of spread of dystonia to other body parts. In general, young-onset dystonia tends to begin in a limb and become generalized whereas adult-onset dystonia tends to be craniocervical and remain focal or become segmental.

2) Anatomic distribution

The topographic characteristics of dystonia are useful in defining the severity of the dystonia and guiding treatment. Focal dystonia affects a single body part. Virtually any part of the body can be involved in dystonia and many types of focal dystonia have specific names: blepharospasm (dystonic eye closure), spasmodic torticollis (Fig. 9.10) and writer's cramp (focal hand dystonia). When dystonia involves two or more contiguous body regions, it is referred to as segmental dystonia. Multifocal dystonia refers to the involvement of two or more noncontiguous body parts. Generalized dystonia represents a combination of crural dystonia (one or both legs plus trunk) and any other area of the body (Fig. 9.11).

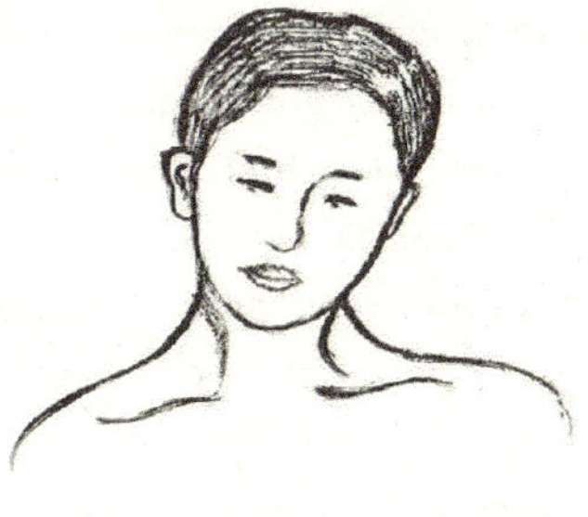

Fig. 9.10 Spasmodic torticollis

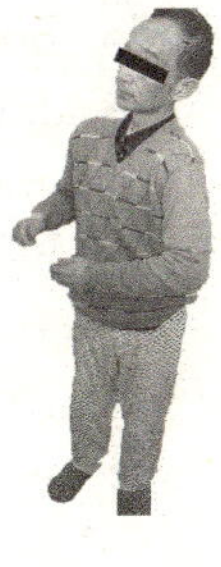

Fig. 9.11 Generalized dystonia

3) Etiology

There are essentially two broad categories: primary and secondary dystonia.

a. Primary dystonia: Primary dystonia are characterized by pure dystonia and most primary dystonia are sporadic with onset in adulthood and a focal or segmental presentation. The most common focal dystonia presenting to movement disorders clinics is cervical dystonia. The involuntary con-traction in the neck muscles results in abnormal head movements, abnormal head position and neck pain. After cervical dystonia, the most common focal dystonias are blepharospasm, spasmodic dysphonia, oromandibular dystonia, and hand dystonia. Blepharospasm is an uncommon problem where the eyes close involuntarily. This can be sufficiently severe to render the patient blind. Spasmodic dysphonia is rare. Speech is variable and often has a high-pitched strangled quality. It may be tremulous. Oromandibular dystonia affects the mouth and tongue, and the jaw may close on the protruded tongue. A minority of primary dystonias have an identified genetic etiology. Perhaps the best studied of the primary dystonias is DYT1 dystonia, or Oppenheim's dystonia, a generalized torsion dystonia that usually begins in childhood affecting the limbs first.

b. Secondary dystonia: Secondary dystonia encompasses a broad clinical category that includes inherited degenerative disorders, degenerative disorders of unknown etiology, acquired dystonias (i.e., drug-induced, structural lesions, trauma), and psychogenic dystonia. Patients with secondary dystonia frequently display associated clinical abnormalities, including other movement disorders besides tremor (i.e., Parkinsonism), dementia, spasticity, ataxia, weakness, reflex changes, eye movement abnormalities, or seizures. Other historical and clinical features that suggest secondary dystonia include history of trauma, perinatal anoxia, toxin or drug exposure, onset of dystonia at rest, and hemidystonia. A number of heredodegenerative disorders may present with dystonia. Autosomal dominant disorders (Huntington's disease, spinocerebellar ataxia type 3, neuroferritonopathy), autosomal recessive disorders (Wilson's disease, pantothenatekinase associated degeneration), X-linked recessive disorders (DYT3 or Lubag), and mitochondrial disorders (Leigh disease) have been described.

c. Dystonia-plus syndromes are a rare group of inherited nondegenerative diseases that include dopa-responsive dystonia (DRD), myoclonus-dystonia (MD), and rapid-onset dystonia-Parkinsonism (RDP). These diseases are considered neurochemical disorders because they are due to biochemical defects that are not associated with neuronal loss. Dystonia is associated with Parkinsonism in DRD and RDP and with myoclonus in MD.

(2) Treatment

Treatment of dystonia is determined by etiology and anatomic region(s) involved. All children and young adults presenting with dystonia should be given a trial of levodopa. The first-line treatment for cervical dystonia, blepharospasm, focal limb dystonia, and spasmodic dysphonia is botulinum toxin. Botulinum toxin and baclofen can be beneficial for oromandibular dystonia. In addition to medications, physical therapy is an important adjunct in the treatment of dystonia. For patients with generalized dystonia, trihexyphenidyl at high doses (about 90 mg/d) can provide some benefit. Baclofen may also be tried for generalized dystonia and can also be given at high doses. The benzodiazepines may provide adjunctive benefit. Variable results have been found for diphenhydramine, carbamazepine, dopamine agonists and dopamine antagonists. Tetrabenazine can be helpful, especially in tardive dystonia. For medication-refractory dystonia, surgery can be considered. Peripheral denervation surgeries such as rhizotomy have produced variable results. More recently, deep brain stimulation (DBS) of the globus pallidus has been performed in patients with medication-refractory dystonia.

9.2.4 Motor Neuron Disease

Motor neuron disease (MND) is a progressive, neurodegenerative disorder that mainly attacks the human motor system, leading to significant disability and ultimately death. The incidence of MND in Western populations is about 2~3 per 100 000, with a male predominance.

The disorder usually occurs sporadically but may be familial in 5% ~ 10% of cases. As there remains no test for MND, diagnosis is based on clinical findings. Given that MND is clinically and pathologically heterogeneous, therapeutic and neuroprotective targets are difficult to identify.

(1) Etiology and pathogenesis

The cause of sporadic MND is unknown. As with other neurodegenerative diseases, it is hypothesized that MND may result from the dual insult of genetic susceptibility and environmental injury. An autosomal dominant familial MND (with upper and lower motor neuron signs) is related in some cases to muaions of the copper/zinc superoxide dismutase gene on the long arm of chromosome 21 (21q22.1 ~ q22.2) whereas an autosomal recessive form maps to 2q33 ~ q35. A recently identified MND mutation occurs in the TDP-43 gene. Non-amyloid, structurally modified TDP-43 is recognized as a major constituent of the ubiquitinated inclusions found in cortical neurons of patients with both sporadic and familial forms of frontotemporal lobar degeneration. There is degeneration of the motor cortex and anterior horns of the spinal cord with chromatolysis of the motor neurons, which may contain inclusion bodies, and degeneration of the corticospinal tracts and peripheral motor axons.

(2) Clinical feature

1) Clinical manifestation

There are four main patterns of disease. All are progressive and evolve at different rates. They overlap significantly and in the late stages tend to merge into a diffuse, combined upper motor neurone (UMN) and lower motor neurone (LMN) disorder. The differential diagnosis depends on the pattern of presentation. Sensation must be normal to make the diagnosis.

① Amyotrophic lateral sclerosis (ALS)

This phenotypes represents 70% of cases. The signature of anterior horn cell loss is painless weakness and atrophy, hypoactive or absent deep tendon reflexes, and fasciculations. In ALS, muscle weakness due to LMN dysfunction occurs in a segmental (myotomal) distribution and spreads in a regional fashion. This commonly presents with stiffness, atrophy, and weakness of the hands, muscle cramps and discomfort (Fig. 9.12). In some cases, onset may be proximal, resembling a plexopathy or with foot drop, simulating peroneal nerve palsy. Over the following months, more widespread, patchy weakness appears that may affect any muscle, except the extraocular muscles. Weakness becomes more diffuse and spreads to the truncal and bulbar muscles. The hands appear severely wasted and there are often fasciculations in the interossei and sometimes other muscle groups. It may be necessary to observe the patients' trunk and limb muscles for 30 s or more in order to see the fasciculations. Tongue atrophy, fasciculation, and weakness are perhaps the most frequently occurring and recognized manifestations of LMN involvement of cranial nerves. It is important to observe for fasciculations when the tongue is relaxed on floor of the mouth (Fig. 9.13).

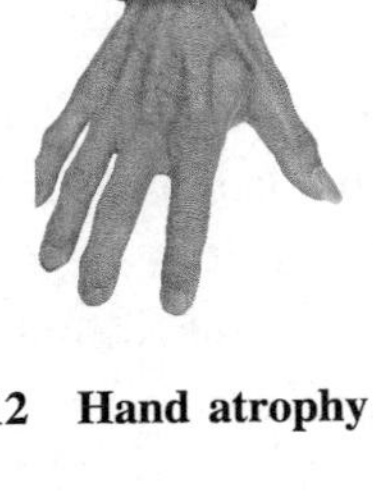

Fig. 9.12 Hand atrophy in ALS

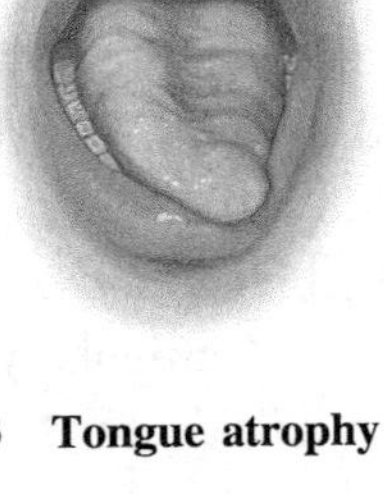

Fig. 9.13 Tongue atrophy in ALS

② Progressive bulbar palsy (PBP)

PBP accounts for 25% of cases. This presents with progressive dysarthria until speech becomes unintelligible. Swallowing becomes difficult and patients spend hours trying to eat each day. They lose weight rapidly and may suffer repeated aspiration pneumonia. Emotional lability is common in this form and 10% of patients develop dementia later in the course of the illness. The tongue is usually wasted and fasciculating but moves stiffly suggesting spasticity. The facial muscles sag and the jaw jerk and facial jerks are brisk. Most patients with this form of MND die within 3 years.

③ Progressive muscular atrophy (PMA)

PMA is very uncommon. There is slowly progressive wasting, which is usually symmetrical in both hands. It progresses to more proximal muscles and to the legs over several years. Fasciculations may be present but there are no UMN signs. Prognosis is best in patients aged under 50, with 72% surviving 5 years.

④ Primary lateral sclerosis (PLS)

PLS is a slowly progressive disorder of the UMNs and comprises 4% of motor neuron disease cases. PLS often presents with four-limb spasticity, often beginning in the lower limbs symmetrically; although a minority of patients have a bulbar-onset presentation with dysarthria, dysphagia, and pseudobulbar affect. Examination reveals spasticity, hyperreflexia, and pathologic reflexes. Urinary urgency often develops, and ocular movement abnormalities may be seen. Weakness may develop, although patients will often maintain antigravity strength. Mild denervation may be seen on EMG. The mean onset age is around 59 and the 10-year survival rate is 71.1%.

2) Diagnostic investigation

There is no single test for MND. Investigations can exclude other causes and support the diagnosis but do not confirm it. Normal nerve conduction studies are used to exclude a neuropathy and electromyography to confirm denervation and show fasciculations in muscles not thought to be affected clinically. MRI may be needed to exclude other causes, depending on the site of clinical involvement: brain for bulbar symptoms and neck for LMN arm features. An MRI brain scan may show corticospinal degeneration.

(3) Diagnosis

The World Federation of Neurology Research Group on Motor Neuron Diseases released revised diagnostic criteria (also known as the El Escorial and Airlie House criteria) for ALS in 2000. The diagnosis of ALS requires:

The presence of a. evidence of LMN degeneration by clinical, electrophysiological or neuropathologic examination; b. evidence of UMN degeneration by clinical examination; c. progressive spread of symptoms or signs within a region or to other regions.

The absence of a. electrophysiological or pathological evidence of other disease processes that might explain the signs of LMN and/or UMN degeneration; b. neuroimaging evidence of other disease processes that might explain the observed clinical and electrophysiological signs.

(4) Differential diagnosis

The differential diagnosis of ALS is largely that of other disorders of anterior horn cells, myopathies, disorders of neuromuscular transmission, motor predominant polyneuropathies and myelopathies. With bulbar onset and predominantly LMN features, myasthenia gravis, inflammatory myopathy particularly inclusion body myositis X-linked bulbospinal muscular atrophy (Kennedy disease), oculopharyngeal muscular dystrophy, multiple cranial neuropathies, or infiltrative head and neck cancers are the primary considerations.

(5) Treatment and prognosis

Treatment is supportive and involves most of the paramedical disciplines: physiotherapy (to optimize function, the best use of walking aids and to advise about positioning); occupational therapy (to optimize the environment); nursing; and speech therapy (to advise about swallowing and provide communication aids). Psychological support for the patient and relatives is important in a difficult, relentlessly progressive disease. Depression is common and can be treated. Some patients with respiratory weakness but otherwise good function may benefit from nocturnal or diurnal respiratory support.

Some drug therapy and other medical interventions are useful. Spasticity can be treated with baclofen. Patients with bulbar involvement may benefit from percutaneous insertion of a gastrostomy tube (percutaneous endoscopic gastrostomy, PEG). Two medications are FDA-approved for the treatment of ALS. Riluzole was approved in 1995 and is administered orally twice daily. While the exact mechanism of action is unknown, its neuroprotective effect is attributed to inhibition of glutamate release, inactivation of voltage-gated sodium channels and interference with intracellular response to excitatory receptor activation. The most common side effect of riluzole is gastrointestinal upset. Liver enzymes are monitored routinely to evaluate for hepatotoxicity. The second medication, edaravone, was approved in 2017. Edaravone is a free radical scavenger believed to prevent motor neuron degeneration by reducing oxidative stress. It is administered as an intravenous infusion.

The overall prognosis is poor; death is usually due to respiratory complications from bulbaror respiratory muscle weakness. 50% of ALS patients die within 3 years and 90% by 6 years. A small number have a slower progression and survive over a decade.

Case

History of present illness: Patient, male, 63 years old. Limb involuntary shaking with movement retardation for 3 years. Three years ago, the patient involuntarily shook his right hand and right upper limbs without obvious inducement, the symptom increased after tension, and disappeared during sleep. After a few months, involving the right lower limb, the left upper limb and left lower limb were gradually affected and accompanied by slow movement. In the past two years, patients often feel tired and depressed. There was no previous special medical history.

Physical examination: Consciousness, mask face, body forward, upper limb swing disappeared, panic gait, slow turn when walking; brain nerve examination found no positive signs, static tremor of limbs, increased muscle tension, tendon reflex (+), muscle level 5, pathological characteristics (−); normal deep feeling and cortical perception; no positive signs in other neurological examination.

Auxiliary examination: No abnormalities were detected in the blood, CSF, and cranial CT and MRI tests.

Question: What diagnosis, differential diagnosis and treatment should be made for the patient?

References

[1] JONES H R Jr. Netter's neurology[M]. 2nd ed. Philadelphia: Elsevier Publishing, 2011.

[2] GERAINT F, MARK M. Neurology[M]. 3rd ed. Beijing: Elsevier Publishing, 2010.

[3] GREENBERG D A, AMINOFF M J, SIMON R P. Clinical neurology[M]. 8th ed. New York: McGraw-Hill Professional Publishing, 2012.

[4] MCKHANN G M, KNOPMAN D S, CHERTKOW H, et al. The diagnosis of dementia due to Alzheimer's disease: recommendations from the National Institute on Aging-Alzheimer's Association workgroups on diagnostic guidelines for Alzheimer's disease [J]. Alzheimer's & Dementia, 2011,7(3):263-269.

[5] MCKEITH I G, BOEVE B F, DICKSON D W, et al. Diagnosis and management of dementia with Lewy bodies: fourth consensus report of the DLB consortium[J]. Neurology, 2017,89(1):88-100.

[6] O'BRIEN J T, THOMAS A. Vascular dementia[J]. Lancet, 2015,386(10004): 1698-1706.

[7] GORNO-TEMPINI M L, HILLIS A E, WEINTRAUB S, et al. Classification of primary progressive aphasia and its variants[J]. Neurology, 2011,76(11):1006-1014.

[8] RASCOVSKY K, HODGES J R, KNOPMAN D, et al. Sensitivity of revised diagnostic criteria for the behavioural variant of frontotemporal dementia[J]. Brain, 2011,134(9):2456-2477.

[9] POSTUMA R B, BERG D, STERN M, et al. MDS clinical diagnostic criteria for Parkinson's disease[J]. Movement disorders, 2015,30(12):1591-1601.

[10] GILMAN S, WENNING G K, LOW P A, et al. Second consensus statement on the diagnosis of multiple system atrophy[J]. Neurology, 2008,71(9):670-676.

[11] BROOKS B R, MILLER R G, SWASH M, et al. El Escorial revisited: revised criteria for the diagnosis of amyotrophic lateral sclerosis[J]. Amyotrophic Lateral Sclerosis and Other Motor Neuron Disorders, 2000,1(5):293-299.

[12] TABRIZI S J, FLOWER M D, ROSS C A, et al. Huntington disease: new insights into molecular pathogenesis and therapeutic opportunities [J]. Nature Reviews Neurology, 2020,16(10):529-546.

[13] FERENCI P, CZLONKOWSKA A, STREMMEL W, et al. EASL clinical practice guidelines: Wilson's disease[J]. Journal of Hepatology, 2012,56(3):671-685.

(Yu Ming, Chen Xiaopeng)

Chapter 10

Muscle and Muscular Connector Diseases

Neuromuscular junction diseases refer to diseases caused by dysfunction of neuromuscular junction transmission, which mainly include myasthenia gravis, Lambert-Eaton myasthenia syndrome and so on. Muscle diseases refer to skeletal muscle diseases, mainly including periodic paralysis, polymyositis, progressive muscular dystrophy, tonic muscular dystrophy, mitochondrial myopathy and so on.

(1) Pathogenesis

Skeletal muscle consists of two types of muscle fibers, type Ⅰ is red muscle fiber, also called slow twitch fiber, which has high oxidase activity, low glycogen hydrolase activity and high lipid content. It mainly obtains energy through aerobic metabolism and accounts a high proportion in the muscles that maintain postures, such as erector spine muscle and other trunk muscles. Type Ⅱ is white muscle fiber, also called fast twitch fiber. In contrast to type Ⅰ muscle fiber, it has low oxidase activity and high glycogen hydrolase activity. It obtains energy through anaerobic metabolism of glycogen, and accounts a high proportion in muscles directly related to exercise. Skeletal muscles are innervated by motor nerves. Motor unit refers to the range that a motor neuron innervates, including the cell body of motor nerve cells of spinal cord and brain stem, peripheral motor nerve, nerve-muscle joint and muscle fiber innervated. It is the smallest unit of the motor system. Different muscles consist of different numbers of motor units.

Abnormal membrane potential of muscle cells, such as periodic paralysis, ankylosing muscular dystrophy, and congenital myotonia, which can cause membrane depolarization block due to the decrease of end plate potential. Energy metabolism disorders, such as mitochondrial myopathy, lipid metabolic myopathy, and glycogen accumulation disease, affect muscle energy metabolism to induce onset. Myocyte structural lesions, such as various muscular dystrophy, congenital myopathy, secretory myopathy, inflammatory myopathy and ischemic myopathy, are also causes of muscle diseases.

Nerve-muscle junction consists of presynaptic membrane, postsynaptic membrane and synaptic cleft. Nerve endings are unsheathed and are divided into thin branches with clubbing terminals, which take up choline of extracellular fluid through "cytosis" and then compose acetylcholine (ACh) to store at synaptic vesicles. Acetylcholine receptors (AChR) are located on the cristae of the postsynaptic membrane, which is the endplate of the sarcomere. The synaptic cleft is filled with extracellular fluid containing acetylcholinesterase to degrade ACh. The transfer process of the neural-muscle junction is a complex process that combines electrical and chemical transfer. The electrical impulse travels from the axon to the nerve terminal, the voltage-gated calcium channel opens, and the influx of calcium ions fuses the synaptic vesicle with the presynaptic membrane. The ACh in the vesicle is released into the synaptic cleft in quantum form. The release of ACh follows the all-or-nothing principle.

ACh synthesis and release disorders are induced by presynaptic membrane lesions, such as botulism and hypermagnesia, which prevent calcium from entering nerve endings and induce ACh release disorders; aminoglycoside drugs and carcinoma-like Lamhert-Eatonmyasthenic syndrome can reduce ACh synthesis and release. Acetylcholinesterase activity and amount are abnormal in synaptic cleft, for example, organophosphorus poisoning decreased acetylcholinesterase activity to induce excessive post-synaptic membrane depolarization. Post-synaptic membrane AChR lesions, for example, myasthenia gravis are caused by the production of AChR autoantibodies that destroyed AChR; American dart binds to AChR to prevent ACh from binding to its receptor.

(2) Clinical manifestation

1) Muscular dystrophy

It refers to a reduction in the volume of skeletal muscle due to a reduction in the number or size of muscle fibers.

2) Myasthenia

It refers to a loss of muscle strength. The distribution of myasthenia varies with different types of neuromuscular diseases. Myasthenia caused by muscle diseases and neuromuscular junction diseases are usually bilaterally symmetric and the range involved often cannot be explained by damage of one group or one nerve.

3) Intolerance fatigue

It refers to the decrease of the athletic load capacity that reaches fatigue, fatigue occured after walking for a short distance and alleviated after resting. It can be seen in myasthenia gravis, mitochondrial myopathy, lipid deposition myopathy and so on.

4) Muscle hypertrophy and pseudohypertrophy

Muscle hypertrophy is divided into functional and pathological hypertrophy. Certain muscle groups in weightlifters and manual workers of specific types of work are particularly developed, resulting in hypertrophy of muscle volume and increased muscle strength, which is physiological (functional) hypertrophy, and the relevant occupational history can provide diagnostic evidence. Pathological muscle hypertrophy can be seen in the following occasions.

a. Myopathy: Patients with congenital myotonic disease are accompanied with muscle hypertrophy, but the muscle strength is weakened. Hypertrophic muscular dystrophy can manifest muscle hypertrophy such as gastrocnemius muscle, which is caused by reactive hyperplasia of fat and connective tissue resulting from the destruction of muscle fibers, thus it is called pseudohypertrophy. Hypertrophia musculorum vera is a rare disease that occurs in children, in which the muscle hypertrophy of the limbs develops progressively until it stops on its own.

b. Endocrine disorders: Hypothyroidism can induce myxedema, increasing the body shape. Acromegaly manifests muscle hypertrophy in the early stage and atrophy in the late stage.

c. Congenital unilateral hypertrophy: It mainly manifests hypertrophy on the side of the face, or hypertrophy on one side of the face and ipsilateral half body.

5) Muscle pain and tenderness

They are most common in inflammatory myopathy. Active pain refers to muscle pain during activity, which can be seen in ischemic tibialis anterior syndrome after long march, mitochondrial myopathy, lipid deposition myopathy and so on. Type Ⅴ glycogen accumulation disease manifests spasmodic pain after activity, known as painful spasms.

6) Myotonia

It refers to involuntary and continuous muscle contractions, relief of symptoms after warmed or activity due to muscle contraction or mechanical stimulation caused by changes in the excitability of muscle membrane, which is seen in congenital myotonia and myotonic muscular dystrophy.

7) Involuntary muscle movement

It refers to the involuntary contraction and twitch of muscles at rest. Fasciculation refers to a transient involuntary contraction of muscle bundles that is visible to naked eyes but does not induce limb movement. It occurs in the damage of anterior horn or root of the spinal cord. Fibrillation cannot be found with naked eyes and only can be seen on EMG. Myokymia refers to slow, persistent, irregular flutter of a group or a piece of muscle at rest, which is visible to naked eyes. It occurs in idiopathic myokymia.

(3) Diagnosis

The correct diagnosis of muscular diseases and neuro-muscular junction diseases must be based on the organic combination of complete and accurate clinical data and relevant auxiliary examinations. The diagnosis and differential diagnosis of muscle diseases can be determined according to the onset age, progression rate, whether it is paroxysmal, distribution, genetic pattern, course and prognosis of muscle atrophy and muscle weakness, which is also combined with laboratory biochemical tests, electromyography, muscle pathology and gene analysis.

(4) Treatment

Etiological treatment firstly indicates removal of the cause or treatment according to the pathogenesis. For example, after thymusectomy, 70% of patients with myasthenia gravis can improve or recover from clinical symptoms. The symptomatic treatments include pyridostigmine bromide alleviates symptoms of myasthenia gravis through inhibiting the hydrolysis of acetylcholine in the synaptic cleft by cholinesterase; phenytoin sodium alleviates muscle rigidity through stabilizing myolemma potential; patients with periodic paralysis of hypokalemia can take 10% potassium chloride orally to improve muscle weakness; and cataracts of ankylosing muscular dystrophy can be treated by surgery to restore vision.

10.1 Myasthenia Gravis

Myasthenia gravis (MG) is an acquired autoimmune disease with transmission dysfunction of the neuromuscular junction. It is mainly caused by damage of AChR in the postsynaptic membrane of the nerve-muscle junction. The main clinical manifestations are partial or systemic skeletal muscle weakness and extreme fatigue. The symptoms are aggravated after activity and relieved after rest or treatment with cholinesterase inhibitors (ChEI). The incidence is (8~20)/100 000, and the prevalence is 50/100 000. The incidence is relatively high in south China. This disease occurs at any age, ranging from a few months to 70~80 years old. There are two peaks in the age of onset. The number of female patients of 20~40 years old is more than that of male patients (the ratio is about 3 : 2). The incidence of 40~60 years old is more common in male, which are mostly accompanied with thymoma. A few patients have a family history. Factors that can worsen MG include infection, surgery, mental trauma, systemic disease, excessive fatigue, pregnancy, childbirth, and sometimes even the myasthenia gravis crisis.

(1) Pathogenesis

The pathogenesis of myasthenia gravis is associated with AChR damage of the postsynaptic membrane mediated by autoantibodies. The main basis are as follows. a. Animal experiments found that an experimental autoimmune animal model of myasthenia gravis could be made by injecting purified AChR and the antibody of AChR could be detected in the serum with a reduced number of AChR in the postsynaptic membrane significantly. b. Myasthenia-like symptoms and electrophysiological changes occur after injection of serum from patients with myasthenia gravis into mice. c. Serum AChR antibodies can be detected in 80% ~ 90% of patients with MG, whose myasthenia symptoms can be temporarily improved by plasma exchange treatment. d. Patients have thymus changes similar to other autoimmune diseases, 80% of patients have thymus hypertrophy, lymphatic follicular hyperplasia, 10% ~ 20% of patients have thymoma. e. Patients with myasthenia gravis are often associated with hyperthyroidism, thyroiditis, systemic lupus erythematosus, rheumatoid arthritis, pemphigus and other autoimmune diseases.

Enhancement of thymus weight, lymphatic follicular hyperplasia and increased germinal centers are seen in 80% patients with mysathenia gravis; 10%~20% of patients are associated with thymoma. Under microscopy, the synaptic cleft widens, the folds of the postsynaptic membrane shallow and the number decreases, the post-synaptic membrane disintegrates, the AChR on the membrane decreases significantly and the deposition of IgG-C3-ACHR binding immune complex can be observed. Change of muscle fiber itself is not obvious, sometimes muscle fiber coagulation, necrosis, swelling occurs. For few patients, the infiltration of lymphocytes around muscle fibers and small blood vessels can be seen, which is known as "lymphatic overflow". Muscle atrophy can be seen in chronic disease.

(2) Clinical feature

1) Clinical manifestation

Onset is insidious, the whole course of disease has fluctuation, remission alternates with recurrence. Advanced patients cannot fully recover after rest. The courses of most cases are prolonged for years to decades, which are sustained by drugs. Natural remission occurs in few cases. Severe weakness and even paraplegics occur after successive muscle contractions. Symptoms can be relieved after rest. Muscle weakness aggravates in the afternoon or evening due to fatigue, and alleviates in the morning or after rest. Skeletal muscle all over the body can be involved, most of which are the muscles innervated by the cranial nerve. Muscle weakness usually begins with a group of muscles and develops in scope. The first symptom is usually paralysis of one side or bilateral external eye muscles, such as ptosis (Fig. 10.1), strabismus and diplopia, and the serious patients manifest limited eye movement, or even fixed eyeball, but the pupil sphincter is not involved. When the facial muscles and oropharyngeal muscles are involved, the expression becomes indifferent and wry, and continuous chewing weakness, cough when drinking water, difficulty in swallowing occur; also speaking with nasal voice, articulation disorder occur; when involving sternocleidomastoid muscle and trapezius muscle, it is manifested as soft neck, difficult to raise the head, turn the neck, and weak shoulder. When involving muscle of the limbs, it is manifested as heavy proximal weakness, difficulty in arm lifting, combing hair,

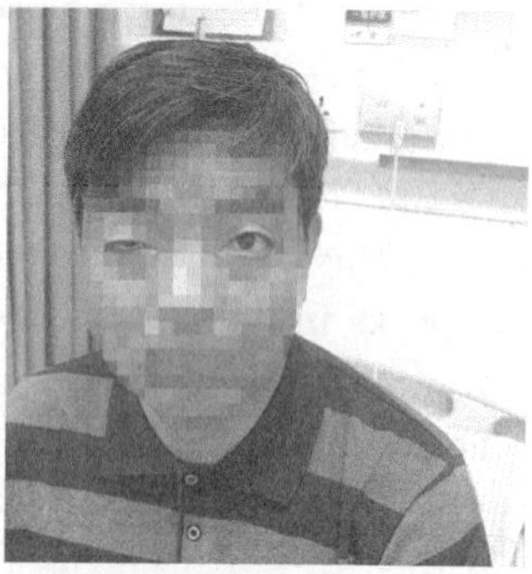

Fig. 10.1 Right eyelid dropped

climbing stairs; tendon reflex is usually not affected, feeling normal.

Myasthenia gravis crisis refers to cough weakness or even dyspnea when respiratory muscles are involved, and it is the main cause of death that ventilator is required to assist breath. Patients with oropharyngeal muscle weakness and respiratory muscle weakness are prone to develop crisis. The inducing factors include respiratory tract infection, surgery (including thymectomy), mental tension, systemic diseases and so on. Myocardial involvement may occasionally cause sudden death. Efficacy of cholinesterase inhibitors is a significant clinical feature of myasthenia gravis.

Modified osserman classification has been frequently recommended and widely used over the past several decades in China. Although it is based on clinical symptoms, impact on work and daily life, course of disease and treatment response, it is extremely challenging to take into account the prognosis and disability of patients. Moreover, this classification does not contain MG-associated auto-antibodies and low-frequency repetitive nerve stimulation (RNS) tests (Tab. 10.1).

Tab. 10.1 Clinical classification (Osserman subtype)

Classification	Character
Ⅰ. Eye muscle type (15%~20%)	Lesions are limited to the extraocular muscle, and manifests ptosis and diplopia
ⅡA. Mild systemic type (30%)	It may involve the muscles of eyes, face and limbs, and patients can take care of themselves in most cases, there is no obvious pharynx muscle involvement
ⅡB. Moderate systemic type (25%)	The muscle groups of extremities are obviously involved. In addition to the external eye muscle paralysis, there are more obvious symptoms of throat muscle weakness, such as slurred speech, dysphagia, coughing when drinking water, and continuous chewing weakness, but the respiratory muscle involvement is not obvious
Ⅲ. Acute severe syndrome (15%)	The onset is acute, it usually involves medulla oblongata, limb-band, trunk and respiratory muscles within a few weeks, and manifests severe muscle weakness and even myasthenia gravis crisis, which requires tracheotomy and has high mortality
Ⅳ. Delayed severe syndrome (10%)	Disease course lasts for more than 2 years, which is often developed from type Ⅰ, ⅡA, ⅡB, the symptoms are same with type Ⅲ. It is often associated with thymoma, and manifests poor prognosis
Ⅴ. Muscular atrophy	Few patients manifest muscle weakness accompanied with muscular atrophy

2) Diagnostic investigation

Blood, urine and cerebrospinal fluid tests are normal. Routine EMG examination is basically normal. Nerve conduction velocity is normal. Repeating nerve electric stimulation (RNES) is a common diagnostic method. This should be done within 17 hours after discontinuation of neostigmine, otherwise a false negative would occur. This method refers to repeated stimulation of motor nerves such as ulnar nerve, median nerve and accessory nerve at low frequency (3~5 Hz) and high frequency (more than 10 Hz). The typical change of MG is that the ratio of the fifth wave to the first wave decreases by more than 10% at low frequency stimulation or more than 30% at high frequency stimulation. Myasthenia gravis with positive sign at low frequency stimulation accounts 90% of patients, and it is related to the severity of the disease. Single fiber electromyography (SFEMG) measures whether the time of action potential in the motor unit is prolonged to reflect the function of the nerve-muscle junction through the special single-fiber needle electrode. Detection of AChR antibody titer has characteristic significance for the diagnosis of myasthenia gravis. Serum AChR antibody concentration is significantly increased in more than 85% of patients with systemic myasthenia gravis, but it is not significantly increased in patients with ocular myasthenia gravis, and the level of antibody titer is not completely consistent with the severity of clinical symptoms. A proportion of people without antibodies against AchR have antibodies against MuSK protein. Antibody to low-density lipoprotein receptor-related protein 4 (LRP4) is also a pathogenic agent of myasthenia gravis. CT and MRI examinations of thymus can find thymus hyperplasia and hypertrophy. 5% of patients with myasthenia gravis have hyperthyroidism, showing elevated T_3 and T_4. Some patients are positive for antinuclear antibody and thyroid antibody.

(3) Diagnosis

Distribution of involved muscle of MG patients and muscle weakness after a motor nerve damage is not consistent, clinical characteristics manifest weakness of involved muscle after the activity, and rest or cholinesterase inhibitor treatment can alleviate it, muscle weakness characterized by fluctuation of "light in the morning and severe in the evening", combined with drug trial, electromyography and immunology examinations can diagnose this disease. In addition, thymus CT and MRI should also be conducted to determine whether there is thymic hyperplasia or thymoma, and to determine whether there are other autoimmune diseases according to the history, symptoms, signs and other immunological tests. The following tests are helpful in the diagnosis of MG. a. Fatigue test (Jolly test): Ask patients to continuously see the upper to manifest ptosis or lift flatly to manifest upper arm droop, which recovers after rest, then the test is positive. b. Anticholinesterase drug test includes neostigmine test (after intramuscular injection of 0.5 ~ 1 mg neostigmine, the symptoms of muscle weakness are significantly relieved 20 minutes later. Atropine 0.5 mg can be injected simultaneously to counter the muscarinic reaction of neostigmine) and tensilon test (10 mg tensilon is diluted to 1 mL water for injection, and 2 mg is injected intravenously, then observe for 20 seconds. If there are no adverse reactions such as sweating, increased salivary, another 8 mg is given. Symptoms are improved within 1 minute, which is positive, and returned to normal state after 10 minutes).

(4) Differential diagnosis

a. Lambert-Eaton myasthenia syndrome is a group of autoimmune diseases in which the target organs of autoantibodies are the calcium channel in the presynaptic membrane of peripheral nerve endings and the ACh vesicle release zone. It is more common in males, and about 2/3 patients are accompanied with cancer, especially oat cell bronchial lung cancer, and other autoimmune diseases. The clinical manifestations are muscle weakness in the proximal extremities, which should be differentiated from myasthenia gravis. Although the patient feels fatigue after the activity, the muscle force after short exert oneself forcibly contractile augments instead, and the fatigue state is shown again after continuous contractile, the muscle that cerebral nerve innervates is rarely involved. In addition, about half of the patients manifest autonomic symptoms, such as dry mouth, sweating, constipation, impotence. Neostigmine test may be positive, but is not as sensitive as myasthenia gravis. The amplitude of repeated stimulation at low frequency does not change significantly, but the amplitude of repeated stimulation at high frequency increased more than 200%. Serum AChR antibody is negative. Treatment with guanidine hydrochloride increases ACh release and improves symptoms. These features can be distinguished from myasthenia gravis.

b. Botulism: Botulinum toxin acts on the presynaptic membrane and blocks the transmission function of the neuro-muscle junction, manifesting symmetrical cerebral nerve damage and skeletal muscle paralysis. However, most of the patients have an epidemiological history of botulism and the neostigmine tests or ethanol-ammonium chloride tests of them are negative.

c. Muscular dystrophy: It has more insidious onset without fluctuations in symptoms. The situation is aggravated with significant muscle shrinkage and elevated blood muscle enzymes, while Neostigmine test is negative and anticholinesterase therapy is ineffective.

d. Bulbar palsy: Laryngeal muscle weakness appears in the posterior group due to cerebral nerve damage caused by bulbar medulla, but there are other signs of nerve localization, progressive aggravation without fluctuation, fatigue test and neostigmine test are negative, and anti-cholinesterase drug treatment is ineffective.

e. Polymyositis: It manifests muscle weakness in the proximal extremities, which is accompanied by muscle tenderness, no fluctuation that light in the morning and severe in the evening, the disease gradually progresses, serum creatinase significantly increases. Neostigmine test is negative and anticholinesterase drug therapy is ineffective.

(5) Treatment

1) Thymus treatment

Thymectomy: It removes the initiating antigen of the patient's autoimmune response and reduce T cells, B cells and cytokines involved in the white body immune response. The treatment applies to patients with thymus hypertrophy and high AChR antibody titer, patients with various types of myasthenia gravis with thymoma, systemic MG in young women, or patients with unsatisfactory response to anticholinesterase drug treatment. About 70% of patients with postoperative symptoms can be relieved or cured. Co radiotherapy of deep thymus is feasible for patients who are not suitable for thymectomy.

2) Drug treatment

a. Cholinesterase inhibitors: ACh hydrolysis can be reduced through inhibiting cholinesterase, and transmission between nerve and muscle joints can be improved. It is advisable to start with a small dose and gradually increase the dose to maintain daily life. Pyridostigmine bromide for adults, oral 60 ~ 120 mg, 3 ~ 4 times per hour. It should be taken 30 ~ 40 minutes before meals, and the peak time is 2 hours after oral administration. The working time is 6 ~ 8 hours. The effect is mild and stable, and the adverse reaction is light. Neostigmine bromide for adults, oral 15 ~ 30 mg, 3 ~ 4 times per hour. It can be taken 15 ~ 30 minutes before meals, with fast release, and reaches peak after 30 ~ 60 minutes, the working time is 3 ~ 4 hours, adverse reactions are muscarinic reactions, against which atropine can be used. Adjuvant drugs such as potassium chloride and ephedrine can enhance the efficacy of cholinesterase inhibitors.

b. Adrenal corticosteroids can inhibit the autoimmune response, reduce the production of AChR antibodies, promote the regeneration and repair of the motor end plate, and improve the transmission function of the nerve-muscle joint. It is suitable for all types of MG. Impact therapy is suitable for hospitalized critical cases, patients who are intubated or used ventilator. Methylprednisolone (MPL), 1 000 mg intravenously, once a day for 3 ~ 5 days, followed by 10 ~ 20 mg dexamethasone intravenous infusion once a day for 7 ~ 10 days, after stable improvement of clinical symptoms, dexamethasone should be discontinued and prednisone 60 ~ 100 mg should be taken every other day. When the symptoms basically disappear, the dosage should be gradually reduced to 5 ~ 15 mg for long-term maintenance, lasting at least one year. If the condition fluctuates, the dose should be adjusted at any time. Prednisone can also be taken orally at the beginning with 60 ~ 80 mg per day till gradual relief of symptoms after 2 weeks, and usually peak efficacy occurs several months later, followed by gradual reduction. Note the aggravation and even crisis of high dose steroid treatment at the beginning. Small-dose increasing method starts from a small dose, 20 mg prednisone should be taken every morning, and increased by 10 mg every week until 60 ~ 80 mg every morning. After stable improvement of symptoms for 4 ~ 5 days, the dosage can be reduced gradually to 5 ~ 15 mg every other day and maintain it for several years. This method can avoid aggravation of initial condition of medication. Long-term steroid users should note the adverse reactions, such as gastric ulcer bleeding, elevated blood glucose, Cushing syndrome, femoral head necrosis, and osteoporosis.

c. Immunosuppressant is suitable for people with poor efficacy or intolerance of adrenal glucocorticoid, or people who cannot use adrenal glucocorticoid due to hypertension, diabetes, ulcer disease. Note the adverse reactions, such as peripheral blood leukopenia, thrombocytopenia, alopecia, gastrointestinal reaction, hemorrhagic cystitis, liver, and kidney damage. Cyclophosphamide: for adult, oral 50 mg each time, 2 ~ 3 times a day, or 200 mg, intravenous injection for 2 ~ 3 times a week; for children, oral 3 ~ 5 mg/(kg · d). Azathioprine: for patients with poor efficacy of steroid treatment, oral 25 ~ 100 mg, twice a day. Cyclosporine A: it can inhibit cellular immunity and humoral immunity and reduce the production of AChR antibody; oral 6 mg/(kg · d), for 12 months. Adverse reactions include glomerular ischemic necrosis, nausea, palpitation and so on.

d. Forbidden and cautious drugs: Aminoglycoside antibiotics, neomycin, polymyxins, paromomycin and other drugs can aggravate the transmission disorder of neuro-muscle junction; quinine, quinidine and other drugs can reduce the membrane excitability; in addition, morphine, diazepam, phenobarbital, phenytoin sodium, propranolol and other drugs are also prohibited or should be used with caution.

3) Plasmapheresis

The AChR antibody, complement and immune complex in MG patients' plasma can be cleared by replacing the plasma with that of normal people or plasma substitutes. Each exchange capacity is about 2 000 mL, 1 ~ 3 times per week, 3 ~ 8 times in succession. It shows rapid onset, but the duration of efficacy is short, only 1 week to 2 months, with the increase of antibody level, symptoms relapse and adverse reactions, only suitable for crisis and refractory myasthenia gravis.

4) High dose intravenous immunoglobulin

Exogenous IgG can interfere with the binding between AChR antibody and AchR to protect AChR from being blocked by antibodies. IgG 0.4 g/(kg · d) Ⅳ infusion. A course of treatment lasts for 5 days, which is used as an adjunctive treatment to alleviate the disease.

5) Crisis treatment

Crisis refers to the sudden severe dyspnea of MG patients under the effect of some factors, or even life-threatening. There are three types of crises summaried in Tab. 10.2. No matter what kind of crisis, note to ensure that the respiratory tract is unobstructed. When the condition does not improve after early treatment, endotracheal intubation or tracheotomy should be treated immediately, and artificial breathing apparatus should be used to assist breathing. Discontinue anticholinesterase drugs to reduce tracheal secretions. To block the nerve-muscle joint to control pulmonary infection, effective and sufficient antibiotics and intravenous medication such as corticosteroids or high doses of gamma globulin can be used. Plasmapheresis can be used when necessary. Myasthenia gravis patients generally have a good prognosis but its crisis has a relatively high mortality rate.

Tab. 10.2 Crisis and treatment

Crisis	Treatment
Myasthenic crisis	It is the most common crisis that caused by the development of the disease itself and mostly due to insufficient anticholinesterase drugs. The diagnosis can be made if the symptoms are relieved after injection of edrophonium or neostigmine
Cholinergic crisis	It is very rare and is caused by an overdose of anticholinesterase drugs. Patients develop significant adverse effects of cholinesterase inhibitors, such as muscle bundle fibrillation and muscarinic reactions. Intravenous injection of 2 mg edrophonium can be used. If symptoms worsen, anticholinesterase drugs should be stopped immediately, and the dose can be readjusted after drug exclusion
Brittle crisis	If the patient with severe dyspnea is insensible to anticholinesterase drugs and has no response to edrophonium test, anticholinesterase drugs should be stopped. Patients with endotracheal intubation or incision can be treated with large doses of steroid hormone, and the anticholinesterase drug dose can be adjusted after the function of the motor end plate recovered

10.2 Periodic Paralysis

Periodic paralysis is a group of muscle diseases characterized by repeated flaccid paralysis of skeletal muscles and related to abnormal potassium metabolism. According to the serum potassium concentration attack, it can be divided into three types: low potassium type, high potassium type and normal potassium type. The low potassium type is more common in clinic. Secondary periodic paralysis is caused by hypokalemia due to hyperthyroidism, aldosteronism, kidney failure, and metabolic diseases. This section focuses on periodic paralysis of hypokalemia.

Hypokalemic periodic paralysis is an autosomal dominant disease, and its caustic gene is mainly located in the long arm of chromosome 1 (1q31–q32), which codes the L type calcium channel protein that is sensitive to dihydropyridine in muscle cells, and it is part of the dihydropyridine complex receptor and located in the transverse canal system. Regulating the release of calcium ions from the sarcoplasmic reticulum affects excitation-contraction coupling of muscles. Muscle weakness is most likely to occur at rest after a full meal or after strenuous activity, and can be triggered by factors that promote the transfer of potassium into the cell, such as injections of insulin, epinephrine or large amounts of glucose. The detailed pathogenesis is still unclear, which may be related to the fluctuation of potassium ion concentration in and outside the membrane of skeletal muscle. The myocyte membrane of patients with this disease is often in a state of mild depolarization, which is more unstable, and the potential changes slightly, namely, the pathway of sodium ion production on the membrane is blocked, leading to the transmission disorder of electrical activity. During an attack, the affected muscles fail to respond to any electrical stimulation and become paralyzed. The main pathological changes are vacuolation of muscle sarcoplasmic reticulum, which contains clear fluid and few single or multiple glycogen particles. It is located in the center of the muscle fiber or even occupies the whole muscle fiber, as well as muscle tubules accumulate. Under electron microscopy, the vacuoles are caused by expansion of the sarcoplasmic reticulum terminal cistern and transverse duct system. The condition during the interval of attacks can be recovered, but not completely, so the number of small vacuoles between muscle fibers can still be seen.

(1) Clinical feature

1) Clinical manifestation

Patients at any age can occur, most are 20 ~ 40 years old male, the number of attacks decreases with the increase of age. Common inducements include fatigue, full meal, cold, alcoholism, mental stimulation and so on. There are symptoms occurred before onset, including limb pain, abnormal feeling, thirst, sweating, little urine, flushing, lethargy, nausea and so on. When sleeping at night or getting up early in the morning after a full meal, different degrees of weakness or complete paralysis can be found in the symmetry of limb muscles. Lower limbs are heavier than upper limbs, and proximal extremities are heavier than distal extremities. The upper limbs can also be gradually involved from the lower limbs. Muscle tone of paralyzed limbs is low and tendon reflexes are weakened or disappeared. It also can be accompanied by limbs acid distension, needling. Innervated muscles are generally not involved, and vesicorectal sphincter function is rarely involved. A few serious cases can manifest respiratory muscle paralysis, urine retention, tachycardia or bradycardia, arrhythmia, blood pressure drop and other symptoms which will endanger life. The duration of the attack ranges from several hours to several days. The frequency of the attack is also different, usually a few weeks or months, a few cases suffer the attack every day, or a few years or even only once a lifetime.

2) Diagnostic investigation

Serum potassium is usually lower than 3.5 mmol/L in the attack stage and normal in the interval. The ECG shows typical change of hypokalemia, U wave appears, T wave is flattened or inverted, P-R interval and Q-T interval are prolonged, ST segment is decreased, QRS wave is widened. EMG shows short duration of motor potential, low amplitude of wave, loss of motor unit potential and no response to electrical stimulation when complete paralysis exists. The membrane resting potential is lower than normal.

(2) Diagnosis

It is not difficult to diagnose based on autosomal dominant inheritance or sporadic, sudden flaccid paralysis of limbs, proximal mainly, muscle damage without cerebral nerve innervation, unconscious disorders and sensory disorders, reaching peak within a few hours to one day, also examination found decreased blood potassium, electrocardiogram hypokalemia changes and muscle weakness quickly relieved after potassium supplement treatment.

(3) Differential diagnosis

1) Periodic paralysis with high potassium

The disease generally occurs before the age of 10, and the frequency of attack is higher after daytime exercise. The duration of myasthenia symptom is short, the blood potassium increases when attacked, and the ECG shows the change of high blood potassium, which can be relieved by itself and improved after reducing blood potassium treatment.

2) Periodic paralysis with normal blood potassium

It is rare and occurs before the age of 10 years old. It often attacks at night, muscle weakness lasts longer, there is no muscle tonic performance. Blood potassium is normal, symptom aggravates after potassium, symptom alleviates after taking sodium.

3) Myasthenia gravis

Subacute onset, limbs and muscles innervated by cranial nerves are involved. The symptom shows fluctuation, which means the patients are often strongest in the morning after a full night's sleep and weakest in the evening. Fatigue test and neostigmine test are positive. Serum potassium is normal, amplitude caused by repeated nerve electric stimulation decreases, positive anti-acetylcholine receptor antibody can be distinguished.

4) Guillain-barre syndrome

This disease manifests flaccid paralysis of limbs, the distal is heavier than the proximal, and it can have peripheral sensory disorders and brain nerve damage, cerebrospinal fluid protein-cell separation phenomenon. EMG shows neurogenic damage, which can be distinguished with periodic paralysis with low potassium.

5) Secondary hypokalemia

Sporadic cases should be distinguished from diseases that may cause recurrent hypokalemia, such as hyperthyroidism, primary aldosteronism, tubular acidosis, potassium loss nephritis, diarrhea, drug-induced hypokalemia paralysis (thiazide diuretics, corticosteroids and so on). But all the above diseases have other special symptoms of the primary disease that can be distinguished.

(4) Treatment and prognosis

During the attack, 40~50 mL of 10% potassium chloride or 10% potassium citrate can be taken orally within 24 hours, with a daily total of 10 g. Potassium chloride solution may also be administered intravenously to correct hypokalemia. For patients with frequent attacks, potassium salt can be taken orally at the inter-attack stage of 1 g, 3 times a day; 200 mg of spironolactone should be taken twice a day to prevent attacks. At the same time, avoid all kinds of causes such as avoid overwork, cold and mental stimulation, low sodium diet, avoid excessive intake of high carbohydrate. Severe patients with respiratory muscle paralysis should be assisted to breath, serious arrhythmia should be actively corrected. The prognosis is good and the attack number tends to decrease along with the increase of age.

10.3 Polymyositis and Dermatomyositis

Polymyositis (PM) and dermatomyositis (DM) are a group of diffuse inflammatory diseases of skeletal muscle caused by multiple etiologies, the onset of which is associated with abnormal cellular and humoral immunity. The main pathological features are skeletal muscle degeneration, necrosis and lymphocyte infiltration. It is clinically manifested as acute or subacute onset, symmetrical muscle weakness mainly in the proximal extremities with pressure pain, increased serum muscle enzymes, increased sedimentation. The electromyography is myogenic damage. The glucocorticoid treatment is effective. PM lesions are limited to skeletal muscle, while DM involves both skeletal muscle and skin.

(1) Pathogenesis and pathology

The occurrence of PM and DM may be related to viral infections, and most patients have a history of influenza A and B, HIV, ECHO, and coxsackievirus infection before the disease. Genetic factors may also increase the susceptibility to PM and DM. About half of PM patients are associated with HLA-DR3, while HLA-DR52 is seen in almost all PM patients. The pathogenesis is related to immune dysregulation. Jo-1 antibody, SRP antibody, Mi-2 antibody, anti-nuclear antibody and other antibodies can be detected in the serum of some PM and DM patients, and muscle pathology reveals the infiltration of activated lymphocytes in muscle tissue, peripheral blood lymphocytes are sensitive to muscle antigens and have obvious cytotoxic effects on cultured myocytes, all of which indicate that this disease is an autoimmune disease. The inflammatory cells in PM are mainly $CD8^+$ T lymphocytes, monocytes and a small number of B lymphocytes, mostly distributed in the endomysium, but also located in the myofascia and perivascular area.

(2) Clinical feature

1) Clinical manifestation

The onset of the disease is acute or subacute, and the age of onset is not limited, but it is more common in children and adults, and more in women than men, with the disease gradually worsening and peaking in a few weeks or months. The disease may be preceded by a history of low-grade fever or cold. The first symptom of muscle weakness is usually weakness of the proximal extremities, often starting from the pelvic girdle muscle and gradually involving the shoulder girdle muscle, manifesting as difficulty in going upstairs, squatting, inability to raise the arms, difficulty in combing the hair, etc.; weakness of the cervical muscle shows difficulty in erecting the neck; weakness of the pharyngeal muscle shows difficulty in making sounds and swallowing; respiratory muscle involvement shows chest tightness and shortness of breath. It is often accompanied by joint and muscle pain. The extraocular muscles are usually not involved. Muscle weakness can last for several years. On examination, muscle weakness and pressure pain in the proximal extremities can be seen, and muscle atrophy and joint contracture are present in the advanced stage. Skin lesions can be seen in patients with DM, and the rash usually appears before or at the same time as muscle weakness. The typical rash is an edematous mauve spot around the orbit and upper and lower eyelids and Gottron's sign, which refers to edematous erythema on the extensor surfaces of extremity joints. Other manifestations of GI tract involvement include nausea, vomiting, and crampy abdominal pain. Cardiac involvement may include syncope, arrhythmia, and heart failure. Renal involvement may include proteinuria and red blood cells. In a few cases, other autoimmune diseases such as rheumatoid arthritis, systemic lupus erythematosus, and progressive systemic sclerosis are combined. A few cases may be associated with malignant tumors, such as breast tumors, lung cancer, ovarian cancer and gastric cancer.

2) Diagnostic investigation

In the acute stage, the peripheral blood leukocytes are increased, the sedimentation is increased, and the C-reactive protein is increased. Serum CK is significantly increased, which can reach more than 10 times of normal. Myositis-specific antibodies (MSAs) Jo-1 and PL-7 are elevated. 1/3 of patients have positive rheumatoid factors and antinuclear antibodies, and immunoglobulin and anti-myosin antibodies are elevated. Urine tests have increased 24-hour urine creatine, an indicator of active myositis. Some patients may have myoglobinuria. EMG shows increased spontaneous fibrillation potentials, positive sharp waves and polyphasic waves, which are indicative of myogenic damage. The nerve conduction velocity is normal. 52%~75% of patients have ECG abnormalities with QT prolongation and ST segment decrease.

(3) Diagnosis

According to the clinical features: a. acute or subacute muscle weakness in the proximal extremities and pelvic girdle with pressure pain, weakened or absent tendon reflex; b. significant increase in serum CK; c. myogenic damage on EMG; d. typical myositis pathology on biopsy;

e. typical skin damage. The diagnosis of PM is made if the first four criteria are present, and DM is made if three or more of the first four criteria are present and the fifth one is present at the same time. Malignant tumors should be excluded in patients over 40 years old.

(4) Differential diagnosis

a. Somatic myositis needs to be differentiated from polymyositis because of inflammatory muscle damage and dysphagia. However, the muscle weakness in inclusion body myositis is asymmetric, and involvement of distal muscle groups is common, such as wrist and finger flexion weakness and foot drop. Normal or mildly elevated serum CK, eosinophilic inclusion bodies found on muscle pathology and ineffective hormonal therapy can be differentiated from polymyositis.

b. Limb-girdle myotonic dystrophy is differentiated from polymyositis by weakness and atrophy of the proximal extremities and the pelvic and scapular girdles, and by increased muscle enzymes. However, limb-girdle myotonic dystrophy often has a family history, no myalgia, and a slower disease course, and the muscle pathology is characterized by muscle fiber degeneration, necrosis, atrophy, and adipose tissue replacement without significant inflammatory cell infiltration.

c. Myasthenia gravis polymyositis is bedridden in the late stage, with difficulty in dysarthria and swallowing, which should be differentiated from this disease. Myasthenia gravis can be excluded based on the absence of significant fluctuations in the former condition, insensitivity to anticholinesterase drug therapy, and increased serum enzyme activity.

(5) Treatment

Adrenal glucocorticoid is the drug of choice for polymyositis. The common method is: prednisone 1~1.5 mg/(kg · d), the maximum dose of 100 mg/(kg · d). Generally after 4~6 weeks, clinical symptoms improve, CK drop close to normal. The dose will be gradually reduced, generally by 5 mg every 2 weeks to 30 mg/(kg · d), and then by 2.5~5 mg every 4~8 weeks, finally reaching a maintenance dose of 10~20 mg/(kg · d) for 1~2 years. Special attention should be paid to the fact that the symptoms of myositis are not easily controlled when the amount of hormone is insufficient, and the symptoms are easily fluctuated if the amount is reduced too quickly. In acute or severe cases, high-dose methylprednisolone 1 000 mg can be used for 3~5 days, and then the dose can be gradually reduced. Long-term adrenal glucocorticosteroid treatment should be prevented by giving a low-sugar, low-salt and high-protein diet, protecting the gastric mucosa with antacids, paying attention to potassium and Vitamin D supplementation, and treating patients with tuberculosis accordingly. Immunosuppressants are added when hormonal therapy is unsatisfactory. The first choice is methotrexate, followed by thiotrexate, cyclophosphamide and cyclophilin A. During the drug administration, attention should be paid to leukopenia and regular liver and kidney function tests. Immunoglobulin is more effective when used in combination with other treatments in the acute phase. Immunoglobulin 1 g/(kg · d) for 2 days; or 0.4 g/(kg · d) intravenous drip for 5 days per month, 4 months as a course of treatment.

Supportive treatment includes high protein and vitamin diet, physical exercise and physiotherapy, and prevention of joint contracture and disuse muscle atrophy in severe cases. Patients in the acute stage should rest in bed, appropriate physical therapy should be given to maintain muscle function and avoid contractures, and attention should be paid to prevent complications such as pneumonia. The prognosis for children is good. Half of the patients with polymyositis can be cured basically. Elderly patients with tumors, especially those with significant lung, heart, and gastrointestinal involvement, have a poor prognosis.

10.4 Progressive Muscular Dystrophy

Progressive muscular dystrophy (PMD) is a group of hereditary muscle degenerative diseases, characterized by slowly progressive symmetric muscle weakness and atrophy without sensory impairment. It is mainly inherited in autosomal dominant, recessive and X-linked recessive forms. According to the genetic pattern, age of onset, distribution of the atrophied muscles, the rate of progression and prognosis, progressive myotonic dystrophy can be divided into at least nine types: Duchenne-type myotonic dystrophy (Duchenne muscular dystrophy, DMD) and Becker-type dystrophy (Becker muscular dystrophy, BMD), facioscapulohumeral muscular dystrophy (FSHD), limb girdle dystrophy (LGD), pseudohypertrophy muscular dystrophy (LHD), Emery-Dreifuss muscular dystrophy (EDMD), congenital muscular dystrophy (CMD), oculopharyngeal muscular dystrophy (OPMD), ocular muscular dystrophy (OMD), and distal muscular dystrophy. Among these types, DMD is the most common, followed by BMD, FSHD and LGD. In fact, each type is an independent genetic disease.

(1) Pathology

In all types of PMD, muscle pathology is characterized by degeneration, necrosis, atrophy and regeneration of muscle fibers, and increased inward migration of myofibrillar nuclei. As the disease progresses, the size difference of myocytes increases under light microscopy, some atrophy, some compensatory enlargement, in a mosaic distribution; there is a large number of adipocytes and fibrous connective tissue proliferation between the atrophied muscle fibers. Various types of specific protein alterations need to be detected with corresponding antibodies, such as immunohistochemical staining of muscle biopsy specimens from patients with DMD and EDMD with anti-myasthenic protein antibodies and emerin antibodies respectively, which reveal the absence of anti-myasthenic and emerin proteins and are decisive for diagnosis.

(2) Clinical feature

1) Clinical manifestation

① Large muscles pseudohypertrophy

It is caused by accumulation of large amounts of fat and fibrous connective tissue within the muscle bundle. According to the presence or absence of hydrophobic peptide of anti-myasthenic protein and the degree of protein spatial structure change and function loss, this type can be divided into two types.

a. Duchenne muscular dystrophy (DMD): DMD is the most common X-linked recessive myopathy in China, with an incidence of about 30/100 000 male infants. 1/3 of affected children are caused by new mutations in the DMD gene. Females are carriers of the causative gene and their new-born boys have a 50% probability to get this disease. It has no significant geographic or racial differences. The insidious appearance of muscle weakness in the pelvic girdle at the age of 3 to 5 is manifested by slow walking, toe landing and easy falling. Difficulty in going upstairs and standing in squatting position is due to weakness of skeletal lumbar muscles and quadriceps. The weakness of the back extensors causes the lumbar vertebrae to be excessively anteriorly convex when standing, and the weakness of the gluteus medius causes the pelvis to swing up and down on both sides when walking, showing a typical duck gait business. Due to the weakness of the abdominal and skeletal lumbar muscles, firstly, the child must turn over to a prone position when rising from a supine position, bend the knee and medullary joints to support the trunk with the hands into a prone kneeling position. Secondly, after supporting the trunk with both hands and legs together, press the knee with the hands to assist the muscle strength of the quadriceps till the body in a deep bowing position. Finally, stand up slowly with the hands attached to the lower limbs. Usually, the child's face will turn red due to great effort. The above actions are called Gowers' sign, which is the characteristic manifestation of DMD. The child with DMD sits on the floor with his hands crossed over his shoulders and cannot stand up, while the normal child can easily stand up. The scapularis and upper arm muscles are often involved at the same time, but to a lesser extent. Free shoulder is formed due to scapular band relaxation. The inner side of the scapula is far away from the chest wall when the arm is raised, and the two scapulae are winged and erected on the back, which is called winged scapula. 90% of children have pseudohypertrophy of the muscles, which is tough to touch and is one of the first symptoms. The gastrocnemius muscle is the most obvious, and the deltoid, gluteus, quadriceps, infraspinatus and triceps can also occur.

In children with DMD, serum creatine kinase is significantly elevated, up to 30 ~ 100 times the normal value; serum creatine tincture is significantly decreased. Most of the patients have myocardial damage, such as arrhythmia, high R waves in the right anterior chest leads and deep Q waves in the left anterior chest leads; enlarged heart and incomplete closure of the heart valves. The electromyography shows myogenic damage. About 30% of children have varying degrees of mental retardation. Smooth muscle damage may include gastrointestinal dysfunction, such as vomiting, abdominal pain, diarrhea, malabsorption, and megacolon. The facial muscles, eye muscles, swallowing muscles, sternocleidomastoid muscles and sphincter muscles are not involved.

With the aggravation of symptoms, significant achilles tendon contracture, foot drop and difficulty walking on flat ground appear. These symptoms help to distinguish DMD from BMD (patients with BMD can walk around the age of 12). In the advanced stage, the muscles of the lower extremities, trunk, upper extremities, medulla and shoulders are significantly atrophied, and tendon reflexes are absent, resulting in contracture of the knees, elbows and medulla. The knees, elbows, and medulla can not be straightened due to muscle contracture, scoliosis, and horseshoe inversion of both feet. The majority of patients die at the age of 20 ~ 30 due to respiratory infection and heart failure.

b. Becker muscular dystrophy (BMD): Clinical manifestations are similar to those of DMD with an incidence of 1/10 that of DMD. BMD differs from DMD in the following aspects: a slightly later age of onset (5 ~ 15 years old), slow progression, milder disease, ability to walk after 12 years of age, minimal cardiac involvement (more severe once involved), normal intelligence, and survival close to normal life span.

② Facioscapulohumeral muscular dystrophy (FSHD)

FSHD is an autosomal dominant inheritance. Most often it starts in adolescence. The muscles of the face and scapular girdle are the first to be affected, with little facial expression, weak eyelid closure or exposed sclera, difficulty whistling and cheek puffing, gradually extending to the scapular girdle, deltoid, biceps, triceps, and upper part of the pectoralis major. Scapular girdle and atrophy of the arm muscles is very pronounced and often asymmetric. The lips are thickened and slightly curved due to pseudohypertrophy of the orbicularis oris muscle, which is called "myopathic face". Pseudohypertrophy of the coracobrachialis muscle can be seen. The disease progresses slowly and gradually involves the muscles of the trunk and pelvic girdle, with pseudohypertrophy of the gastrocnemius muscle, retinopathy and hearing impairment (neurological deafness). Electromyography is myogenic and serum enzymes are normal or mildly elevated. The diagnosis can be confirmed by blot hybridization DNA analysis to determine the number of long, terminal 3.3 kb/KpnI repeat fragments on chromosome 4.

③ Limb-girdle muscular dystrophy

Limb-girdle muscular dystrophy is inherited autosomally recessive or dominant, and disseminated cases are more frequent. Compared with dominant inheritance, patients with recessive inheritance are more common, more symptomatic, and have an earlier onset of 10~20 years old. The first symptoms are mostly pelvic girdle muscle atrophy, lumbar lordosis, duck walk, proximal weakness of the lower limbs and difficulty in going upstairs, and there may be pseudohypertrophy of the gastrocnemius muscle. Gradually, atrophy of the scapular band muscles occurs, with difficulty in raising the arm and combing hair, and pterygoid scapula. Facial muscles are generally not involved. The knee reflex disappears earlier than the ankle reflex. Serum enzymes are markedly elevated, electromyography is myogenically impaired, and electrocardiography is normal. The disease progresses slowly, with an average of about 20 years of incapacity after the onset of disease.

④ Oculopharyngeal muscular dystrophy (OPMD)

OPMD is an autosomal dominant disorder that begins around the age of 40 with symmetrical ptosis and ocular motility disorders as the first symptoms. Mild facial and ocular muscle weakness and atrophy, dysphagia, dysphonia, and proximal limb weakness gradually appear. Serum CK is normal or mildly elevated.

⑤ Emery-Dreifuss muscular dystrophy (EDMD)

EDMD is an X-linked recessive disorder with a slow onset at the age of 5 to 15. The clinical features of EDMD are flexion contracture of the elbow and shortening of the achilles tendon early in the disease, limitation of forward neck flexion, and difficulty in bending and turning due to spinal ankylosis. The affected muscles are mainly biceps, triceps, peroneus brevis and anterior tibialis, followed by weakness and atrophy of the pelvic girdle muscles and proximal muscles of the lower extremities. Intelligence is normal. Cardiac conduction dysfunction is manifested by bradycardia, syncope, atrial fibrillation, etc. The heart is enlarged and myocardial damage is evident. Serum CK is mildly elevated. The disease progresses slowly, and patients often die from heart disease.

⑥ Other types

a. Ocular muscle type: Also known as Kiloh-Nevin type, it is rare. It starts slowly at the age of 20 to 30 and initially presents with bilateral eyelid ptosis with head tilt and frontal muscle contraction, and later involves the extraocular muscles. There is no limb muscle atrophy or loss of tendon reflexes in this type.

b. The distal type: It is less common, autosomal dominant and starts at the age of 10~50, muscle weakness and atrophy begins in the distal extremities, around the wrist and ankle joints and the small muscles of the hands and feet, such as the large and small fissure muscle atrophy. The extensor muscles are significantly involved and may progress proximally. There is no sensory impairment or autonomic damage. The common subtypes are Welander, Finnish, Nonaka, and Miyoshi types.

c. Congenital myotonic dystrophy: The disease begins at birth or in infancy and presents with severe generalized muscle weakness, hypotonia, and bony joint contractures. The facial muscles may be mildly involved, the pharyngeal muscles are weak, the cry is weak, and the sucking power is weak. There may be extraocular muscle paralysis, and the tendon reflexes are weak or absent.

2) Diagnostic investigation

Serum enzyme tests include creatine kinase (CK), lactatedehydrogenase (LDH), and creatine kinase-MB (CK-MB). Abnormal and significantly elevated (20 ~ 100 times normal) values are seen in DMD, BMD, Miyoshi subtype of distal muscular dystrophy, and LGMD types 2C, 2D, 2E, and 2F. Mild to moderate elevations of other types of myokines are seen. In the late stages of DMD and LGMD2, serum CK values may be significantly decreased due to severe muscle atrophy in patients. Other serum enzymes such as glutamate oxaloacetate aminotransferase and glutamate pyruvate aminotransferase can be mildly-moderately elevated in the progressive stage.

Electromyography has typical signs of myogenic impairment. When the quadriceps or deltoid muscle is examined with a needle electrode, fibrillation waves and positive sharp waves are seen at rest; during light contraction, the time frame of motor unit is shortened, wave amplitude is reduced, and polyphasic waves are increased; during vigorous contraction, tonic-like discharges and pathological interference phases are seen. The nerve conduction velocity is normal.

Muscle biopsies of patients with most types of progressive muscular dystrophy show a commonality of muscle necrosis and regeneration, interstitial fat and fibrous connective tissue hyperplasia. Conventional staining methods cannot distinguish between the various types, but the presence of specific proteins in myocytes can be detected by immunohistochemistry, using specific antibodies to identify the various types of muscular dystrophy. For example, DMD and BMD can be detected with anti-myoglycan antibodies, LGMD2C with 7-sarcoglycan antibodies, LGMD2D with a-myoglycan antibodies, LGMD2E with 6-myoglycan antibodies and EDMD with Emerin antibodies.

Genetic testing using PCR, MLPA, blot hybridization, DNA sequencing and other methods can detect genetic mutations for genetic diagnosis. Other tests such as X-rays, ECG, and echocardiogram can provide early detection of the extent of cardiac involvement in patients with progressive muscular dystrophy.

(3) Diagnosis

Based on clinical presentation, genetic pattern, age of onset, family history, serum enzyme measurement, electromyography, muscle pathology and genetic analysis, it is not difficult to make a diagnosis. If the genetic test is negative or it is difficult to detect all mutation points, immunohistochemical testing of muscle tissue with specific antibodies can clarify the diagnosis.

(4) Differential diagnosis

a. Juvenile proximal spinal muscular atrophy, which starts in adolescence, has a symmetrical distribution of proximal muscle atrophy of the extremities and needs to be differentiated from limb-girdle muscular dystrophy. However, the disease is mostly associated with myotonic tremor; the EMG is neurogenic damage with huge potentials; and the pathology is neurogenic myasthenia gravis, which can be differentiated.

b. Chronic polymyositis is differentiated from limb-girdle muscular dystrophy because of symmetrical proximal limb weakness. However, there is no genetic history of this disease, and the disease progresses rapidly, often with myalgia, increased serum muscle enzymes, muscle pathology consistent with myositis, and effective treatment with adrenal glucocorticoids, so it is not difficult to differentiate.

c. Amyotrophic lateral sclerosis needs to be differentiated from distal muscular dystrophy because of the weakness and atrophy of small muscles in the hands. However, in addition to myasthenia gravis, this disease also has muscle jumping, high muscle tone, hyperactive tendon reflexes and positive pathological reflexes, which are easy to differentiate.

d. Myasthenia gravis is mainly distinguished from oculopharyngeal type and oculomotor type. Myasthenia gravis is characterized by easy fatigue and fluctuation, positive neostigmine test, and low frequency repetitive electrical stimulation of electromyography can also be distinguished.

(5) Treatment and prognosis

PMD has no specific treatment so far, only symptomatic treatment and supportive treatment, such as increasing nutrition and proper exercise. Physiotherapy and orthopedic treatment can prevent and improve spinal deformity and joint contracture, especially early correction of ankle contracture, which is important to maintain walking function. Drugs can be used such as ATP, inosine, Vitamin E, and Chinese medicine can be selected. Since there is no effective treatment yet, it is especially important to detect carriers, perform prenatal diagnosis, and abort the affected fetus. First of all, the genotype of the affected child should be determined, and then determine whether the mother is a carrier. When the carrier is pregnant, we will determine whether the fetus is a male or female, perform prenatal genetic diagnosis on the male fetus, and terminate the pregnancy if it is a diseased fetus to prevent the birth of the affected child.

Patients with DMD die of respiratory failure or heart failure in their 20s; patients with LGMD2C, 2D, 2E, 2F also have a poor prognosis; patients with FSHD, BMD, oculopharyngeal and distal myotonic dystrophy have a better prognosis, and some patients can live close to normal life years.

10.5 Mitochondrial Myopathy and Mitochondrial Encephalomyopathy

Mitochondrial myopathy and mitochondrial encephalomyopathy are a group of disorders in which defects in mitochondrial DNA (mtDNA) or nucleus DNA (nDNA) cause mitochondrial. The common features are extreme fatigue and weakness after mild activity, which improves after rest; muscle biopsy reveals broken red fibers (ragged red fiber, RRF). If the lesion mainly invades skeletal muscle, it is called mitochondrial myopathy; if the lesion also involves the central nervous system, it is called mitochondrial encephalomyopathy. The cause of mitochondrial myopathy and mitochondrial encephalomyopathy is the mutation of mtDNA so that the enzymes or carriers necessary to encode mitochondria in the process of oxidative metabolism are impaired. The mitochondrial disease is caused by a lack of energy to maintain normal physiological functions of the cell and induce apoptosis.

(1) Pathology

RRF caused by a large number of degenerated mitochondrial aggregates, can be seen in frozen sections of muscle biopsies by Gomoritrichrome (GT) staining. It is mainly seen in type Ⅰ muscle fibers, and oil red staining and glycogen staining also reveal fat and glycogen accumulation. Positive SDH staining of the vascular wall within the muscle tissue helps to diagnose mitochondrial encelhalomyopath with lactic acidosis and stroke-like episodes (MELAS). The lesions of the cerebral brain are complex and diverse, with extensive involvement. Patients with MELAS also have focal softening of the parieto-occipital cortex, cortical atrophy and calcification of the basal nuclei, intracranial multifocal necrosis with small vessel proliferation and astrocytosis, and focal or laminar sponge-like changes. The nuclei of myoclonus epilepsy ragged-red fibers (MERRF) patients may have dentate nuclei, red nuclei and pale globules, etc.

(2) Clinical feature

1) Clinical manifestation

The disease can occur at any age, with chronic progression, and can involve multiple systems, with complex and diverse clinical manifestations. Skeletal muscle and brain are the most susceptible to symptoms due to their rich mitochondrial content and high energy demand. The clinical picture is divided according to the tissue involved.

① Mitochondrial myopathies

Mitochondrial myopathies most often start in the early 20s, and also in children and middle-aged people. It is often characterized by muscle weakness and inability to tolerate fatigue, which is often felt after mild activity and improves after rest, often accompanied by muscle pain and pressure, without the phenomenon of "strongest in the morning after a full night's sleep and weakest in the evening".

② Mitochondrial encephalomyopathies

Mitochondrial encephalomyopathies mainly include:

a. Chronic progressive external ophthalmoplegia (CPEO): It can develop at any age, with more cases starting in childhood. The first symptom is eyelid ptosis and ocular muscle paralysis, which slowly progresses to total ophthalmoplegia and ocular motility disorders. Some patients may have pharyngeal muscle and limb weakness. They are not sensitive to neostigmine.

b. Kearns-Sayre syndrome (KSS): The disease usually starts before the age of 20 and presents with a triad of symptoms, such as CPEO, retinitis pigmentosa, and heart block. Other neurological abnormalities include cerebellar ataxia, cerebrospinal fluid protein elevation, neurological deafness and mental retardation. The disease progresses rapidly and most patients die of heart disease before the age of 20.

c. MELAS syndrome: The disease starts before the age of 40 and is more common in childhood. Clinical manifestations include stroke-like episodes with hemiparesis, hemianopia or cortical blindness, migraine, nausea and vomiting, recurrent seizures, mental retardation, short stature, and neurological deafness. The disease progressively worsens, and cranial CT and MRI show mainly occipital cerebral softening with lesions that are not consistent with the distribution of major cerebral vessels. Lactate levels in blood and cerebrospinal fluid increase.

d. MERRF syndrome: The main features are myoclonic seizures, cerebellar ataxia, often combined with mental retardation, hearing impairment and proximal limb weakness, mostly in childhood, with a clear family history, and some families with multiple symmetrical lipomas.

2) Diagnostic investigation

Lactate and pyruvate minimal exercise test: about 80% of patients are positive, i.e., blood lactate and pyruvate still cannot return to normal after 10 minutes of exercise. CSF lactate level is also increased in cerebral myopathy. Mitochondrial respiratory chain complex enzyme activity is decreased. Serum CK and LDH levels are elevated in about 30% of patients.

Muscle biopsies are described earlier in the pathology. Imaging cranial CT or MRI shows white matter encephalopathy, calcification of the basal nucleus, cerebral softening, cerebral atrophy and ventricular enlargement (Fig. 10.2). Electromyography is myogenic in 60% of patients, with a minority showing neurogenic damage or both.

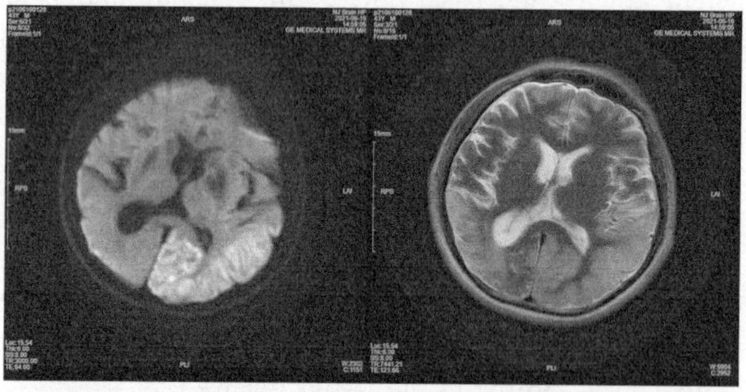

(a)

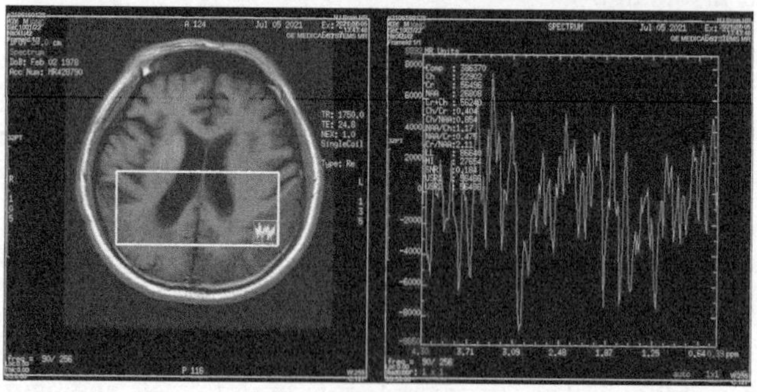

(b)

(a) MRI shows softing lesion in the right parietal-temporal-occipital lobe (mismatching to flow irrigation) with long-T_2, short-T_1 and slightly higher-DWI signals; new lesion in the left part with both long-T_2, -T_1 and markedly higher-WDI signals. Ventricle system enlargement and cerebellar atrophy also are obvious. (b) MRS shows lactate peaks and necrosis peaks in the lesion.

Fig. 10.2 A 32-male patient of MELAS syndrome for 2 years

Mitochondrial DNA analysis is decisive for diagnosis. Both CPEO and KSS syndromes are deletions of mtDNA fragments, which may occur at the time of egg or embryo formation. 80% of patients with MELAS syndrome are due to a point mutation in mtDNA tRNA leucine locus 3243. MERRF syndrome is mainly due to a point mutation at mtDNA tRNA lysine locus 8344.

(3) Diagnosis

The diagnosis can be made based on family history, typical clinical manifestations, combined with positive blood lactate and pyruvate minimum motility tests, a large number of abnormal mitochondria found on muscle histopathological examination, abnormal mitochondrial biochemical tests and mtDNA pathogenic mutations found by genetic testing.

(4) Differential diagnosis

Mitochondrial myopathy is mainly differentiated from myasthenia gravis, lipid deposition myopathy, polymyositis, and limb-girdle muscular dystrophy. In addition to the above diseases, mitochondrial encephalomyopathy should also be differentiated from multiple sclerosis, acute disseminated encephalomyelitis, cerebrovascular disease, cardiomyopathy, myoclonic epilepsy, vascular dementia, etc. However, lactate and pyruvate levels in the blood are not high in the above diseases, and muscle biopsy and mitochondrial biochemical function assay can be used to differentiate them.

(5) Treatment and prognosis

There is no specific treatment, but mainly symptomatic treatment. The main measures are as follows. Diet therapy can reduce the production of endogenous toxic metabolites. A high-protein, high-carbohydrate, low-fat diet can compensate for impaired gluconeogenesis and reduce lipolysis. Other physiotherapy can reduce pain, and pacemakers can be used for severe heart block in KSS patients. The most fundamental treatment is pending gene therapy which is under investigation. Drug therapy may include intravenous ATP 80~120 mg and coenzyme A 100~200 U once a day for 10~20 days, followed by oral ATP. Edibenone, coenzyme Q10 and a large number of B vitamins may reduce blood lactate and pyruvate levels. Levocarnitine can promote lipid metabolism and improve energy metabolism. Corticosteroid therapy may be an option if the serum muscle enzyme profile is significantly elevated. Symptomatic treatments for seizures, increased cranial pressure, heart disease, or diabetes mellitus may be essential. In addition, Chinese herbal medicines such as Huang Ying, Radix Codonopsis and Fructus Lycii can also improve the symptoms.

The prognosis is closely related to the age of onset and clinical manifestations. The earlier the age of onset and the more clinical symptoms, the worse the prognosis.

References

[1] LOUIS E D, MAYER S A, ROWLAND L P. Merritt's neurology[M]. New York: Lippincott Williams and Wilkins, 2015.

[2] DUBOWITZ V. Muscle disorders in childhood[M]. London: Saunders, 1995.

[3] MERIGGIOLI M N, HOWARD J F, HARPER C M. Neuromuscular junction disorders [M]. New York: Marcel Dekker, 2004.

(Han Wei, He Yue)

Chapter 11
Neurogenetic Diseases

Genetic disease is a disease caused by abnormalities of genetic material or determined by genetic factors. About 80% of hereditary diseases involve the nervous system, in which the disease with main clinical manifestation of neurological impairment is called genetic diseases of the nervous system. Genetic diseases of nervous system include mono-gene disease, polygene disease, chromosomal disorder and mitochondrial disease. The prevalence of mono-gene diseases of nervous system in China is about 109.3/100 000, such as Duchenne muscular dystrophy, hereditary ataxia, spinal muscular atrophy, and tuberous sclerosis. Neurogenetic diseases can occur at any age, but most start in childhood or adolescence and have familial and lifelong characteristics. The etiology and pathogenesis of many diseases have not been clarified, whose disability, teratogenic and idiotic rate are very high, and they have great harm and are difficult to treat.

(1) Pathogenesis

According to the change mode of the structure of the involved genes, the affected site, the changed form of the protein expressed by the gene and so on, the etiology and pathogenesis of the currently clear neurological genetic diseases are divided as follows.

1) Trinucleotide repeat expansion

It is a disease caused by trinucleotide repeated amplification, which results in unstable meiosis replication and abnormal gene expression products, such as Huntington's disease, partial spinocerebellar ataxia, tonic muscular dystrophy, fragile X syndrome, and Kennedy syndrome.

2) Channelopathies

Ion channel disease is a disease caused by gene mutations encoding ion channel protein subunits, which results in changes in the function of calcium, sodium, potassium, and chlorine channels, such as hypokalemic periodic paralysis, familial hemiplegic migraine, partial hereditary ataxia, benign neonatal familial convulsion and primary epilepsy.

3) Inherited metabolic disorders

Genetic metabolic disease is a disease caused by the reduction or lack of enzyme activity caused by gene mutation, thus the normal metabolic process of organic acids, sugars, fats, electrolytes, hormones and other substances can not be completed, such as the lack of metabolic end products, accumulation of substrates, increase of intermediate metabolites, and the accumulation of additional products in the body to result in toxic effects, such as glycogen disease, lipid metabolic disease, mucopolysaccharidosis, and glycoprotein disease.

4) Deposition of abnormal protein product

Extracellular deposition of amyloid plaques, caused by amyloid precusor protein (APP) gene mutations, is associated with familial Alzheimer's disease. α-synuclein gene mutation, which causes accumulation of this protein in the cytoplasm of neurons to form Lewy bodies, is associated with familial Parkinson's disease.

5) Metal ion transport disorder

Both Menkes disease and Wilson's disease are copper ion transport metabolic disorders, which are caused by the deposition or deficiency of copper ion in different tissues and organs due to different genes mutation of the metal transporter family of P-type ATPase, which results in neurological deficits.

(2) Classification

Genetic disorders of the nervous system can be divided into four main categories according to the genetic material involved, including monogenic disease, polygenic discase, chromosomal disorder and mitochondrial disease.

1) Monogenic disease

It is a disease caused by base substitution, insertion, deletion, duplication or dynamic mutation of single gene, which is inherited in Mendelian single-gene manner. Heredity includes autosomal dominant inheritance, such as Huntington's disease, hereditary spinocerebellar ataxia, and Charcot-Marie-Tooth disease; autosomal recessive inheritance, such as hepatolenticular degeneration, and spinal muscular atrophy; X-linked recessive inheritance, such as duchenne muscular dystrophy; X-linked dominant inheritance is rare.

2) Polygenic disease

It is a disease caused by the co-effect of addictive effect of multiple genes and environmental factors, also known as multifactorial disease. Epilepsy, migraine, Parkinson's disease and Alzheimer's disease are common neurological polygenic diseases. Most of polygenic diseases are sporadic, only a small part (5%~10%) is inherited in single gene manner, such as familial Parkinson's disease and familial Alzheimer's disease.

3) Chromosomal disorder

It is a disease caused by abnormal chromosome number or structure. Chromosomal abnormalities can be found directly through microscope, for example, an extra chromosome 21 can be found in patients with congenital idiopathic syndrome.

4) Mitochondrial disease

It is a disease caused by mitochondrial DNA mutation, which is inherited from the mother, including mitochondrial myopathy, mitochondrial encephalomyopathy and so on.

(3) Clinical feature

The symptoms and signs of genetic diseases of the nervous system are various, which can be divided into the common characteristics that most diseases have, the characteristic symptoms of certain diseases, and non-specific symptoms such as dystonia, muscle weakness, muscle atrophy, and paresthesia.

1) Universal characteristics

a. Early onset age. Although the onset age varies greatly, this disease is more common in children and young adults. Diseases with older onset are often related to minor functional changes caused by genetic mutations or the involvement of environmental factors, such as some types of hereditary ataxia and Wilson's disease.

b. Progressive aggravation. Defects and dysfunction caused by gene mutations tend to show characteristic of progressive aggravation.

c. Family aggregation. Dominant genetic diseases tend to have an obvious family history, while recessive genetic diseases have a history of atavism, non-immediate relatives and inbreeding.

d. Cognitive, behavioral and developmental abnormalities. It includes intellectual insufficiency, dementia, behavioral abnormalities, facial abnormalities, facial deformity, spina bifida, arcuate foot, finger (toe) deformity, skin and hair abnormalities and so on.

e. Dyskinesia. It includes language disorder, involuntary movement, ataxia, paralysis, clumsy action and so on.

f. Multi-system, multi-organ and multifunctional disorders. Mutations of single gene can affect multiple organs, leading to multifunctional disorders, such as mitochondrial encephalomyopathy.

2) Characteristic symptoms

The characteristic symptoms of certain neurological genetic diseases can be used as diagnostic basis or important hints for diagnosis, for example, the K-F ring of cornea suggests hepatolenticular degeneration, the cherry erythema of fundus suggests amaurosis and so on.

(4) Diagnosis

When finding common characteristics of the above clinical manifestations through history, symptoms, signs and routine auxiliary examinations, the possibility of genetic disease should be considered firstly, and then the diagnosis should be proposed and confirmed according to genetic special diagnosis methods, such as pedigree analysis, chromosome examination, DNA and gene product analysis. Detailed methods are as follows.

a. Clinical data collection. Note onset age, disease progression, multisystem and multifunctional disorders and unique symptoms and signs, and the possibility of neurogenetic diseases should be preliminarily proposed.

b. Pedigree analysis. Perform detailed family investigation, according to the family tree, judge whether it is hereditary disease, distinguish whether it is mono-genetic, multi-genetic or mitochondrial inheritance, dominant or recessive inheritance, and predict whether it is dynamic mutation disease according to the presence or absence of genetic premature phenomenon.

c. Routine auxiliary examination. Biochemical examinations can reveal enzyme and protein changes caused by specific genetic defects, such as increased serum creatine kinase in patients with DMD, decreased serum copper and ceruloplasmin and increased urinary copper excretion in patients with Wilson's disease. Imaging examination can detect changes in specific neural structures, such as head imaging examination of tuberous sclerosis, spinocerebellar ataxia. Pathological examination can detect characteristic changes and has diagnostic value for some neurogenetic diseases, such as Charcot-Marie-Tooth disease.

d. Detection of genetic material and gene products. It tends to achieve the diagnosis of the disease. Chromosome number detection detect chromosome number abnormalities and structural aberrations, such as congenital syndromes and chromosome diseases. DNA mutation diagnosis is widely used that mainly for mono-genetic diseases, such as the detection of Duchenne muscular dystrophy, familial amyotrophic lateral sclerosis, hereditary ataxia and other diseases. It is suitable for symptomatic patients, pre-symptomatic patients, gene carriers, fetuses at risk (prenatal diagnosis) and so on. Gene product detection mainly targets the analysis of specific proteins of genetic diseases with known gene products. For example, the dystrophin content of muscle membrane can be measured by immunohistochemical method in patients with Duchenne muscular dystrophy.

(5) Prevention and treatment

The treatment principles of this disease include alternative treatment, symptomatic treatment, rehabilitation and surgical correction, that are applied to improve patients' quality of life, neuronutrition and protective treatment is used to delay the progression of the disease. It is worth noting that early diagnosis and timely treatment can alleviate symptoms and even delay the occurrence of the disease for those preclinical patients with neurogenetic diseases. Gene therapy is being tested to cure genetic diseases by replacing, supplementing or correcting faulty genes. There is no effective treatment for most of genetic diseases of nervous system yet. Thus it is the most fundamental measure to prevent the birth of children patient and the occurrence of genetic diseases by avoiding consanguineous marriage, implementing genetic counseling, genetic testing of carriers, prenatal diagnosis and selective abortion.

11.1 Hereditary Ataxia

Hereditary ataxia is a group of genetic degenerative diseases that are characterized by chronic progressive ataxia, manifesting obvious familial genetic background and pathological changes dominated by cerebellar lesions. In addition to the involvement of cerebellum and its conduction fibers, these diseases often affect the posterior cord, pyramidal tract, pontine nucleus, basal ganglia, cranial nucleus, spinal ganglion, autonomic nervous system and so on. Clinically, they are often companied with complex and variable symptoms and signs caused by other system damage, and even patients in the same family can show high degree of clinical heterogeneity. According to different genetic modes and pathogenic genes and loci, it can be divided into: a. Autosomal dominant cerebellar ataxia (ADCA), such as spinocerebellar ataxia (SCA), dentatorubral-pallidoluysian atrophy (DRPLA); b. Friedreich type ataxia, ataxia-telangiectasia (A-T), ataxia with Vitamin E deficiency and so on; c. Sexually linked hereditary ataxia; d. Ataxia with mitochondrial disease.

Friedreich ataxia (FRDA) is the most common type of autosomal recessive hereditary ataxia, which was first reported by Friedreich (1863). It is common in Europe and America, but rare in East Asia (including China), whose prevalence rate reaches 2/100 000.

(1) Pathogenesis and pathology

In most cases, Friedreich ataxia is due to amplified mutations of the GAA trinucleotide sequence in the intron region of frataxin gene on chromosome 9 long arm 9q13 ~ q21.1. The number of GAA repeats in normal is less than 42 times, while in patients with Friedreich type ataxia, the number or length of repeats reached 66 to 1 700 copies, forming abnormal spiral structures to suppress gene transcription. The number of repeated amplifications is significantly related to the severity of the disease. The more repeated amplifications, the more severe the symptoms, and the earlier the onset age. About 4% of cases are caused by compound heterozygous mutations, that is, GAA amplification on one allele and nonsense or missense mutations on the other. Either form of the mutation results in reduced frataxin protein expression and loss of function. Frataxin is a mitochondrial matrix protein that regulates the internal environment of iron in mitochondria, whose deficiency causes the accumulation of iron in mitochondria, increasing the sensitivity of mitochondria to oxidative stress and mediating cell death through free radical release.

It manifests thinning of spinal cord, especially in the thoracic segment, degeneration of the posterior cord, spinal cerebellar tract, and corticospinal tract, loss of myelinated fibers, and glial proliferation. The nerve cells of dorsal root ganglion, especially in lumbosacral ganglion and Clarke's column, are lost and the posterior root is thinned. Peripheral nerves involved are extensive and a large number of myelinated fibers are lost. But the corticospinal tract is usually uninvolved above the craniocervical junction. The cell numbers of facial nerve, vagus nerve and sublingual nerve nucleus decreased, the nerve cells of cerebellum dentate nucleus decreased slightly to moderate, and the middle foot and upper foot of cerebellum decreased. Loss of nerve cells can be found in the vermis and lower olivary nucleus of the cerebellum. Myocardial fibers manifest hypertrophy with iron-positive particles and fibrous connective tissue hyperplasia.

(2) Clinical feature

1) Clinical manifestation

Onset age is usually 4~15. It occasionally occurs in infants and adults more than 50 years old. The first symptom is generally progressive gait ataxia, usually both lower limbs involved at the same time, manifesting standing instability and walking difficulties. When the symptoms are obvious, there are sensory and cerebellar ataxia coexist. The patients appear widened foot distance when standing, swaying from side to side, positive Romberg sign, wavering when walking, and frequent tremor of head. After months or years, ataxia developed in both upper limbs, with motor and intentional tremors. Finally, dysarthria, slow speech, slurred, violent, and even difficulty understanding speech occurred. It can be accompanied by deafness, vertigo, optic nerve rhomboid and facial muscle mild weakness. Breathing and swallowing can also be affected by ataxia. Mild muscular atrophy can be seen in late progress. Sphincter function is usually not involved. Intelligence is generally normal. Neurological examination may have horizontal nystagmus, unrestricted eye movements and pupillary reflexes. In the early stage, the position and vibration sense decreased, and in the later stage, the sense of touch, pain and temperature decreased slightly. Almost all patients have early disappearance of tendon reflex, positive Babinski sign and flexor spasm, and retained abdominal wall reflex. Clawfoot and kyphoscoliosis can be seen.

Cardiomyopathy occurs in more than half of patients and is a prominent characteristic of Friedreich type ataxia. Many patients died from arrhythmias or congestive heart failure. Kyphoscoliosis can induce restrictive respiratory dysfunction and is a cause of death. In addition, it also accompanied with diabetes or abnormal glucose tolerance.

Friedreich ataxia with retained reflexes (FARR) is a variant of Friedreich ataxia. Patients retain tendon reflexes, even hyperactivity, accompanied by limb spasm, have no scoliosis or heart disease and their prognosis are good. Another variant is late-onset Friedreich ataxia (LOFA), which starts after the age of 25 with a low incidence of skeletal deformity, normal visual evoked potential, and slow progression of the disease. There are also very-late-onset Friedreich ataxia (VLOFA) after 40 years old, and the amplification frequency of these variants is generally less than 600 times.

2) Diagnostic investigation

ECG can find ventricular hypertrophy, arrhythmia and heart block. Echocardiography can find symmetry, centripetal and hypertrophic cardiomyopathy. X-rays can manifest heart size and spinal deformity. MRI manifests thinning of the spinal cord, usually without significant cerebellar atrophy. Neuroelectrophysiological examination shows that the conduction velocity of sensory nerve is normal and the amplitude decreases significantly or even disappeares. Abnormal visual evoked potentials suggest involvement of optic nerve. The number of amplifications of FRDA gene GAA can help to diagnose.

(3) Diagnosis

According to the child or adolescent onset, autosomal recessive, progressive ataxia developed from lower to upper limb, obvious deep feeling obstacle, tendon reflex disappearance and so on, it usually can be diagnosed. If there are dysarthria, stretch after plantar reflex, scoliosis, or protrusion deformity, clawfoot, cardiomyopathy, spinal cord atrophy on MRI and the FRDA gene GAA amplification can diagnose this disease.

(4) Differential diagnosis

Atypical cases need to be distinguished with the following diseases.

a. Familial atrophy of cerebellar cortex: The onset age is late and the progress is slow, showing progressive cerebellar ataxia. Many patients have active or hyperactive tendon reflexes.

b. Charcot-Marie-Tooth disease: It is genetic peripheral neuropathy, with weak atrophic distal limbs as the main characteristic, it also can appear clawfoot.

c. Roussy-Lévy Syndrome (hereditary ataxia with myasthenia gravis): It usually occurs in infancy and has a relatively benign course, manifesting sensory ataxia (difficulty standing with eyes closed), clawfoot, loss of reflexia, and no manifestations of cerebellar involvement (dysarthria, tremor, nystagmus).

d. Vitamin E deficiency: It induces ataxia, which is difficult to distinguish from that caused by FRDA, but the absence of dysplasia, bone or heart abnormalities helps to make diagnosis of Vitamin E deficiency and further test for serum Vitamin E levels can be conducted.

e. Chronic inflammatory demyelinating polyneuropathy (CIDP): Ataxia with absent reflexes may occur in childhood onset, but the absence of dysarthria and Babinski sign can be used to distinguish from FRDA.

(5) Treatment and prognosis

At present, treatments of this disease include coenzyme Qm and other antioxidants (ubiquinone and idebenone), which have been shown to improve bioenergy metabolism of myocardium and skeletal muscle and slow down the progression of the disease in previous studies. Light cases can be treated with supportive therapy, functional training, and surgery can be used for spinal and foot deformities.

Patients may be unable to walk independently within 5 years after symptom onset, bedridden within 10~20 years, the average age of death is about 35. Survivors can effectively prolong their lives by treating heart failure, arrhythmias and diabetes and preventing complications caused by long-term disability.

11.2 Spinocerebellar Ataxia

Spinocerebellar ataxia (SCA) is the main type of hereditary ataxia that affects the cerebellum and spinal cord but without restriction. It is a highly genetic heterogeneous disease with autosomal dominant inheritance (except SCA24) and mostly appears in adults. The majority of SCA are SCA 1, 2, 3, 6, 7 and 8 subtypes. Symptoms of each subtype are generally similar but have their own characteristics. Genetic pre-mature phenomenon is a typical feature of SCA, which manifests that the onset age is advanced and the symptoms are aggravated generation by generation in the same family. SCA is related to races. SCA1 and SCA2 are common in Italy and the United Kingdom, and SCA3 is common in Japan, China, Germany, Portugal, and the United States.

(1) **Pathogenesis and pathology**

The most characteristic gene defect of autosomal dominant spinocerebellar ataxia is CAG amplification, which leads to polyglutamine diseases (polyQ diseases). The more CAG amplification, the earlier the onset. Another characteristic of CAG amplification is meiosis instability. In parental transmission, the number of repeats would change, especially in patronymic transmission, the number of repeats would increase obviously. Thus the phenomenon of early emergence is more prominent in patronymic transmission. The pathogenesis of SCA can be divided into the following: transcriptional abnormalities (SCA7/SCA17), calcium signal deficiency (SCA6), phosphorylation deficiency (SCA12/SCA14), ubiquitination and proteasome function deficiency (SCA3) and protein misfolding and chaperonin deficiency (SCA1).

The main manifestations are degeneration and atrophy of cerebellum, brainstem and spinal cord, but each subtype has its own characteristics. For example, SCA1 mainly damages spinal cerebellar bundle and posterior cord, and rarely involves substantia nigra, basal ganglia and anterior horn cells of spinal cord. SCA2 severely damages the inferior olivary nucleus, pons and cerebellum. SCA3 mainly damages pons, spinal cerebellar tracts, substantia nigra and anterior horn cells. SCA7 mainly manifests degeneration of retinal nerve cells.

Q: What are polyQ diseases?

A: Polyglutamine (polyQ) diseases are a group of neurodegenerative disorders caused by expanded cytosine-adenine-guanine (CAG) repeats encoding a long polyQ tract in the respective proteins. To date, a total of nine polyQ disorders have been described: five spinocerebellar ataxias (SCA) types 1, 2, 6, 7, 17; Machado-Joseph disease (MJD/SCA3); Huntington's disease (HD); dentatorubral pallidoluysian atrophy (DRPLA); and spinal and bulbar muscular atrophy, X-linked 1 (SMAX1/SBMA). PolyQ diseases are characterized by the pathological expansion of CAG trinucleotide repeat in the translated region of unrelated genes. The translated polyQ is aggregated in the degenerated neurons leading to the dysfunction and degeneration of specific neuronal subpopulations.

(2) **Clinical feature**

1) Clinical manifestation

The common manifestations are occult onset at the age of 30~40, the progress is slow, and there are also patients with onset in childhood or around the age of 70. Lower extremity ataxia occurs as the first symptom, which manifests wobbly walking, wide step base, easy to fall. Upper limb ataxia and dysarthria are also early symptoms. The patients will show clumsy hands and intentional tremor, poor distance discrimination. Active tendon reflex is seen in early stage, diminished tendon reflex as well as sensory disorder are seen in late stage. Ocular symptoms include eye tremors, slow saccades, dementia, dystonia, Parkinson-like symptoms, tremor of facial muscle bundles, peripheral neuropathy and muscle atrophy of distal limbs, but the frequency of these features varies in different SCA subtypes. Inability to walk usually occurs 10~20 years after onset.

2) Diagnostic investigation

CT or MRI can manifest cerebellar atrophy, and sometimes brain stem atrophy. Abnormalities of brainstem evoked potentials can occur. EMG may show peripheral nerve damage. Cerebrospinal fluid test is normal. Diagnosis of SCA and differential subtypes can be determined by molecular genetic testing.

(3) Diagnosis

According to the history and family history of ataxia, dysarthria, pyramidal tract signs and other associated symptoms and signs, combined with the data of neuroimaging, a clinical diagnosis can be determined. Besides, molecular genetic examination is helpful for the diagnosis.

(4) Differential diagnosis

Differential diagnosis needs to consider the causes of non-hereditary, acquired ataxia, such as alcoholism, multiple sclerosis, primary or metastatic tumors, paraneoplastic syndromes, and vascular diseases.

(5) Treatment

There is no specific treatment for this disease yet, symptomatic treatment can only relieve the symptoms. Amantadine can improve ataxia symptoms. Levodopa can relieve extrapyramidal symptoms such as tetania. Rehabilitation training, physical treatment and assisted walking may help improve the quality of life. Genetic counseling can be beneficial to the understanding of condition of the next generation.

11.3 Peroneal Muscular Dystrophy

Peroneal muscular dystrophy, also known as Charcot-Marie-Tooth disease (CMT), hereditary motor sensory neuropathy (HMSN) is a group of genetically heterogeneous diseases with the same clinical phenotype. CMT was first reported by Charcot, Marie and Tooth and is the most common type of hereditary peripheral neuropathy. The mode of inheritance is mainly autosomal dominant, but can also be autosomal recessive or X-linked. The distinctive features of this disease are symmetric, slowly progressive peripheral nerve myelin loss and axonal degeneration, resulting in muscle atrophy and weakness in the distal limbs. 60%~70% of CMT is caused by PMP22 repeat mutation in 17pll.2 (CMT1A), and 10%~20% is caused by GJB1 mutation in Xql3. 1 (CMTX). In addition, more than 40 CMT-causing genes or loci are identified. Clinically, CMT is usually classified into demyelinating type (CMT1) and axonal degeneration type (CMT2).

(1) Clinical feature

1) Clinical manifestation

Peroneal muscular dystrophy usually starts in childhood or adolescence, but can also start in middle age. It mainly presents with chronic progressive, symmetrical muscle weakness and atrophy of the distal limbs, sensory impairment, and decreased or absent tendon reflexes. Muscle atrophy and weakness usually begins in the foot and lower leg, and patients may develop foot drop, walk with a cross-threshold gait, have difficulty in running and walking, and be prone to tripping. Muscle atrophy of the foot can lead to bowed feet (Fig. 11.1) and hammertoe deformity. When muscle atrophy involves all of the calf muscles and the lower third of the thigh, the entire lower extremity takes on the shape of an inverted champagne bottle,

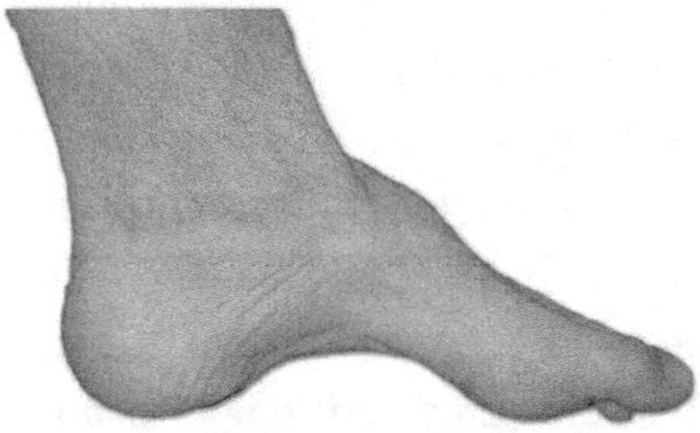

Fig. 11.1 Bowed foot

(https://www.orthobullets.com/pediatrics/)

called "crane leg". CMT muscle atrophy rarely exceeds the middle 1/3 of the elbow and thigh. Although CMT can involve sensory nerves, the symptoms of limb pain and sensory disturbance are often not prominent. Deep and superficial sensory hyperalgesia tend to show glove/sock-like sensory changes. In general, the autonomic nerves and cerebral nerves are not involved. CMT1 can palpate thick peripheral nerves, especially the greater auricular nerve and ulnar nerve. The severity of clinical manifestations of CMT patients varies widely. Some patients may have only bowed feet, or even no clinical symptoms, and only occasional neurophysiological examination may reveal abnormalities.

2) Diagnostic investigation

In CMT1, there is a significant decrease in nerve conduction velocity without conduction block, and the wave amplitude of compound muscle action potential and sensory nerve action potential is normal or decreased, while in CMT2, the nerve conduction velocity is approximately normal or slightly decreased, and the wave amplitude of compound muscle action potential and sensory nerve action potential is significantly decreased. Peripheral nerve biopsies may reveal varying degrees of demyelination and/or axonal degeneration. Genetic tests are useful in diagnosing and typing the disease. PMP22 repeat mutations and GJB1 mutations are most common in CMT and can be used as routine screening genes.

(2) Diagnosis

The diagnosis is based on the onset of the disease in childhood or adolescence, with slowly progressive symmetric bilateral lower extremity weakness, as well as "crane legs", foot drop, bowed feet, associated sensory deficits, diminished or absent tendon reflexes, slowed motor nerve conduction, demyelination and/or axonal degeneration on nerve biopsy, a positive family history, and abnormalities in genetic testing. Family history is important for the diagnosis of CMT. In patients without a clear family history, a neurological examination of the family members, especially the parents, may be helpful even if minor peripheral nerve damage or only abnormal EMG changes are found.

(3) Differential diagnosis

CMT usually progresses slowly. For peripheral neuropathy that progresses relatively quickly, other diagnoses should be considered. The sensory symptoms of CMT are often not prominent, but a careful sensory examination is still needed. CMT needs to be differentiated from the following diseases.

Distal myotonic dystrophy with progressive upward development of muscle weakness and atrophy in the distal extremities, with onset in adulthood, myogenic changes on EMG, and normal motor nerve conduction velocity. The distribution and course of myasthenia in distal spinal muscular atrophy is similar to that of CMT2. Extensive anterior horn cell damage such as fibrillation, fasciculation and giant action potentials are seen on EMG, and extensive denervation of paraspinal muscles and analogous lingual or facial muscles suggest spinal muscular atrophy. The slowly progressive course of Roussy-Lévy syndrome has peroneal muscle atrophy, bowed feet, loss of reflexes, slowed nerve conduction velocity, and nerve biopsies with demyelination and onion head structures, which are similar to CMT1, but with loss of vibriodynia and position sense, sensory ataxia, and postural tremor. CIDP progresses relatively quickly, with increased protein levels in the cerebrospinal fluid and effective hormone therapy. CIDP should be considered if the EMG shows long latency or conduction block of compound muscle action potential.

(4) Treatment and prevention

Patients with CMT usually do not lose the ability to walk and can wear orthopedic shoes for foot drop or foot deformity; when severe foot deformity causes pain or walking difficulties and conservative treatment is not effective, surgical treatment should be considered. In order to reduce walking difficulties, obesity should be avoided; drugs that may cause nerve damage, such as vincristine, should be avoided. Genetic diagnosis can be used to determine the genotype of the preexisting patient, and fetal genotype can be analyzed using fetal chorion, amniotic fluid or umbilical cord blood to determine prenatal diagnosis and terminate the pregnancy.

References

[1] ROPPER A H, SAMUELS M A, KLEIN J. Adams and Victor's principles of Neurology[M]. 10th ed. New York: McGraw-Hill Education, 2009.

[2] ROWLAND L P, PEDLEY T A. Merritt's Neurology[M]. New York: Lippincott Williams and Wilkins, 2009.

[3] HAUSER S L. Harrison's Neurology in clinical medicine[M]. New York: McGraw-Hill Education, 2009.

(Tong Xuezhi, Han Wei)

Chapter 12
Neurological Complications

Many internal medicine diseases have nerve injury more or less. The more common ones are ischemic and hypoxic neuropathy caused by heart and lung diseases of various reasons, hepatic encephalopathy, myelopathy and peripheral neuropathy caused by liver diseases, uremic encephalopathy, peripheral neuropathy, blood system diseases, metabolic diseases and tumors caused by kidney diseases. Due to the limitation of space, only some common medical diseases in department of neurology are selected here.

12.1 Diabetic Neuropathy

Diabetic neuropathy is a group of clinical syndromes caused by different pathophysiological mechanisms and diversified manifestations. It is the most common chronic complication of diabetes. The common types of diabetic neuropathy are distal symmetric polyneuropathy (DSPN) and autonomic neuropathy. DSPN is the most common type. With the increasing understanding of the nervous system damage and the widespread application of new examination methods (such as MRI, PET, electromyography and neuromuscular biopsy), the detection rate of diabetic nervous system complications increases significantly, reaching more than 50%, which is the most common complication of diabetes.

Diabetic neuropathy is the most common chronic complication of type 1 diabetes mellitus (T1DM) and type 2 diabetes mellitus (T2DM), and about 50% of diabetic patients will eventually develop DSPN. Research shows that the prevalence of DSPN through clinical diagnosis is about 45%, but when more sensitive nerve conduction assay is used for diagnosis, the prevalence of DSPN increases to 60% ~ 75%. At present, there are few epidemiological studies on autonomic neuropathy. Some studies show that the prevalence rates of T1DM and T2DM patients are 61.6% and 62.6% respectively.

(1) Etiology and pathogenesis

The etiology and pathogenesis of diabetic neuropathy have not been fully elucidated. At present, it is believed to be mainly related to a series of pathophysiological changes, including polyol pathway, glycolysis pathway, hexose amine pathway, advanced glycation end products pathway, and Toll like receptor-4 signaling pathway, resulting from abnormal blood glucose, lipid metabolism and abnormal insulin signaling pathways. Oxidized low density lipoprotein receptor-1 signaling pathway, alone or together, led to the down-regulation of cell sodium-potassium pump expression, endoplasmic reticulum stress, mitochondrial dysfunction, DNA damage, enhanced inflammatory signal and increased level of inflammatory factors.

1) Distal symmetric polyneuropathy

DSPN is the most common complication of diabetic nervous system. The lesions are usually symmetrical. The lower extremities are heavier than the upper limbs. The sensory and autonomic symptoms are the main symptoms, while the motor nerves are mild.

① Clinical feature

It is a chronic progressive disease, most of which occur symmetrically. Atypical patients can develop from one side to the other. The subjective feeling is obvious and the objective signs are not obvious. Sensory symptoms usually begin at the distal end of the lower limb, mainly including burning sensation, acupuncture sensation and electric shock sensation. They are severe at night, and sometimes the pain is severe and unbearable, affecting sleep. There can also be sensory abnormalities such as limb numbness and ant walking, which can improve after activity, and there can be glove/sock-like hypoesthesia or allergy. Autonomic nerve symptoms are more prominent. Postural hypotension may occur. In addition, the skin, pupils, cardiovascular, sweat glands and peripheral blood vessels, gastrointestinal, urogenital system can be involved. Limb weakness is mild or absent, generally without muscle atrophy. During physical examination, the deep and shallow sensation and tendon reflex of lower limbs are weakened or disappeared.

② Diagnosis

DSPN is a kind of exclusive diagnosis, and its diagnostic criteria are as follows: a. having a clear history of diabetes mellitus; b. neuropathy in the diagnosis of diabetes or after diagnosis; c. with clinical symptoms of neuropathy, such as pain, numbness, paresthesia, any abnormalities in the five examinations (ankle reflex, vibration sensation, pressure sensation, temperature sensation, acupuncture pain sensation); without clinical symptoms, any two abnormalities in the five examinations; d. except neuropathy caused by other reasons. If the diagnosis cannot be made according to the above examination and differential diagnosis is required, neuroelectrophysiological examination can be performed.

2) Autonomic neuropathy

Autonomic neuropathy includes cardiovascular autonomic neuropathy, gastrointestinal autonomic neuropathy and urogenital autonomic neuropathy.

a. Cardiovascular autonomic neuropathy can be asymptomatic in the early stage, and can only be detected by reducing heart rate variability (HRV) through deep breathing. Due to the dysfunction of cardiac vagus nerve and sympathetic nerve, the late stage can be characterized by resting tachycardia and orthostatic hypotension. Patients with orthostatic hypotension can also have the disappearance of diurnal changes of blood pressure, supine hypertension and postprandial hypotension at night, as well as exercise intolerance, syncope, asymptomatic myocardial infarction, cardiac arrest and even sudden death. HRV, blood pressure measurement during posture change, 24-hour ambulatory blood pressure monitoring and other methods can be used to assist diagnosis.

b. The main clinical manifestations of gastrointestinal autonomic neuropathy include esophageal motility disorder, gastroesophageal reflux, gastroparesis, diarrhea, fecal incontinence and constipation. Gastroparesis is mainly manifested by nausea, vomiting, early satiety, abdominal distention and upper abdominal pain.

c. Urogenital autonomic neuropathy shows sexual dysfunction and bladder dysfunction. Sexual dysfunction in men can lead to erectile dysfunction (ED) (or) reverse ejaculation. In women, it is characterized by decreased sexual desire, increased pain during sexual intercourse, decreased sexual arousal ability and decreased vaginal lubrication. Bladder dysfunction is manifested as nocturnal, urinary frequency, urgency, low flow rate, urinary retention and urinary tract infection.

3) Mononeuropathy

Diabetic mononeuropathy is a single nerve involvement, which can encroach on the cranial nerves. It can also invade the spinal nerves. If more than two nerves are involved, it is called multiple mononeuropathy. The main cerebral nerves are oculomotor nerve, abducent nerve, trochlear nerve and facial nerve. Spinal nerves often invade the superficial peroneal nerve, sural nerve, common peroneal nerve, median nerve, ulnar nerve, radial nerve and axillary nerve, and a few can invade the phrenic nerve and obturator nerve. Most of the patients are acute or subacute onset. The clinical manifestations are sensory and motor disorders in the corresponding innervated areas of the damaged nerves. The electromyography examination is mainly slow nerve conduction velocity. The course of disease can last for weeks and months, and the treatment is the same as that of multiple peripheral neuropathy.

(2) Treatment

The risk of diabetic neuropathy is huge, but there is no special treatment for diabetic nerve injury. In addition, the early clinical manifestations of diabetic neuropathy are often hidden and easily overlooked. When clinical diagnosis is made, it is often in an irreversible stage. Therefore, active prevention and early intervention of diabetic neuropathy is particularly important. It mainly includes the control of blood glucose and the change of living habits.

At present, the treatment of diabetic neuropathy is to control blood glucose, nourish nerve, resist oxidative stress, inhibit aldose reductase activity and improve microcirculation. In addition, patients with painful DSPN need to be treated with some analgesic drugs and electrical stimulation.

12.2 Neurological Complications of Thyroid Diseases

12.2.1 Nervous System Diseases of Hyperthyroidism

Hyperthyroidism, refers to the hypermetabolic syndrome involving multiple systems caused by the enhancement of thyroid function and excessive secretion of thyroid hormone. The affected systems include circulatory system, digestive system, nervous system, etc. The mechanism of nervous system damage in hyperthyroidism is unclear. It may be caused by the massive release of thyroid hormone, which accelerates the oxidation process of mitochondria in nerve cells, consumes a lot of energy, and leads to cell hypoxia and energy deficiency. The onset of the disease can be urgent or slow, and acute is common. It can coexist with hyperthyroidism crisis, mostly induced by irregular medication or withdrawal, or it can exist independently. On the basis of hyperthyroidism or hyperthyroidism crisis symptoms, fever with central nerve damage and mental abnormalities can occur, including the following four types.

a. Thyrotoxic encephalopathy can have different degrees of consciousness disorder, a large number of illusions and hallucinations and obvious psychomotor excitement, and the patient can quickly enter a coma state. It can also be manifested as decortication, seizures, bulbar paralysis, pyramidal tract involvement, spinal thalamic tract involvement, extrapyramidal system involvement, etc. Mental disorders can be excited or depressed. Cerebrospinal fluid is colorless and transparent, the number of cells is normal, and there may be increased pressure and protein. EEG shows moderate and severe abnormalities, mainly diffuse high amplitude slow waves. In the early stage of brain CT, most of them are normal, and there are uneven low-density lesions in frontotemporal region, semioval center and basal nucleus. Abnormal signals of long T_1 and long T_2 in corresponding parts can be seen on head MRI.

b. Acute thyrotoxic myopathy is rare, which is characterized by rapidly developing muscle weakness. In severe cases, soft paralysis can occur within a few days. It often invades pharyngeal muscles and causes dysphagia and dysphonia, and even involves respiratory muscles, causing respiratory paralysis. For some patients, it can invade the muscles dominated by eye muscles and other brain nerves. Tendon reflex often decreases or disappears, muscle atrophy is not obvious, sphincter function is preserved, and there is no sensory impairment.

c. Chronic thyrotoxic myopathy is very common, especially in middle-aged and elderly men, and rare in children. It is characterized by progressive muscle atrophy and decreased muscle strength, while the symptoms of hyperthyroidism are not obvious. It is easy to invade the proximal muscle, and the extensor muscle is more vulnerable than the flexor muscle. For some patients, it can invade the distal muscle and facial muscle at the same time, but there is no simple distal muscle atrophy. Generally, the degree of muscle atrophy is consistent with that of muscle weakness, but there are also those with obvious decline in muscle strength but no obvious atrophy, especially female patients. The disease often invades both sides at the same time, and a few can be mainly unilateral. Tendon reflexes are normal or excessive. Some patients with atrophic muscles can be accompanied by bundle fibrillation.

d. The probability of thyroid toxic periodic paralysis is 1.9% ~ 6.5%, common in men. The attack characteristics are the same as those of familial periodic paralysis, that is, limb soft paralysis often occurs suddenly at night or in the quietness of the day, mainly involving the proximal muscles, and rarely involving the trunk, head and neck. It can be accompanied by autonomic nerve disorders, such as bradycardia or tachycardia, hypotension, vomiting, thirst, hyperhidrosis, paralysis, edema and decreased blood potassium, but potassium supplementation did not improve muscle strength.

12.2.2 Hypothyroid Neuropathy

Hypothyroidism induced brain damage is mainly manifested in varying degrees of neuropsychiatric symptoms such as mild memory loss, slow reaction, mental depression, apathy, mild intellectual impairment, etc; severe cases include unstable gait, ataxia, lethargy, dementia, insanity, and even hypothyroid coma. Hypothyroidism, if congenital or occurring in the early postnatal period, can cause mental dysplasia and mental retardation.

Hypothyroid cerebral neuropathy includes olfaction, taste, vision and hearing loss, true vertigo, blurred vision and visual field defects. Visual changes are generally believed to be caused by compression of the optic nerve by pituitary enlargement secondary to hypothyroidism. In addition, there can also be trigeminal neuralgia and facial paralysis.

Hypothyroid spinal neuropathy is more common, which is characterized by sensory abnormalities in the distal extremities, such as tingling, numbness and burning sensation. Some patients are accompanied by sensory symptoms, such as tremor, pain and tactile disorders; some patients have glove/sock-like sensory impairment.

In addition, hypothyroidism can easily lead to obstructive sleep apnea hypopnea syndrome

(OSAHS), resulting in dizziness, drowsiness and impaired cognitive function.

After thyroxine treatment, most of the clinical symptoms can disappear quickly and the prognosis is good.

12.2.3 Hashimoto Encephalopathy

Hashimoto encephalopathy (HE) is an encephalopathy associated with autoimmune thyroid diseases. Acute or subacute onset, which can show a variety of clinical symptoms such as epilepsy, stroke like attack and mental disorder, and is a recurrent remission or progressive disease. The thyroid function of patients can be normal, hyperthyroidism or hypothyroidism. It is characterized by increase of antithyroid antibody in blood. It is sensitive to hormones. After application of adrenocortical hormone, it can have a significant therapeutic effect.

(1) Etiology and pathogenesis

At present, the etiology and pathogenesis of HE are not clear. Most scholars believe that HE is a disease caused by autoimmune reaction involving CNS. Some scholars put forward the theory of angiogenic edema: multiple focal edema or diffuse brain edema in the brain caused by damage of blood-brain barrier due to immune inflammatory reaction, which can involve the brain stem and cortex, resulting in clinical symptoms such as focal neurological loss or coma, and can be rapidly relieved with the application of cortical hormone. The most common symptom is mild lymphocytic inflammatory infiltration around small blood vessels in brain parenchyma, followed by demyelination, and gray matter gliosis such as cortex, basal ganglia, thalamus and hippocampus.

(2) Clinical feature

1) Clinical manifestation

The clinical manifestations of HE are diverse and lack of specificity. HE mainly occurs in women. The gender distribution is similar to Hashimoto thyroiditis. It can be found in adults and children. The age is between 8 and 86, with an average age of 46. The age ratio is similar to that of autoimmune thyroid disease.

a. Consciousness and mental symptoms. Consciousness disorder is the most common, including the change of consciousness level and consciousness content. The change of consciousness level ranges from mild to severe, and most of them are vague. At the same time, it is accompanied by mental symptoms such as hallucination, abnormal behavior, agitation and depression.

b. Seizures. It can be manifested as complex partial seizures, focal motor seizures, myoclonic seizures, tonic seizures and generalized tonic clonic seizures; among them, generalized tonic clonic seizures secondary to complex partial seizures are common.

c. Extrapyramidal symptoms. Involuntary movement is common, myoclonus and tremor often appear in the distal ends of bilateral upper limbs. A few of them had strabismus eye clonus, choreographic movement, rhythmic myoclonus, soft palate tremor and eyelid spasm. There may be cerebral cortex symptoms such as aphasia, apraxia and dyslexia.

d. Others. It shows stroke like attack, which is a specific symptom and can occur repeatedly. A few patients may have extrapyramidal symptoms similar to Parkinsonism, auditory hypersensitivity, neuropathic muscular atrophy and demyelinating peripheral neuropathy.

2) Diagnostic investigation

a. Laboratory examination. The serum anti thyroidperoxidase antibodies (anti-TPO) and/

or antithyroglobulin antibodies (anti TG) are significantly increased, which could be more than 30 times higher than normal; anti thyroid stimulating hormone (TSH) receptor antibody increases slightly; anti MBP antibody is positive; other immunological tests and routine laboratory tests show no abnormalities. Thyroid function is normal.

b. Cerebrospinal fluid examination. The pressure of cerebrospinal fluid can be high, the protein is mostly slightly or moderately increased, the oligoclonal band is also mostly abnormal, and the number of lymphocytes in some patients increases slightly.

c. Electroencephalogram (EEG). Most of the EEG show nonspecific abnormalities, such as diffuse slow wave or focal slow rhythm (mostly in temporal lobe and frontal lobe), triphasic wave, epileptic activity and light source paroxysmal response. EEG abnormalities are often related to the clinical process of the disease, which can judge the progress of the patient's condition.

d. Cranial MRI. Cortical and/or subcortical changes can occur, the most common brain atrophy, diffuse white matter abnormalities and meningeal enhancement are also reported, but they are nonspecific.

(3) Diagnosis

Due to the diversity of clinical symptoms and the lack of specific diagnostic criteria, the diagnosis of HE is often difficult. At present, according to the clinical manifestations of nervous system involvement, the serum antithyroid antibody (especially anti-TPO) is increased, the CSF protein is high, and there is no specific finding on brain CT and MRI. HE can be diagnosed after excluding other encephalopathy that can cause similar symptoms.

(4) Treatment

HE is an autoimmune disease, so its treatment is mainly immunomodulatory treatment. The most commonly used is adrenocortical hormone. The disease is relieved in about a week. The response to hormone at the time of recurrence is the same as that at the beginning. Other immunosuppressants such as azathioprine and methotrexate can also be used. And immunoglobulin or plasma exchange therapy can also be tried.

12.3 Systemic Lupus Erythematosus Encephalopathy

Systemic lupus erythematosus (SLE) is an immune disease that produces a variety of autoantibodies due to cellular and humoral immune dysfunction, involving the central nervous system. When neuropsychiatric symptoms occur, it is called neuropsychiatric systemic lupus erythematosus (NPSLE).

The occurrence and development of NPSLE is immune injury caused by multiple factors on the basis of SLE. NPSLE with diffuse higher cortical dysfunction is mostly related to anti neuronal antibody and anti ribosomal protein antibody; NPSLE with focal neurolocalization signs may be accompanied by positive antiphospholipid antibody or systemic vasculitis and obvious disease activity.

(1) Clinical feature

a. Headache. It is the most common symptom of NPSLE, mainly migraine, followed by tension headache. Migraine can occur alone before the diagnosis of SLE. Epilepsy can occur in the early stage of the disease, and most commonly in the late stage of the disease. Its inducement is due to the invasion of blood vessels in the motor center of the anterior central gyrus of the cerebral cortex, hypertension, uremia, brain edema, increased intracranial pressure, etc.

b. Cerebral vascular disease. The incidence rate is 7.5%~15%, manifested as hemiplegia, aphasia, visual field loss and so on. The causes of the disease are small vessel vasculitis, blood vessel occlusion, bleeding, low platelet, intracranial or intracerebral hemorrhage, hypertension, uremia, hypertensive encephalopathy, cerebral edema and cerebral hemorrhage.

c. Intracranial hypertension. There are no other signs of nerve localization except optic papilledema. During CSF inspection, only the pressure increases, C4 decreases, and the rest are normal.

d. Cranial nerve paralysis. The manifestations are vision loss, double vision, eyelid ptosis, eye position deviation, facial numbness, mouth eye deviation, salivation, hearing loss, dysphagia, drinking water choking cough, abnormal pronunciation, etc.

e. Myelopathy. The incidence rate is 3%~4%, myelopathy often occurs in the active phase of SLE. The lesion often occurs in the thoracic segment. It often presents with weakness of the lower extremities, even paraplegia. Transverse myelitis has a poor prognosis and often dies of secondary infection.

f. Mental symptoms. Patients may have psychotic reactions, such as hallucinations, delusions, numbness, fear and a sense of control; emotional disorders and neuroticism, such as mania, depression, anxiety, hysteria, and hypochondriasis; and organic encephalopathy syndrome, such as cognitive impairment, disorientation, inattention, poor memory and abnormal behavior.

(2) Diagnosis

At present, there is no unified classification and diagnostic standard for the diagnosis of NPSLE. It is generally believed that the diagnosis can be made with clinical manifestations such as epilepsy, mental symptoms and local brain signs suddenly appear in the course of systemic lupus erythematosus. Imaging shows brain parenchymal damage and excludes other diseases.

(3) Treatment

a. General treatment. Stay in bed and keep urine unobstructed; control the amount of liquid and pay attention to the balance of water and electrolyte; for those with severe headache, excitement and irritability, choose analgesic sedatives as appropriate; pay attention to protecting brain cells, especially those in coma, and give drugs to promote brain cell metabolism and body recovery, such as adenosine triphosphate, coenzyme A, cytochrome C, cerebrolysin, cytidine diphosphate choline, B vitamins, etc.

b. Treatment of SLE. Hormone shock therapy, such as methylprednisolone intravenous drip. Intrathecal injection of dexamethasone and methotrexate can effectively alleviate the symptoms and control the condition of patients with lupus encephalopathy.

c. Treatment of neurological symptoms. Anticoagulant therapy can be used when patients are in hypercoagulable state, such as cerebral infarction due to thrombosis; patients with epilepsy should be given antiepileptic drugs, and patients with mental symptoms should be given antipsychotic drugs. In case of intracranial hypertension, 20% mannitol, 50% glucose solution, hypertonic saline, etc. can be used.

12.4 Subacute Combined Degeneration of Spinal Cord

Subacute combined degeneration (SCD) of spinal cord is a degenerative disease of the central and peripheral nervous system caused by insufficient intake, absorption, binding, transport or metabolism of vitamins. The lesions mainly involve the posterior funiculus, lateral funiculus and peripheral nerves. The clinical manifestations are deep sensory loss of both lower extremities, sensory ataxia, spastic paralysis and peripheral neuropathy, often accompanied by clinical signs of anemia.

(1) Pathogenesis and pathology

The disease is related to vitamin B_{12} deficiency. Vitamin B_{12} deficiency leads to insufficient synthesis of nuclear proteins, which affects the methylation of the central nervous system, resulting in demyelination and axonal degeneration. Because vitamin B_{12} is also involved in the synthesis of hemoglobin, the disease is often accompanied by malignant anemia. Atrophic gastritis, subtotal gastrectomy and congenital defects of endocrine factors lead to the lack or deficiency of internal factors. Ileal resection and localized enteritis affect the absorption of vitamin B_{12}. Deficiency of adenosine cobalamin transporter in the blood can lead to the disturbance of vitamin B_{12} metabolism. As folic acid metabolism is related to vitamin metabolism, folic acid deficiency can also produce corresponding symptoms and signs.

The lesions are mainly in the posterior funiculus and pyramidal tract of the spinal cord, and in severe cases, the white matter, optic nerve and peripheral nerve could be involved in varying degrees. Mild atrophy can be seen in the brain, common peripheral neuropathy, demyelination and axonal degeneration can be seen. Demyelinating changes in white matter can be seen in the spinal cord section. Microscopically, myelin swelling, vacuole formation and axonal degeneration are seen. At first, the lesions are scattered, and then fuse into a spongy necrotic focus with varying degrees of glial proliferation.

(2) Clinical feature

1) Clinical manifestation

Most of the disease occurs after middle age, conceals the onset, and progresses slowly. In the early stage, there is a history of anemia, burnout, diarrhea and glossitis, accompanied by a decrease in serum vitamin B_{12}, which often precedes the appearance of nervous system symptoms. The neurological symptoms are weakness of both lower limbs, stiffness, clumsy movement of both hands, unstable gait, feeling of stepping on cotton, stumbling gait, broadened base, positive Romberg sign and so on. Then there are persistent tingling, numbness and burning sensation at the ends of fingers and toes. The disturbance of vibration sensation and position sensation of both lower limbs are examined, which is obvious at the distal end. The objective examination of limb sensation is more normal, and a few patients have decreased glove/sock-like sensation. In some patients, a touch inductance radiating downward from the back of the spine occurs during neck flexion. Both lower limbs can show incomplete spastic paralysis, which is characterized by increased muscle tone, hyperreflexia of tendon and positive pathological signs. If the peripheral neuropathy is severe, it shows decreased muscle tone and weak tendon reflex, but the pathological signs are often positive. Optic nerve atrophy and central scotoma can be seen in a few patients, suggesting that the white matter and optic nerve are widely involved, rarely affecting other brain nerves. Sphincter dysfunction appears later.

Besides, mental abnormalities such as irritability, depression, hallucinations, insanity, paranoid tendencies, cognitive impairment and even dementia can be seen.

2) Diagnostic investigation

a. Peripheral hemogram and bone marrow smear examination. Examination shows that giant cell hypochromic anemia, decrease of blood reticulocyte count, decrease of vitamin B_{12} content (normal value 220~940 pg/mL), injection of vitamin B_{12} 1 000 μg/d, 10 days after reticulocytosis is helpful for diagnosis. Patients with normal serum vitamin B_{12} content should do Schilling test (oral radionuclide ^{57}Co labeled vitamin B_{12}, determine its excretion in urine and stool), the disturbance of vitamin B_{12} absorption can be found.

b. Gastric juice analysis. Antihistamine-induced gastric acid deficiency could be found by gastric juice analysis after injection of histamine.

c. MRI can show the location of spinal cord lesions, showing striped and patchy lesions with low signal intensity on T_1 and high signal on T_2 (Fig. 12.1). T_2 sequence of C4-T_2 segments shows slightly high signal intensity in the sagittal plane of the spinal cord, and high signal intensity in the axial position of the posterior funiculus and lateral funiculus of the spinal cord, showing a "three-point sign".

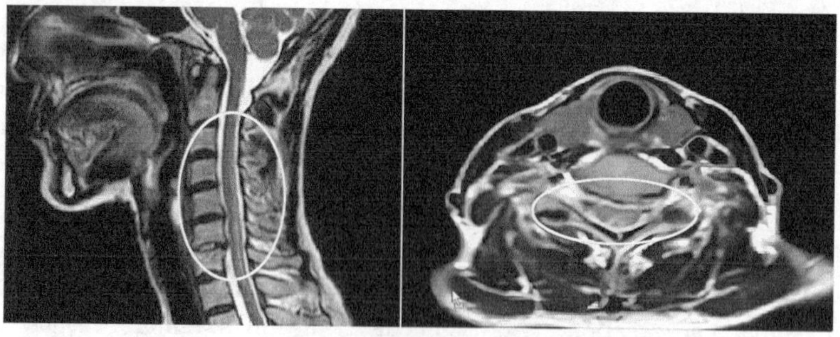

Fig. 12.1 MRI-T_2 findings of SCD in spinal cord

(3) Diagnosis

According to the symptoms and signs of slowly concealed onset, posterior funiculus, lateral funiculus and peripheral nerve damage, vitamin B_{12} deficiency in serum, malignant anemia is not difficult to diagnose. If the diagnosis is not clear, experimental treatment is feasible to assist the diagnosis: in patients with serum vitamin B_{12} deficiency and abnormal increase of serum methylmalonic acid, if the serum methylmalonic acid decreases to normal after vitamin B_{12} treatment, the diagnosis is supported.

(4) Differential diagnosis

a. Combined system disease of non-pernicious anemia type. This is an endogenous spinal cord disease involving the posterior and lateral funiculus of the spinal cord and has nothing to do with malignant anemia. The difference between this syndrome and subacute combined degeneration is that the damage of corticospinal tract appears earlier and more obvious than posterior cord damage in the whole course of the disease, and its progress is slow, and little is known about its pathology and etiology.

b. Spinal cord compression has nerve root pain and sensory disturbance. Cerebrospinal fluid dynamic test shows partial or complete obstruction, and cerebrospinal fluid protein increases, which can be distinguished by myelography and MRI.

c. Multiple sclerosis shows subacute onset, with an obvious history of remission and recurrence, and is generally not accompanied by symmetrical peripheral nerve damage. Most of the first symptoms are visual loss, including nystagmus, cerebellar signs, pyramidal signs and so on. MRI and brainstem evoked potentials are helpful for differentiation.

d. Peripheral neuropathy can be similar to peripheral nerve damage in subacute combined degeneration of spinal cord, but there are no pathological signs, no damage of posterior or lateral funiculus of spinal cord, and no evidence of anemia and vitamin B_{12} deficiency.

(5) Prevention and treatment

Early diagnosis and timely treatment is the key to improve the prognosis of the disease. If the disease can be treated actively within 3 months, most patients can recover completely. If there is still neurological dysfunction after full treatment for 6 months to 1 year, it will be difficult to recover. First, correct or treat the primary causes and diseases leading to vitamin B_{12} deficiency, such as correcting malnutrition, improving dietary structure, giving foods rich in B vitamins, and abstaining from alcohol. Once diagnosed or suspected, the disease should be treated with high-dose vitamin B_{12} immediately. The commonly used dose is 500~1 000 μg/d, intramuscular injection for 2~4 weeks. Then the same dose is given two or three times a week. After 2~3 months, 500 μg is taken orally, twice a day, for a total course of 6 months. People with vitamin B_{12} absorption disorders need to take drugs for life, and the effect of combined use of vitamin B_1 and vitamin B_6 is better. Anemic patients are treated with iron, such as ferrous sulfate 0.3 ~ 0.6 g orally, 3 times a day; or 10% ferriamine citrate solution 10 mL orally, 3 times a day. For those with malignant anemia, folic acid is recommended to be used with vitamin B_{12} 3 times a day every time 5~10 mg. Folic acid should not be used alone, otherwise it will lead to aggravation of neuropsychiatric symptoms. Patients with atrophic gastritis with lack of free gastric acid in gastric juice can take pepsin mixture or dilute hydrochloric acid mixture 10 mL 3 times a day before meals. Strengthen the functional exercise of paralyzed limbs, supplemented by acupuncture, physiotherapy and so on.

12.5 Alcoholic Encephalopathy

Alcoholic encephalopathy includes acute and chronic alcoholic encephalopathy. Chronic alcoholic encephalopathy refers to a chronic and recurrent brain disease caused by the effect of alcohol on brain tissue caused by long-term drinking, and it is a serious poisoning of the central nervous system caused by long-term excessive drinking. The cause of chronic alcoholic encephalopathy is the deficiency of ammonium sulfate (vitamin B_1) caused by gastrointestinal malabsorption. Since the beginning of the 21st century, the incidence of alcoholic neuropsychiatric disorders has continued to rise, and it has become a prominent and even the first neuromental health problem in many areas.

(1) Clinical feature

According to the clinical manifestations, onset and duration of the disease, chronic alcoholic encephalopathy can be divided into six syndromes: Wernicke encephalopathy, Korsakov's syndrome, chronic alcoholic dementia, alcoholic tremor-delirium, alcoholic epilepsy, alcoholic mental and behavioral disorders.

1) Wernicke's encephalopathy

Patients with typical Wernicke encephalopathy have three groups of characteristic symptoms: ophthalmoplegia, mental abnormality and ataxia. Ophthalmoplegia is one of the characteristic manifestations of this disease and vomiting and nystagmus are the earliest symptoms. Ataxia dyskinesia usually occurs after eye symptoms. The symptoms of most patients are so severe at the beginning that they develop into difficulty in standing and walking within a few days. Mild patients show cerebellar ataxia and are easy to fall when walking. Individual patients can also be accompanied by vague speech, incoherent pronunciation and other phenomena. More than 80% of patients have psychiatric symptoms which are sometimes hidden and need to be carefully examined by doctors.

Abnormal density and signal shadow can be seen in the third and fourth ventricles and periaqueductal papillary body, quadrigeminal body, thalamus and other parts of the head CT (Fig. 12.2). Low density changes in the aqueduct area of the midbrain (Fig. 12.2a); abnormal density and signal shadow in the third and fourth ventricles and periaqueductal papillary body, quadrigeminal body and thalamus, and slightly low density changes along the third ventricular wall (Fig. 12.2b). The low signal intensity of the white matter around the third ventricle (arrow) can be seen in the T_1WI sequence of the skull MR, while the high signal intensity can be seen on the FLAIR sequence (Fig. 12.3). Low signal intensity of white matter around the third ventricle could be seen on MRI-T_1WI axis. The MRI-FLAIR sequence shows obvious high signal intensity.

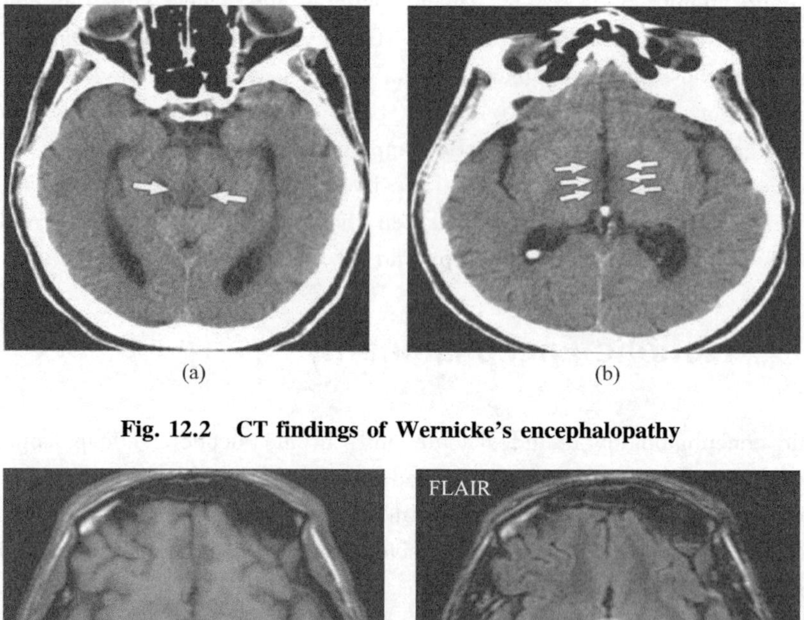

(a) (b)

Fig. 12.2 CT findings of Wernicke's encephalopathy

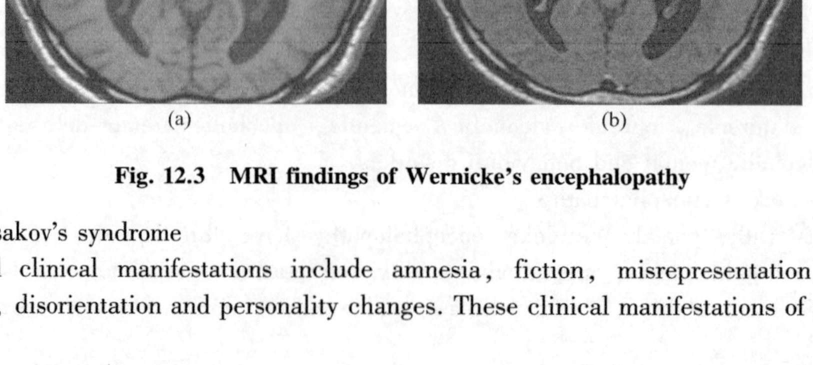

(a) (b)

Fig. 12.3 MRI findings of Wernicke's encephalopathy

2) Kosakov's syndrome

Typical clinical manifestations include amnesia, fiction, misrepresentation, cognitive dysfunction, disorientation and personality changes. These clinical manifestations of patients are often based on cognitive dysfunction, decreased learning ability and personality changes. Patients are often unable to retain new information and show signs of forgetting, but in order to fill this gap, patients describe events that happened in the past as happening at present, or fill in what he has forgotten with a paragraph of absurd, changeable, rich and varied fictional facts, and firmly believe in it. In addition, patients often show apathy in personality, lack of initiative, lack of active will and concern for the surrounding personnel, but sometimes appear selfish and stubborn, cheerful and superficial, or mood swings are very violent.

3) Chronic alcoholic dementia

Obvious cognitive impairment caused by chronic alcoholism can develop from Wernicke's encephalopathy or Kosakov's syndrome, with a significant decline in personal living ability, untidy appearance, poor personal hygiene, and the need for alcohol is more than anything else. Late speech function is also seriously damaged, only a few words, and finally bedridden, urinary incontinence, mostly died of various complications.

4) Alcoholic tremor-delirium

The disease can be promoted by trauma, infection and other factors that weaken the alcoholic's resistance. The typical prodromal symptoms are insomnia, fear and tremor. The classic triad is delirium with vivid hallucinations or delusions, behavioral disorders and obvious tremors. Tremor is mostly gross tremor, especially in fingers, face, tongue and other parts, sometimes lack of regularity, showing as swing tremor. Delirium occurs within a few days, and the patient loses orientation, accompanied by a variety of vivid hallucinations, mainly visual hallucinations, often accompanied by misrepresentation and fiction, delusions of being killed, and even suicide, self-injury or attack, impulsive performance. The disease usually lasts for several days, and the patient usually has no recollection of the experience during the disease. The fatality rate of patients without complications is lower after timely treatment, but once complications occur (such as pneumonia, heart failure), the mortality is significantly increased.

5) Alcoholic epilepsy

The clinical manifestations are many types of seizures, of which generalized tonic-clonic seizures are more common, and status epilepticus can be present in severe cases.

6) Alcoholic mental and behavioral disorders

It includes withdrawal reaction caused by long-term alcohol use disorder, and accompanying personality, emotional or mental disorders. Emotional disorders are common manifestations of depression, anxiety and others. Patients present with complex and changeable emotions, poor stability, poor response to drugs, accompanied by personality disorders, hallucinations, sleep disorders or cognitive disorders.

(2) Diagnosis

First of all, there should be a history of long-term drinking, or a history of alcohol dependence. The core symptoms/diagnostic criteria of alcohol dependence are described in DSM-4/ICD-10 as follows ($\geqslant 3$ factors within 12 months): Tolerance to alcohol (need to consume more to achieve pleasure); withdrawal symptoms/reactions after stopping drinking; excessive intake beyond control; a lot of time is spent on seeking, acquiring and ingesting alcohol; a decline in the willingness to engage in social activities; regardless of any adverse consequences (physical/psychological problems).

In view of the fact that the clinical manifestation and severity of patients may also be closely related to the type of alcohol, initial drinking time, alcohol consumption and frequency, whether drinking is accompanied by food and the functional status of the nervous system, therefore, clinicians should make a comprehensive judgment on the basis of the above-mentioned diagnostic criteria, combined with clinical manifestations and imaging features.

(3) Treatment

1) Abstain from drinking

Treatment is generally divided into the abstinence stage and the rehabilitation stage. Active drug treatment can help patients stop their dependence on alcohol and prevent the disease from relapsing.

The first-line drug treatment is as follows. Nalmefen, naloxone or naltrexone, opioid receptor antagonists, can block opioids stimulating the paraventricular nucleus of the hypothalamus and reduce patients' dependence on alcohol. Amphetamine mainly reduces patients' dependence on alcohol psychologically, but has no therapeutic effect on the core symptoms of alcohol dependence. Acarboxylic acid may block the NMDA receptor to alleviate withdrawal symptoms, such as drinking desire, anxiety, and insomnia. But its curative effect is weak, oral bioavailability is low, the curative effect is short, and the frequency of taking medicine is high.

The second-line drug treatment is as follows. Baclofen has a sedative effect in the process of abstinence, and the curative effect may be related to the drug dose and the amount of alcohol consumed before abstinence. Topiramate is effective in preventing the recurrence of alcohol dependence. However, it has certain dose-related side effects, such as abnormal sensation, taste inversion, anorexia, difficulty in concentration and skin itching. Benzodiazepines is often used to treat alcohol withdrawal symptoms such as anxiety and insomnia, and can also be used to prevent and treat seizures and delirium, but attention should be paid to the addiction of these drugs. Tricyclic antidepressants can be used to control anxiety and depression after the end of the abstinence phase. High-dose antioxidants, such as vitamin C, vitamin E, may have a certain protective effect on alcoholic encephalopathy. After drinking a lot of alcohol, ethanol metabolizes in the body to produce a large number of free radicals, and reduced glutathione can be used in the treatment of alcoholism.

2) Etiological treatment

Due to gastrointestinal malabsorption in patients with chronic alcoholic encephalopathy, oral vitamin B_1 is not effective, so intravenous administration is generally chosen. When thiamine storage is seriously insufficient, patients with acute brain injury can be induced by intake of large amounts of carbohydrate fluid, which is characterized by acute attack or aggravation of chronic alcoholic encephalopathy. Therefore, rapid thiamine supplementation in the early stage of chronic alcoholic encephalopathy is expected to be effective. For patients with chronic alcoholic encephalopathy, malnutrition, hypoglycemia and liver disease with cognitive impairment, large doses of vitamin B_1 should be supplemented through the intestinal tract before intravenous infusion of glucose.

3) Correct nutritional disorders

Malnutrition is an important factor that causes and aggravates chronic alcoholic encephalopathy. First of all, intravenous water, electrolytes, vitamin B_1 and vitamin C, etc. should be given. For patients lacking vitamin A, complex vitamin B and vitamin C, carnitine, magnesium, selenium, zinc, as well as essential fatty acids and antioxidants, nutritional supplements, especially B vitamins, contribute to rehabilitation. Secondly, help patients restore their appetite, keep their mouth clean and hygienic, eat less and eat more times, and try to meet the dietary requirements of patients. Patients are encouraged to eat foods rich in vitamins. Patients should avoid eating sugar, or drinking fruit juice, which may contain more sugar than whole fruits; reduce diets with high monosaccharide content, such as white flour and prepared potatoes; and increase the consumption of plant proteins and polysaccharides. These substances are high in cereals, legumes and vegetables.

4) Brain protection therapy

Appropriate and effective neuroprotective treatment is helpful to improve the symptoms of chronic alcoholic encephalopathy. Large doses of vitamin C and B supplements such as mecobalamin, free radical scavengers such as edaravone, mitochondrial protective agents such as coenzyme Q10, and neurotrophic drugs such as oxiracetam can be used.

5) Rehabilitation and other treatments

To maintain a certain ability of daily life and quality of life, timely rehabilitation treatment is very necessary. Acupuncture can reduce the withdrawal symptoms of alcoholics, help to prevent seizures and relapse of alcoholism, and help patients successfully complete the abstinence plan. Hyperbaric oxygen therapy can increase the aerobic metabolism of brain tissue in patients with chronic alcoholic encephalopathy, which is beneficial to accelerate the rehabilitation of patients.

12.6 Delayed Encephalopathy Caused by Acute Carbon Monoxide Poisoning

Worldwide, carbon monoxide (CO) poisoning is one of the main causes of poisoning death. After the recovery of consciousness disturbance in some patients with acute CO poisoning, a series of neurological and mental disorders may appear again after a "false-cure period" of 2~60 days, which is called delayed encephalopathy due to acute carbon monoxide poisoning (DEACMP). It is one of the common complications of acute CO poisoning, with an incidence of 30%~40%. About 25% of the patients can leave behind permanent neurological disorders, which not only significantly affect the quality of life of the patients, but also bring a huge burden to the society and families.

Actively explore the promoting factors of DEACMP in order to prevent the occurrence of delayed encephalopathy. The more serious the disturbance of consciousness in acute CO poisoning, the more likely it is to develop DEACMP. The incidence is significantly higher in patients who are in a coma for more than 12 hours, and nearly 60% in patients who are in a coma for more than 48 hours. The older the age, the higher the incidence of DEACMP. The risk of patients over 60 years old is more than 4 times higher than that of patients under 45 years old, and the prognosis is poor. Hyperbaric oxygen therapy in the early stage of acute CO poisoning can effectively reduce the incidence of DEACMP. It is possible that most patients with cardio-cerebral atherosclerosis tend to develop DEACMP or ischemia and hypoxia due to their greater COHb binding capacity and slower dissociation rate. The typical lesions of CT/MRI in patients with DEACMP show low density or long T_1 and long T_2 signal changes in bilateral white matter, basal ganglia or pallidus. The incidence of DEACMP in patients with low density lesions of pallidus is 3.4 times higher than that in patients with normal CT. After acute CO poisoning occurs in patients with a history of smoking and drinking, the tolerance of the body to hypoxia is weakened, and it is more likely to damage neurons in the brain, resulting in DEACMP. What's more, the increase of serum CRP level is positively correlated with the incidence of DEACMP.

(1) Clinical feature

1) Clinical manifestation

Most of the patients are subacute, and the symptoms reach the peak about 2 weeks after acute CO poisoning, a few patients reach the peak within 2 ~ 3 days, and the onset process of very few patients is more than 4 weeks. The main clinical manifestations are as follows: a. Cognitive impairment of memory, calculation, comprehension, orientation decline or loss, lack of attention, slow response, severe incontinence, patients can not take care of themselves or even show a stiff state. b. Mental symptoms include strange behavior, mania and irritability, hallucinations, speech disorders, indifference, depression and so on. c. Extrapyramidal symptoms include bradykinesia, decreased expression, increased muscle tone of the extremities, resting tremor, abnormal posture and gait. A small number of patients may have chorea. d. Cone system symptoms mainly present paralysis of one or both limbs, increased muscle tone, hyperreflexia of tendons, positive pathological signs, and pseudobulbar paralysis may also occur. e. Focal cerebral cortical dysfunction include cortical blindness, seizures, parietal lobe syndrome (agnosia, apraxia, agraphia, aphasia), motor aphasia, etc.

2) Diagnostic investigation

The results of blood COHb level, arterial blood gas analysis and serum enzyme test are generally normal. Most of them show diffuse slow wave activity, which can recover gradually with the improvement of the condition. The specificity of EEG is poor, and it is generally not regarded as a routine examination item. Visual evoked potential (VEP) examination shows that the latency of P100 is prolonged and improved during the recovery period. Median nerve somatosensory evoked potential (SEP) examination shows that N32 and other medium-and long-latency components are selectively damaged, the abnormal rate is more than 70%, and recovers with the improvement of consciousness. The abnormal results of brainstem auditory evoked potentials (BAEP) are closely related to the degree of disturbance of consciousness and the prognosis of patients with CO poisoning. If the latency of event-related potential P300 is significantly prolonged and the amplitude of event-related potential P300 is significantly decreased in patients with "pseudo-recovery" of acute CO poisoning, it is often indicative of the possibility of delayed encephalopathy.

There are no abnormal changes in the early stage, usually 2 weeks after the appearance of encephalopathy symptoms, the density of bilateral subcortical white matter, globus pallidus and internal capsule decrease symmetrically, and in the later stage, the ventricle is enlarged and the sulcus widens. It shows low signal on T_1WI, high signal on T_2WI and DWI, and mild low signal or equal signal on ADC. The lesions are mainly located in the center of semiovale and the white matter around the lateral ventricle. In severe cases, the lesions could also be found in subcortical white matter, corpus callosum and internal and external capsule. It is usually symmetrical, flaky or diffuse. (Fig. 12.4)

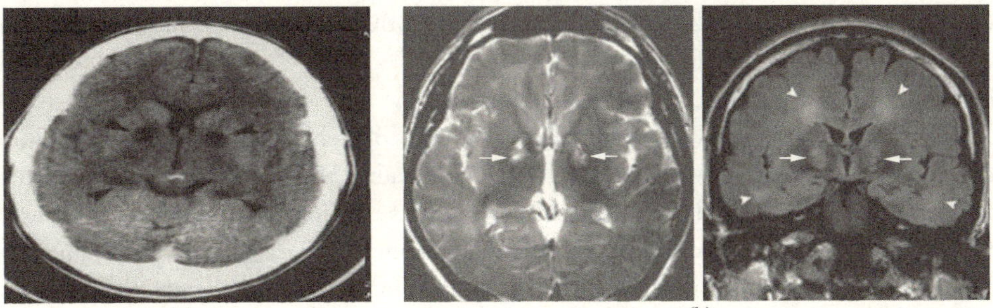

(a) (b)

(a) CT abnormalities are characterized by extensive subcortical low density changes in white matter and focal low density in the basal ganglia. (b) MRI shows bilateral long T_1 and long T_2 abnormal signals, oval in shape, smaller in diameter than 1 cm, and not accompanied by enhancement.

Fig. 12.4 Imaging abnormalities of DEACMP

(2) Diagnosis

The diagnosis requires a clear history of acute CO poisoning and a "false-cure period" after which typical clinical manifestations such as dementia, mental symptoms, hypertonia and tremor paralysis always appear. There are symmetrical T_2 high signal changes in the center of semiovale and white matter around the lateral ventricle in cranial MRI. Rule out encephalopathy caused by other causes.

(3) Prevention and treatment

When acute CO poisoning occurs, patients should be immediately removed from the poisoning site and transferred to areas with fresh air. For coma patients, respiratory secretions should be cleared and respiratory tract should be kept unobstructed. Shortening exposure time can reduce the risk of DEACMP. When hyperbaric oxygen therapy cannot be carried out under limited conditions, normobaric oxygen therapy should be carried out immediately. Nasal catheters, masks and simple respirators can be used to help breathe. Administration of hyperbaric oxygen once or twice within 24 hours and early continuous hyperbaric oxygen therapy for more than 6 days can reduce the risk of DEACMP. The treatment of DEACMP is difficult, the prognosis is poor, and the disability rate is high, which seriously endangers the life and health of patients.

1) Hyperbaric oxygen therapy

Hyperbaric oxygen therapy can promote the rapid replacement of CO in hemoglobin, increase the normal level of oxygenated hemoglobin in red blood cells, increase the level of plasma dissolved oxygen and transport it to the tissue, at the same time, it can also inhibit the adhesion of neutrophils to the damaged cerebral vascular endothelium and reduce tissue edema and lipid peroxidation. Hyperbaric oxygen is effective in improving the clinical symptoms and signs of patients with acute CO poisoning, increasing the cure rate and improvement rate, and can reduce the risk of DEACMP by inhibiting central nervous system ischemia-reperfusion injury. If the COHb of the patient with acute CO poisoning is less than 3% and the clinical poisoning symptoms disappear, hyperbaric oxygen therapy can be terminated.

2) Brain protection therapy

Neuroprotective therapy is helpful to the improvement and recovery of patients' symptoms. Agents that promote brain metabolism and brain cell energizer include citicoline, piracetam, adenosine triphosphate and so on. Free radical scavengers include edaravone, hydrogen-rich saline, lactulose and so on. Neurotrophic drugs include gangliosides and rat nerve growth factor.

Antioxidants include vitamin E and erythropoietin (EPO). Mitochondrial protective agents include idebenone and coenzyme Q10.

3) Symptomatic treatment

Glucocorticoid can effectively reduce the incidence of delayed encephalopathy. However, long-term bedridden patients with delayed encephalopathy have a higher risk of infection, impaired glucose tolerance or diabetes in elderly patients, which also limits the routine use of glucocorticoids. Donepezil hydrochloride and galantamine hydrobromide can improve the cognitive function of patients with DEACMP. Galanthamine seems to increase the blood flow of the whole brain, especially in the frontal lobe of DEACMP patients. In addition, bromocriptine, magnesium sulfate, amphetamine and risperidone have been reported to improve the treatment of cognitive and mental disorders in DEACMP. Sulforaphane, granulocyte colony stimulating factor, EPO and methylene blue may also be potential drugs for treatment of DEACMP.

12.7 Poisoning by Sedative Hypnotics

Sedative hypnotics are central nervous system inhibitors, which have sedative and hypnotic effects. Excessive doses can anesthetize the whole body, including medulla oblongata. A large dose can cause acute sedative hypnotic poisoning. All kinds of sedative hypnotics can produce tolerance and dependence, so they can cause abstinence syndrome, but the mechanism has not been fully elucidated. Long-term use of benzodiazepines reduces the number of benzodiazepine receptors, which is one of the reasons for tolerance. When taking benzodiazepines for a long time, abstinence syndrome occurs due to the increase of benzodiazepine receptor density. Tolerance, dependence and withdrawal syndrome are more serious in barbiturates, non-barbiturates and ethanol.

(1) Clinical feature

1) Clinical manifestation

① Acute poisoning

Benzodiazepine poisoning has mild inhibition of the central nervous system, and the main symptoms are drowsiness, dizziness, fatigue, ambiguity of speech, confusion of consciousness and ataxia. Serious symptoms such as prolonged deep coma and respiratory depression are rare. A large dose of barbiturates causes inhibition of the central nervous system, and the severity of the symptoms is related to the dose. Mild poisoning can be characterized by drowsiness, emotional instability, inattention, memory loss, ataxia, ambiguous pronunciation, unstable gait and nystagmus. Severe poisoning is characterized by progressive central nervous system inhibition, from narcolepsy to deep coma. Respiratory inhibition changes from shallow breathing to slow breathing to respiratory arrest. There may be hypotension or shock, decreased muscle tone, disappearance of tendon reflex, bullous lesions and so on. Long-term coma patients can be complicated with pneumonia, pulmonary edema, brain edema and renal failure.

Although the symptoms of non-barbiturate non-benzodiazepine poisoning are similar to those of barbiturate poisoning, they have their own characteristics. Chloral hydrate poisoning can be manifested as exhaled gas with pear-like smell, pupil narrowing at the initial stage, dilation at the later stage, arrhythmia, pulmonary edema, injury of liver and kidney function, coma and so on. Grummett poisoning can cause periodic fluctuations of disturbance of consciousness. The inhibition of circulatory system is prominent and includes hypotension, shock, anticholinergic nerve symptoms, such as pupil dilation and so on. Mequantel poisoning may have obvious respiratory inhibition and pyramidal signs. Methanate poisoning is similar to barbiturate poisoning, often with a drop in blood pressure. The most common type of phenothiazine poisoning is extrapyramidal reaction, and the clinical manifestations are as follows. Tremor paralysis syndrome, akathisia, and acute dystonia reactions, such as torticollis, dysphagia and dental atresia. It is generally believed that there may be acute poisoning reaction when the single dose of chlorpromazine reaches 214 g. As these drugs have obvious anticholinergic effects, patients often have tachycardia, high temperature and reduced intestinal peristalsis. The blocking effect on α-adrenergic receptor leads to vasodilation and decrease of blood pressure. Because the drug has the stabilization of quinidine-like membrane and myocardial inhibition, the poisoning patients have arrhythmia, prolongation of ECG P-R and Q-T interval, changes of ST segment and T wave. An overdose can also have extrapyramidal symptoms, coma and respiratory depression after poisoning; systemic convulsions are rare.

② Chronic poisoning

With long-term abuse of hypnotic, patients can have chronic poisoning. In addition to mild poisoning symptoms, there are some mental symptoms as follows. a. Disturbance of consciousness and hypomania. There is a state of temporary restlessness or confusion of consciousness. Speech is excited, cheerful, easy to fatigue, accompanied by tremors, unclear articulation and unstable gait. b. Mental disorders are characterized by a significant decrease in memory, calculation and comprehension, and a decrease in work and learning ability. c. Personality change. The patient loses his ambition and sense of responsibility to his family and society.

③ Abstinence syndrome

Abstinence syndrome may occur in patients who take large doses of sedative and hypnotic drugs for a long time and suddenly stop taking drugs or rapidly reduce the dosage. The main manifestations are increased excitability of autonomic nerve and mild and severe neuropsychiatric abnormalities. Anxiety, irritability, insomnia, headache, anorexia, weakness and tremor occur within 1 day or several days after the last medication. It reaches the peak after 2~3 days, with nausea, vomiting and muscle spasm. Seizures occur 1~2 days after sudden withdrawal (for some patients, seizures can also occur 7~8 days after drug withdrawal), sometimes hallucinations, delusions, loss of orientation, high fever and delirium, which recover within a few days to 3 weeks. The symptoms of patients with large dose for a long time and sudden withdrawal are serious. The abusers of barbiturates have more early onset, more epileptic seizures or hypomania after withdrawal and benzodiazepines have a late onset after withdrawal, which may be related to the slow excretion of intermediate metabolites and mild symptoms, mainly anxiety and insomnia.

2) Diagnostic investigation

Make a determination of drug concentration in blood, urine and gastric juice. The concentration of serum benzodiazepines is limited in judging the severity of poisoning because of the difference in the half-life of active metabolites and the rate of personal drug excretion. Blood biochemical tests include blood glucose, urea nitrogen, creatinine, electrolytes and arterial blood gas analysis.

(2) Diagnosis

For acute poisoning, there is a history of taking a large number of sedative hypnotics, disturbance of consciousness and respiratory inhibition and blood pressure drop. Sedative hypnotics or their metabolites are detected in gastric juice, blood and urine. For chronic poisoning, long-term abuse of a large number of hypnotic drugs, mild ataxia and mental symptoms are indications. Withdrawal syndrome presents with tremors, anxiety, insomnia, delirium, psychotic symptoms and epileptic seizures after long-term abuse of sedative hypnotics.

(3) Differential diagnosis

To understand whether there is a past history of essential hypertension, epilepsy, diabetes, liver disease, kidney disease, as well as a history of exposure to poisons such as carbon monoxide, alcohol and organic solvents. Check for head trauma, fever, meningeal irritation, hemiplegia, cyanosis and so on. Combined with necessary laboratory examination, differential diagnosis can be made. Patients with chronic poisoning and hypomania are prone to fatigue, tremor and gait instability, which can be identified in combination with the history of medication. Patients with primary epilepsy generally have a history of seizures. Patients with schizophrenia or alcoholism can have tremor and delirium, but the former has a past history, the latter has a history of alcoholism.

(4) Treatment

Treatment of acute poisoning is illustrated in Fig. 12.5.

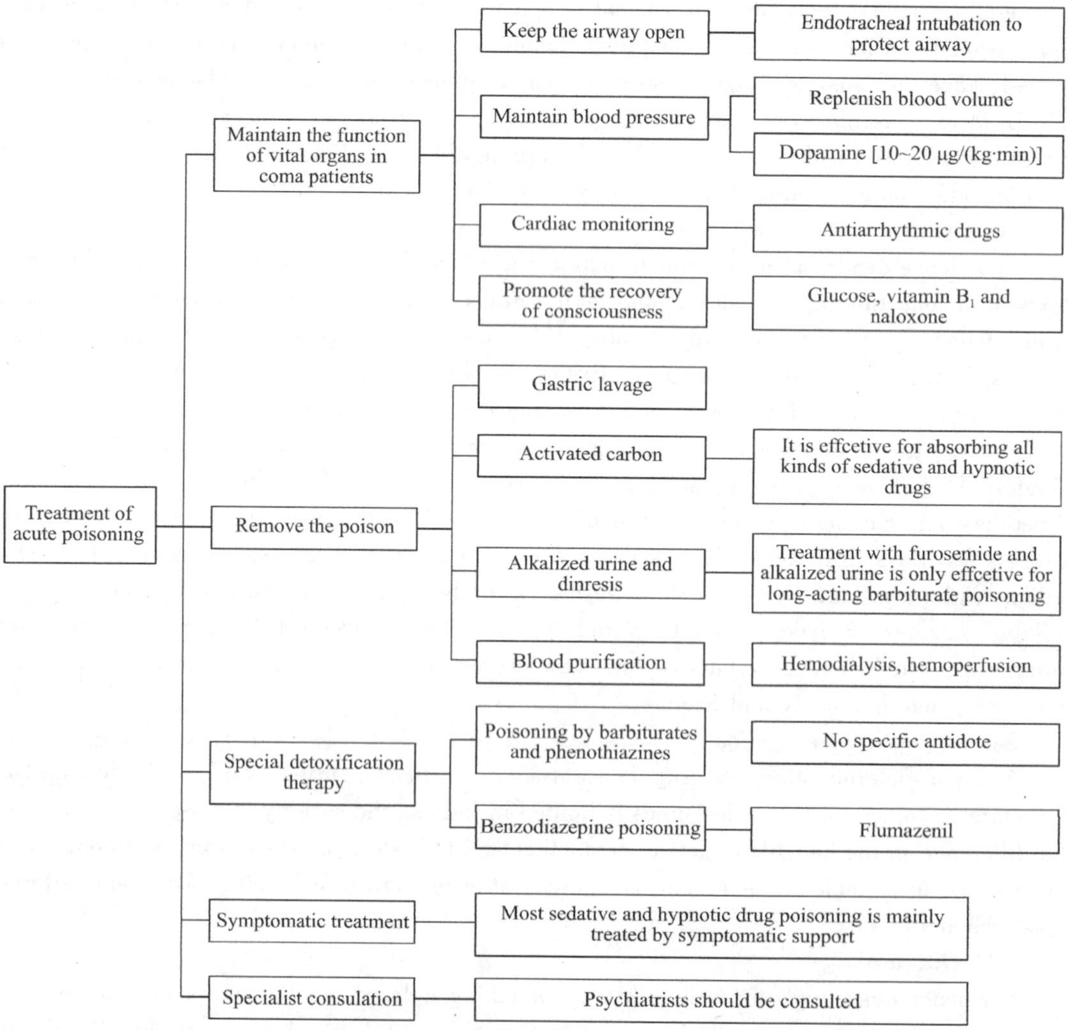

Fig. 12.5 Treatment of acute poisoning

The treatment principles of chronic poisoning are reduction of dose gradually until cease abuse and obtain a consultion with a psychiatrist for psychotherapy.

The treatment principle of abstinence syndrome is to use sufficient sedative hypnotics to control the withdrawal symptoms, and then gradually reduce the dose and even stop the drug after stabilization. The specific method is to replace the original short-acting drugs with long-acting drugs, such as diazepam or phenobarbital. Patients with mild poisoning can recover without treatment. Patients with moderate poisoning can recover within 24 ~ 48 hours after careful nursing and proper treatment. It may take 3 ~ 5 days for patients with severe poisoning to regain consciousness. The case fatality rate is less than 5%.

References

[1] POP-BUSUI R, BOULTON A J, FELDMAN E L, et al. Diabetic neuropathy: a position statement by the American Diabetes Association[J]. Diabetes Care, 2017,40(1):136-154.

[2] SHABEEB D, NAJAFI M, HASANZADEH G, et al. Electrophysiological measurements of diabetic peripheral neuropathy: a systematic review[J]. Diabetes & Metabolic Syndrome, 2018,12(4):591-600.

[3] ALINK J, DE VRIES W T. Unexp lained seizures, confusion or hallucinations: think Hashimo to Encephalopathy[J]. Acta Paediatrica, 2008,97(4):451-453.

[4] RIZOS T, SIEGELIN M, HÄHNEL S, et al. Fullminant onset of cerebral immunocomplex vasculitis as first manifestation of neuropsychiatric systemic lupus erythematosus (NPSLE)[J]. Lupus, 2009,18(4):361-363.

[5] HOCHBERG M C. Updating the American college of rheumatology revised criteria for the classification of systemic lupus erythematosus[J]. Arthritis and Rheumatism, 1997,40(9): 1725.

[6] WALLS M R. Rosen's emergency medicine: concepts and clinical practice[M]. Philadelphia: Elesvier, 2017.

[7] MCPHEE J S, PAPADAKIS M, RABOW W M. Current medical diagnosis and treatment[M]. NewYork: McGraw-Hill, 2017.

[8] GOLDMAN L, SCHAFER A I. Goldman's Cecil medicine[M]. 24th ed. Philadelphia: Elsevier Sauders, 2012.

[9] GAWARAMMANA I B, BUCKLEY N A. Medical management of paraquat ingestion [J]. British Journal of Clinical Pharmacology, 2011,72(5):745-757.

[10] EDWARD W, BOYER M D. Management of opioid analgesic overdose[J]. New England Journal of Medicine, 2012,367(2):146-155.

[11] 贾建平. 神经病学[M]. 北京: 人民卫生出版社, 2013.

[12] 吴江, 贾建平. 神经病学[M]. 北京: 人民卫生出版社, 2015.

[13] 吕传真, 周良辅. 实用神经病学[M]. 上海: 上海科学技术出版社, 2014.

[14] RUPP R, BLESCH A, SCHAD L, et al. Novel aspects of diagnostics and therapy of spinal cord diseases[J]. Der Nervenarzt, 2014,85(8):946-954.

(Cai Zhirong, Zhang Lei)

Chapter 13
Epilepsy

The word epilepsy is derived from Greek words meaning "to seize upon" or "taking hold of". Our predecesors referred to it as the "falling sickness" or the "falling evil". Although a useful medical term to denote recurrent seizures, the word epilepsy may still have unpleasant connotations and should be used advisedly in dealing with patients. In the practice of pediatric neurology, epilepsy is one of the most common disorders. The incidence increases again after the age of 60. For all these reasons, physicians should know something of the nature of seizure disorders and their treatment.

13.1 Seizure and Epilepsy

(1) Definition

A seizure is a paroxysmal electrical discharge of neurons in the brain resulting in changes of function or behavior. One seizure does not signify epilepsy, as up to 10% of people worldwide have one seizure during their lifetime. Epilepsy is defined as a tendency to recurrent seizures. Epilepsy is not a single disease but a symptom of congenital or acquired CNS disease. Different types of epilepsy can be classified according to different features, including seizure type, age of onset, prognosis and cause, and the more appropriate wording is epilepsies (Tab. 13.1). Epilepsy is one of the world's oldest recognized conditions, with written records dating back to 4000 BC. More than 50 million people worldwide have epilepsy, and nearly 80% live in low-income or middle-income countries. Every year, an estimated 2.4 million people are newly diagnosed with epilepsy globally. In china, epilepsy prevalence is approximately 4.6/1 000. An epilepsy syndrome refers to a cluster of features incorporating seizure types, EEG and imaging features that tend to occur together. It often has age-dependent features such as age of onset and remission, seizure triggers, diurnal variation and sometimes prognosis.

The operational definitions of epilepsy are as follows.

a. At least two unprovoked/reflex seizure occurring more than 24 hours apart.

b. One unprovoked/reflex seizure and a probability of further seizures similar to the general recurrence risk (at least 60%) after two unprovoked seizures, occurring over the next 10 years.

c. Diagnosis of an epilepsy syndrome: Epilepsy is considered to be resolved for individuals past the applicable age of an age-depending epilepsy syndrome or those who have remained seizure-free with no seizure medication for the past 10 years.

(2) Classification

Although many concepts outlined in the 1989 ILAE (International League Against Epilepsy) classification remain valid to day, a revision is needed to account for newest scientific discoveries that have fundamentally changed our understanding of the epilepsies as well as our approach to the diagnosis and management over the last few decades. The official definition of epilepsy and classification of seizures (Tab. 13.1) have been updated by ILAE, which is the world's official body of epilepsy professionals.

Tab. 13.1 Classification of seizure type (expanded version) by ILAE

Focal onset • Aware • Impaired awareness	Motor onset	Automatisms, atonic, clonic, epileptic spasms, hyperkinetic, myoclonic, tonic
	Non-motor onset	Autonomic, behavior arrest, cognitive, emotional, sensory
	Focal to bilateral tonic-clonic	
Generalized onset	Motor onset	Tonic-clonic, clonic, tonic, atonic, myoclonic, myoclonic-tonic-clonic, myoclonic-atonic, epileptic spasms
	Non-motor onset (absence)	Typical, atypical, myoclonic, eyelid myoclonia
Unknown onset	Motor onset	Tonic-clonic, epileptic spasms
	Non-motor onset	Behavior arrest
Unclassified	Inadequate information or inability to place in other categories	

1) Classification of seizure

The 2017 classification maintains the primary distinction between seizures that begin focally in one hemisphere of the brain versus those begin apparently generalized (by behavior or EEG) in both hemispheres of the brain. A new category for seizures of unknown onset is served as a placeholder for a few seizure types whose onset is obscure. With further observation, some seizures may move into the focal or generalized onset category. The expanded seizure classification is intended for use by neurologists, neurosurgeons, psychiatrists, and others with special expertise in epilepsy. By knowing and understanding the ILAE classification of seizures, technologists are better equipped to use EEG as a tool to impact the improvement of patients' lives by knowing what signs and symptoms to watch for, assess, and document during EEG testing.

Focal seizures are classified according to the "rule of first." The first symptom or sign determines the name of the seizure, even if other signs and symptoms are more impressive later in the course of the seizure.

① Focal motor onset

Automatisms are robot-like movements, such as saying a stock phrase over and over, picking at the clothes, rubbing, fumbling, lip-smacking, or wandering. These automatisms are commonly not recognized by the public or even some physicians as being part of a seizure. Atonic seizures present with sudden loss of tone on one side of the body or in one limb. Focal clonic seizures involve rhythmical sustained jerking. Epileptic spasms occur in children and present with sudden flexion at the waist and flexion or extension of the arms and legs. They may occur in clusters. Spasms can be focal, generalized, or of unknown onset. Under the age of 1, epileptic spasms are called infantile spasms. Hyperkinetic seizure, previously called hypermotor seizure, entails agitated kicking, thrashing, and peddling during the seizure. Such seizures commonly originate in the frontal lobe. Focal myoclonic seizures may appear similar to clonic seizures but are defined as unsustained, irregular jerking in one part of the face or body. Focal tonic seizure involves stiffening of a limb or the neck.

② Focal non-motor onset

Non-motor onset seizures include those affecting the autonomic nervous system, with gastrointestinal sensations, rising sense, hot/cold feelings, or goose bumps. Focal behavior arrest seizure would show cessation of all activity for duration of the entire seizure. Cognitive seizure can begin with a strangely familiar sensation or hallucinations. It may manifest with a specific type of cognitive disfunction, such as language (aphasia) instead of globally impaired cognitive function. Focal emotional seizures begin with fear, panic, joy, laughing, or crying. Sensory seizures exhibit skin tingling, visual or auditory changes, smell or taste hallucinations, or vertigo.

③ Generalized-onset

A few of these generalized-onset motor seizures are new seizure types. Myoclonic-tonic-clonic seizures are most often seen in patients with juvenile myoclonic epilepsy. There will be a few jerks of the arms, followed by tonic stiffening and then clonic rhythmical jerking. Myoclonic-atonic seizures occur in epileptic encephalopathies, such as Dravet syndrome or Doose syndrome. Non-motor, absence seizures can be typical or atypical. Atypical absence seizure has slow onset or offset, marked changes in tone, or EEG findings of slow spike-waves at less than three per second with a disordered background. Myoclonic-absence seizure presents with a few jerks followed by a staring spell. The arms may jerk rhythmically up into the air for a few seconds. Eyelid myoclonia refers to forced upward jerking of the eyelids, typically precipitated by eye closure. The associated syndromes are Jeavon syndrome, or the sunflower syndrome, in which children will wave fingers in front of a bright light to self-provoke a seizure.

Myoclonic-tonic-clonic seizure **Atypical absence seizure** **Myoclonic-absence seizure**

2) Classification of epilepsy

Epilepsy classification is the key clinical tool in evaluating an individual who is presenting with seizures. The new classification of the epilepsies is a multi-level one, designed to cater for classifying epilepsy in different clinical environments (Tab. 13.2). The epilepsy type includes a new category of "combined generalized and focal epilepsy" in addition to the well-established generalized and focal epilepsies. It also includes an "unknown" category.

Tab. 13.2 ILAE 2017 classification of epilepsy type

Epilepsy type	Seizure onset	Interictal EEG
Focal	Focal aware, focal impaired awareness, focal motor, focal non-motor, focal to bilateral tonic-clonic seizures	Focal epileptiform discharges
Generalized	Absence, myoclonic, atonic, tonic, tonic-clonic seizures	Generalized spike-wave activity
Combined generalized and focal epilepsy	Both generalized and focal seizures	Both generalized spike-wave and focal epileptiform discharges
Unknown	Insufficient information	Unavailable/unreliable

3) Classification of epilepsy syndromes

It is pragmatic to recognizing that the syndromes are multifaceted and defined by an association of clinical, electrophysiological, etiological and comorbid factors. It may have distinctive co-morbidities such as intellectual and psychiatric dysfunction, associated prognostic and treatment implications.

Idiopathic generalized epilepsies (IGEs) is used to describe "no known or suspected etiology other than possible hereditary predisposition". The term "idiopathic" is intentive to remove from the nomenclature of epilepsy classification and replace it with genetic generalized epilepsies (GGEs) where the clinician feels there is sufficient evidence for this classification. IGE will be acceptable specifically for the group of four epilepsy syndromes: childhood absence epilepsy, juvenile absence epilepsy, juvenile myoclonic epilepsy and generalized tonic-clonic seizures alone. Self-limited focal epilepsies typically begin in childhood. The most common is self-limited epilepsy with centrotemporal spikes, called "benign epilepsy with centrotemporal spikes (BECT)". Others include Panayiotopoulos syndrome and the late-onset form by Gastaut syndrome.

4) Epilepsy classification framework

Fig. 13.1 demonstrates framework for epilepsy classification. First of all, the starting point of the framework is the seizure type. The classification starts with the type of seizures, including focal, generalized, or unknown. The second level is that of epilepsy type and assumes that the patient has a diagnosis of epilepsy based on the 2017 definition. The epilepsy type level includes a new category of "combined generalized and focal Epilepsy" in addition to the well-established "generalized epilepsy" and "focal epilepsies". It also includes an unknown category. Many epilepsies include multiple types of seizures. The third level is an epilepsy syndrome diagnosis. The most important categories of etiologies are structural, genetic, infection, metabolic, immune, or unknown. Comorbidities of epilepsy also are of prime importance. Comorbidities include conditions that commonly travel with epilepsy, such as depression, anxiety, and social and economic dislocation. All of these clinical factors are combined to diagnose an epilepsy syndrome. Classification also informs the risks of co-morbidities. Those include learning difficulties, intellectual disability, psychiatric features such as autism spectrum disorder, and mortality risk such as sudden unexpected death in epilepsy (SUDEP).

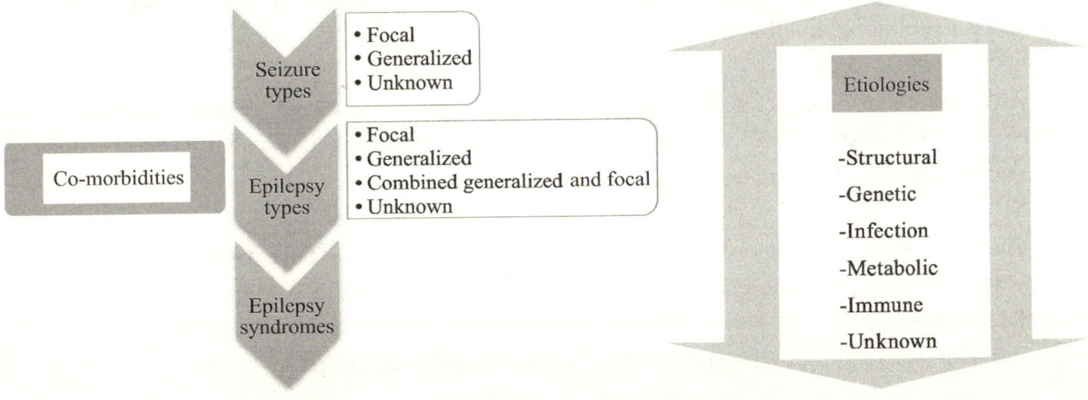

Fig. 13.1 Framework for epilepsy classification

(3) Etiology

A range of etiologic groups has been recognized, which have implications for treatment.

1) Structural etiology

Often neuroimaging should be carried out firstly, ideally MRI where available, to decide if there is a structural etiology. A structural etiology refers to abnormalities visible on structural neuroimaging and can explain the patient's seizures. Structural etiologies may be acquired such as stroke, trauma, infection, and genetic malformations of cortical development. There are well-recognized associations within the epilepsies with a structural etiology. These include the frequent finding of hippocampal sclerosis, hypothalamic hamartoma, Rasmussen syndrome, and hemiconvulsion-hemiplegia-epilepsy.

2) Genetic etiology

It results directly from a known or presumed genetic mutation in which seizures are a core symptom of the disorder. In most cases, the underlying genes have not been known yet. First, the inference of a genetic etiology may be based solely on a family history of an autosomal dominant disorder. Second, a genetic etiology may be suggested by clinical research in populations with the same syndrome such as childhood absence epilepsy or juvenile myoclonic epilepsy. Third, a molecular basis may be identified and may implicate a single gene or copy number variant of major effect. The best known example is Dravet syndrome in which >80% of patients have a pathogenic variant of SCN1A. However, genetic does not equate with inherited but refers to a pathogenic variant (mutation) of significant effect in causing individual's epilepsy.

3) Infectious etiology

It is the most common etiology worldwide actually and refers to a patient with epilepsy, rather than with seizures occurring in the setting of acute infection. Common examples include neurocysticercosis, tuberculosis, HIV, cerebral malaria, subacute sclerosing panencephalitis, cerebral toxoplasmosis, and congenital infections such as Zika virus and cytomegalovirus.

4) Metabolic etiology

Epilepsy results directly from a known or presumed metabolic disorder in which seizures are a core symptom of the disorder. A range of metabolic disorders is associated with epilepsy, for example, porphyria, uremia, cerebral folate deficiency or pyridoxine-dependent seizures. In many cases, metabolic disorders may have a genetic defect, implying to specific therapies and potential prevention of intellectual impairment.

5) Immune etiology

An immune etiology can be conceptualized as where there is identified evidence of autoimmune-mediated central nervous system inflammation, such as anti-NMDA receptor encephalitis and anti-LGI1 encephalitis.

6) Unknown etiology

There are many patients with epilepsy with unknown cause. The extent to which a cause can be found depends on the extent of the evaluation available to the patient.

(4) Diagnosis

Epilepsy is a complex diagnosis without an easy gold standard.

a. A detailed history together with a reliable eyewitness account is the key to diagnosis. The diagnosis of seizures is based on clinical recognition of one of the seizure types described previously. The general physical examination is also important to determine whether the patient has an underlying condition. The neurological examination assesses focal signs that might implicate or localize cerebral pathology.

b. The electroencephalogram can be a helpful confirmatory test in distinguishing seizures from other causes of loss of consciousness. However, a normal or nonspecifically abnormal interictal EEG never excludes the diagnosis of epilepsy. Specific EEG features that suggest epilepsy include abnormal spikes, polyspike discharges, and spike-wave complexes (Fig. 13.2). Now the long-video EEG monitoring is in common use and is of higher sensitivity in patients with surgically removable epileptogenic foci and differentiate an epileptic seizure from a nonepileptic event.

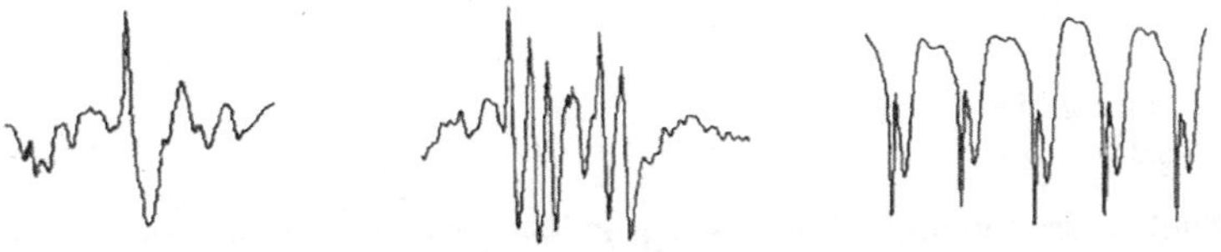

Fig. 13.2 Specific EEG wave

c. Cerebral imaging has come to play a major role in the diagnosis of seizures. MRI is more sensitive for detection of small structural abnormalities underlying epilepsy and must be done with an epilepsy-appropriate protocol comprising at least 1 mm three-dimensional volumetric T_1-weighted imaging, axial and coronal T_2-weighted, and fluid attenuated inversion recovery sequences (including hippocampal angulation) and axial hemosiderin or calcification-sensitive T_2-sequences or susceptibility-weighted sequences. PET images the brain's regional use of glucose with asymmetries suggesting areas of interictal or ictal abnormality. SPECT compares local blood flow discrepancies, information that is most useful when recorded during a seizure. MEG assesses the brain's dynamic electromagnetic fields and can better localize epileptic dipoles, including those tangential to the scalp, which can be missed by conventional EEG.

d. Immunology. The discovery of neuronal antibodies leads to the identification of previously unknown encephalopathies and epilepsies associated with autonomic immune etiology. Encephalitis linked to antibodies targeting glutamic acid decarboxylase (GAD)-65, LGI1, CASPR2, and NMDA receptors seems to be the most common causes.

Metabolic and toxic disorders that can cause seizures should be excluded because they do not require anticonvulsants. Seizures with a clearly focal onset or those begin after the age of 25 require prompt evaluation to exclude the presence of a structural brain lesion. If no cause is found, the decision to begin chronic anticonvulsant therapy should be based on the probability of recurrence.

(5) Differential diagnosis

The conditions most likely to simulate an epileptic seizure are called "epilepsy mimic disorders" (Tab. 13.3), including psychogenic nonepileptic seizures and other paroxysmal events such as panic attack, syncope, TIA, particularly those associated with limb shaking, rapid eye movement (REM), sleep behavior disorder, subarachnoid hemorrhage, migraine, hypoglycemia, cataplexy and some movement disorders, and transient global amnesia.

Tab. 13.3 Epilepsy mimic disorders

Syncope	Vasovagal/neurocardiogenic, arrhythmia, low cardiac output, volume depletion
Migraine	Classic, basilar, confusional, acephalgic
Cerebrovascular	TIA, amyloid angiopathy

Continued

Sleep disorders	REM sleep behavior disorder, narcolepsy, cataplexy, parasomnias
Movement disorders	Tics, nonepileptic myoclonus, tremor
Psychiatric	Panic, dissociation, conversion, malingering

(6) Treatment

The treatment of epilepsy of all types can be divided into four parts: the use of anti-seizure drugs (ASDs), the surgical excision of epileptic foci and other surgical measures, the removal of causative and precipitating factors, and the regulation of physical and mental activity. ASDs are the first-line treatments.

1) Drug therapy

It is important to understand that a seizure is a CNS event present as convulsive or non-convulsive. There are both excitatory neurotransmitters (glutamate, aspartate, and acetylcholine) and inhibitory neurotransmitters (gamma-aminobutyric acid) and mechanisms (calcium ion-dependent potassium ion current and magnesium blockade of NMDA) in the brain that play a role in the genesis and inhibition of isolated seizures. Therefore, drugs used to treat epilepsy work by decreasing the electrical activity of the brain, either by preventing neuronal depolarization or promoting inhibition mediated by GABA. Blocking sodium channels or calcium channels, enhancing potassium channel function, inhibiting excitation mediated by the neurotransmitter glutamate are the pathways of weakening the depolarization. In 1857, Sir Locock discovered the anticonvulsant traits of potassium bromide and began treating his patients. From then on, ASDs had been developed over 150 years and now nearly 40 kinds are used for seizures. Specialists divide them into 3 generations including the older ASDs (phenytoin, phenobarbital, carbamazepine, and valproic acid) and newer ones (vigabatrin, felbamate, gabapentin, lamotrigine, tiagabine, topiramate, levetiracetam, oxcarbazepine, zonisamide, pregabalin, rufinamide, and lacosamide), which have improved tolerability and safety compared to their older counterparts. In 2018, the FDA approved the use of CBD-rich (Epidiolex) for two severe forms of epilepsy in children (Lennox-Gastaut and Dravet syndromes).

The choice and dose of medication depends on many factors including gender, age, other medications as they have manifold interactions with each other and with a wide variety of other drugs. Renal or hepatic dysfunction and psychiatric conditions might be influenced by a particular agent. Nearly all seizure medications have CNS side effects. In clinic, starting in the lower dose range and attempting to provide twice daily or daily administration are favored. The mechanisms, titration rates and maintenance doses (adult) for various available ASDs are listed in Tab. 13.4.

There are four key principles of drug management: a. Establish the diagnosis of epilepsy before starting drug therapy. b. Choose the right drug for the seizure type. Absence seizures, for example, do not respond to most drugs used for focal onset or generalized seizures. Stiripentol, pregabalin, rufinamide, lacosamide, eslicarbazepine, and perampanel are licensed for adjunctive use only. c. Modulate treatment according to seizure control, rather than the serum drug levels. d. Evaluate one drug at a time—the first ASD controls seizures in about 50% of patients; introducing a second ASD achieves control in another 10%~15%, and a third drug is successful in only about 1%. So beginning therapy with multiple drugs may expose patients to increased drug toxicity without increased therapeutic benefit.

Tab. 13.4 Efficacy spectrum of available anti-seizure drugs (ASDs) currently

	Generic name	Mechanism	Starting schedule	Side effects	Broad-spectrum
The first generation	Phenobarbital/PB	GABA protentiation	Start with 100 mg qd. The target serum level is 10~40 mg/mL	Addictive, thinking/memory problems, depression, birth defects, long-term bone problems	√
	Phenytoin/PHT	Sodium channels inhibitor	Typical adult dose is 300 ~ 400 mg/d. The target serum level is 10~20 mg/mL	Cognitive problems; long-term potential cosmetic, osteoporosis; Stevens-Johnson syndrome	√
	Ethosuximide/ESM	T-type calcium channels inhibitor	Start with 500 mg/d and increase by 250 mg/d at 5~7 day intervals to 500~1 500 mg/d	Stevens-Johnson syndrome, drowsy, dizziness, ataxia, anorexia, headache hiccups, Nausea vomiting, abdominal pain	Absence epilepsy (adjunctive use only)
The second generation	Carbamazepine/CBZ	Sodium channels inhibitor	Start with 200 mg bid and increase by 200 mg/d to about 400 mg tid	GI upset, weight gain, blurred vision, low blood counts, hyponatremia, Stevens-Johnson syndrome (Asian with HLA-B 1502 antigen at hight risk)	Partial seizure
	Primidone/U	Chloride channel inhibitor	250 mg at bedtime initiated during the first week and increase by 250 mg/d to 250 mg qid in the fourth week	Sedation, drowsiness, ataxia, diplopia, nystagmus, dizziness, vertigo, epigastric pain, megaloblastic anemia, respiratory depression, polyuria, skin rash, facial edema, QT prolongation	√
	Valproic acid/VPA	Multiple: GABA protetiation; NMDA inhibition; sodium/calcium channels inhibitor	250~500 mg tid	Weight gain, tremor, hair loss, GI upset, blood count decreases, hepatic or pancreatic injury, osteoporosis, birth defects	√
	Clonazepam/CZP	GABA protetiation	0.5~1.0 mg tid	Sedation, thinking impairment, mood changes, addiction	√

Continued

	Generic name	Mechanism	Starting schedule	Side effects	Broad-spectrum
The third generation	Zonisamide/ZNS	Sodium channels inhibitor	Start with 25 mg qd, adding 25 mg bid each week until 100 ~ 300 mg bid	Thinking/memory problems, renal stones, weight loss	√
	Lamotrigine/LTG	Multiple: AMPAblocker; Sodium channels inhibitor	Start at 25 mg, adding 25 mg daily each week until 200 mg bid	Rash, dizziness, fatigue, mild cognitive impairment	√ (Except myoclonic seizures)
	Oxcarbazepine/OXC	Sodium channels inhibitor	Start at 300 mg/d and increase by 150 mg/d each week to target dosage 600 ~ 900 mg bid	Hyponatremia (fewer than carbamazepine)	Partial seizure
	Gabapentin/GBP	GABA protetiation; calcium channels inhibitor	Start at 300 mg daily and increase by 300 mg every 3 days until 300 ~ 600 mg tid	Weight gain, unsteadiness, fatigue, dizziness	Not powerful
	Topiramate/TPM	Multiple: GABA protetiation; AMPA inhibition; sodium/calcium channels inhibitor	Start with 25 mg qd, adding 25 mg each week bid until 150 ~ 200 mg bid	Thinking/memory problems, renal stones, glaucoma, weight loss	√
	Tiagabine	GABA reuptake inhibitor	Start with 4 mg qd and increase by 4 mg at weekly intervals until 16 mg qid	Sdation, impaired speech, agitation, myoclonus, tremors, vomiting, temporary paralysis, respiratory depression	Partial seizures (adjunctive therapy)
	Levetiracetam/LEV	SV2A modulation	Start with 250 mg bid and increase by 250 mg each time at weekly intervals to 500 ~ 1 500 mg bid	No drug interactions, no protein binding, dizziness, fatigue, insomnia, irritability	√
	Pregabalin/PGB	Calcium channels inhibitor	Start 50 mg qd, adding 50 mg each week bid until 150 ~ 300 mg bid	No drug interactions, no liver metabolism, no protein binding, similar to gabapentin	Adjunctive therapy
	Rufinamide/RFN	Sodium channels inhibitor	Start with 5 mg/(kg · d) bid, adding additional 10 mg/kg every two days, until 45 mg/(kg · d)	Headache, dizziness, fatigue, sleepiness, double vision, tremor, short QT syndrome	LGS (add-on treatment)
	Lacosamide/LCM	Sodium channels inhibitor	Start with 50 mg bid and increase each week by 100 mg, to 100 ~ 200 mg bid	Dizziness, headache, nausea or vomiting, double vision, fatigue, memory or mood problems	Partial/secondarily generalized seizures

In fact, there are few firm rules to guide the physician to the withdrawal of medications. One plan, applicable to most forms of epilepsy, is to obtain an EEG whenever withdrawal of medication is contemplated. It is reported that the recurrence rate following ASD discontinuation ranged from 12% to 66%, and reinstatement of treatment is successful in obtaining further remission in 80%. Up to 23% of those discontinuing treatment go on to develop intractable epilepsy. Risk factors for subsequent poor treatment outcome are symptomatic focal epilepsy and cognitive deficits.

2) Surgical treatment

Epilepsy surgery uses neurosurgical procedures to treat epilepsy that causes the following: a. seizures that are resistant to ASDs; b. drug-controlled seizures with intolerable side effects; c. seizures associated with structural lesions that always develop to drug resistance. Each individual case must be evaluated in relation to such factors as age, disease duration, presence of anatomical lesions, and seizure frequency. Resective surgery includes temporal lobe resections, extra temporal resections, laser interstitial thermal therapy, and SEEG-guided thermocoagulation by radio frequency, and laser ablation. Those may remove, disconnect or deactivates the epileptogenic zone (EZ), thereby eliminating seizures. By contrast, a "palliative" approach is aimed at reducing the intensity and frequency of epileptic seizures, but not primarily at eliminating them completely. There are three main types of neuromodulation: vagal nerve stimulation, responsive neurostimulation, and deep brain stimulation for epilepsy. Vagus nerve stimulation (VNS) is the most common therapy involving implantation of a programmable signal generator (neurocybernetic prosthesis, NCP) in the chest cavity, and the stimulating electrodes carry electrical signals from the generator to the left vagus nerve. Deep brain stimulation (DBS) is a safe and efficacious therapy in well-selected patients who are not candidates for resective surgery. The anterior nucleus of the thalamus (ANT), hippocampus and centromedian nucleus of thalamus are the most investigated targets to date. Adverse effects may be surgical-related, hardware-related, or stimulation-related. Infection is the most common complication, followed by lead migration, fracture of the lead or other component of the device, internal pulse generator malfunction and skin erosion without infection.

3) Ketogenic diet

Although many children with epilepsy have seizures controlled with ASDs, a large percentage of patients are refractory to drug therapy and some are not suitable for surgical intervention. Ketogenic diet (KD) or ketogenic diet therapy (KDT) remains a valid option, which refers to a therapy with high fat, low carbohydrate diets designed to mimic a fasting state, first proposed at the beginning of the last century. Over the last decades, different types of KDs have been developed. Currently, there are 4 major KDT with different compositions—the classic ketogenic diet (cKD), the modified Atkins diet (MAD), the medium chain triglyceride ketogenic diet and the low glycemic index treatment. About 70% of children achieve a period of remission of at least 2 years without a seizure. At that time, one can consider stopping medication, especially if there is no identified underlying etiology. Of all patients, 37% have easily controlled seizures from the onset, 25% have refractory seizures from the onset, and 38% have a remitting relapsing pattern.

(7) Complication and prognosis

Epilepsy is a treatable condition, with up to 80% entering prolonged periods of seizure remission and up to 50% continuing to be seizure-free after treatment discontinuation. It is estimated that up to 70% of people living with epilepsy could live seizure-free if properly diagnosed and treated. The risk of premature death in people with epilepsy is up to three times higher than that for the general population. Lifestyle adjustment is a crucial aspect of epilepsy management. Optimizing sleep, improving medication compliance, and reducing stress can significantly improve epilepsy outcome. It is also important to prevent the causes of symptomatic epilepsies, such as head trauma, perinatal injury, and brain infections like neurocysticercosis. Finally, health professionals need to advocate for people with epilepsy. People with epilepsy and their families often suffer from stigma and discrimination because of lack of knowledge and understanding about the condition from the public.

13.2 Status Epilepticus

(1) Definition

Status epilepticus (SE) is defined as a condition resulting either from the failure of the mechanisms responsible of seizure self-limitation or from the initiation of mechanisms which lead to typically prolonged seizures. It is a neurological and medical emergency with high mortality, defined by two operational time dimensions: T_1, the time beyond which seizures are likely to be prolonged and when treatment should be initiated; T_2, the time after which there is increasing risk of irreversible consequences, such as neuronal injury, neuronal death, alteration of neuronal networks and functional deficits. Status epilepticus has several subtypes, including convulsive status epilepticus (CSE), epilepsia partialis continua, and nonconvulsive status epilepticus (NCSE). For CSE including generalized tonic-clonic movements of the extremities and impaired mental status, T_1 is 5 minutes and T_2 is 30 minutes, but for focal status epilepticus or absence status, these time points are different or unknown (Tab. 13.5). Status epilepticus incidence appears to peak at the age of more than 50 (approximately 28.4 per 100 000 per year) and younger than the age of 10 (14.3 per 100 000 per year) and seems to be greater in African-Americans (13.7 per 100 000 per year) compared to whites (6.9 per 100 000 per year) and other races (7.4 per 100 000 per year).

Tab. 13.5 SE operational dimensions with T_1 and T_2

Type of SE	T_1	T_2	Evidence base
Convulsive SE	5 minutes	30 minutes	Animal experiments clinical research
Focal SE with impaired consciousness	10 minutes	60 minutes	Animal experimentation
Absence SE	10~15 minutes	Unknown	No information

Refractory status epilepticus (RSE) is continuous seizure activity not controlled by first-line and second-line ASDs. RSE is seen in approximately 9%~43% of all SE cases, with a reported in-hospital mortality of 15%~33%.

Super-refractory status epilepticus (SRSE) is defined as status epilepticus not controlled by third-line agents, or condition if status epilepticus continues for 24 hours or longer after anesthesia is administered. It is observed that approximately 4%~12% of patients with SE eventually progress to SRSE, with in-hospital mortality reported to be as high as 40%~54%.

New-onset refractory status epilepticus (NORSE) is defined as a "clinical presentation characterized by new onset of refractory status epilepticus, in a patient without active epilepsy or other preexisting relevant neurological disorder (acute strokes, brain masses, drug overdoses, etc.), and without a clear acute or active structural, toxic or metabolic cause" in 2018 by an international group of experts. Febrile infection-related epilepsy syndrome (FIRES) is defined as a subset of NORSE, associated with a prior febrile infection, with fever starting from 24 hours to 2 weeks before the onset of RSE. In contrast, patients with NORSE may or may not be associated with fever before the start of RSE. The most common etiologies include autoimmune and paraneoplastic encephalitis followed by infections. Approximately 50% of patients with NORSE have an unknown etiology despite an extensive workup.

(2) Diagnosis

According to ILAE, SE is classified into different types based on the following four axes: semiology, etiology, EEG correlates, age. The purpose of the diagnostic axes is to provide a framework for clinical diagnosis, investigation, and therapeutic approaches for each patient.

Axis 1: Semiology Semiology refers to the clinical presentation of SE with two main taxonomic criteria: a. The presence or absence of prominent motor symptoms (e.g. CSE, myoclonic SE, focal motor, tonic status, hyperkinetic SE); b. The degree of impaired consciousness.

Axis 2: Etiology The term "known" or "symptomatic" is used for SE caused by a known disorder, while the term "idiopathic" or "genetic" is not applicable to the underlying etiology of SE. There are multiple etiologies for status epilepticus and will be updated periodically: CNS infections; metabolic abnormalities (hypoglycemia, hyponatremia, hypocalcemia, hepatic encephalopathy, and inborn errors of metabolism in children); cerebrovascular accidents; head trauma; drug toxicity; drug withdrawal syndromes (alcohol, benzodiazepines, and barbiturates); hypoxia; hypertensive emergency; autoimmune disorders; CNS tumors; pre-existing epilepsy with breakthrough seizures or non-compliance with anti-epileptic drugs, ethanol withdrawal. Age of the patient and the semiology will be immediately assessable. On the contrary, etiology may take time to be identified and EEG recordings may not be available in many settings, particularly at presentation. However, EEG patterns influence clinical approach, aggressiveness of treatment and prognosis, so it should be performed as early as possible.

So, differential diagnoses of status epilepticus include cute intoxication, early catastrophic brain hypoxia, encephalopathy of toxic and metabolic origin, ischemic stroke, non-epileptic seizures or trauma.

(3) Treatment

Status epilepticus is an emergency that requires immediate treatment in an organized manner. A staged approach to treatment has been advocated, with different drugs used in early (stage Ⅰ), established (stage Ⅱ), refractory and super-refractory status epilepticus (stage Ⅲ). In stage Ⅰ, the first line therapy is benzodiazepines. Stage Ⅱ occurs when there are continued seizures despite benzodiazepine therapy, and treatment in this stage is with Ⅳ ASDs, including phenobarbital. Fig. 13.3 presents a treatment algorithm with details on drug doses used in various stages. All patients with status epilepticus require hospital admission, preferably to the intensive care unit (ICU) and consult a neurologist early in the management. Neurologist may consider withdrawal of life support after discussion with family for those patients whose anaesthetic drugs have failed to wean off over a period of weeks.

(4) Complication and prognosis

The mortality rate for patients with the first episode of generalized convulsive status epilepticus is 16%~20%. Refractory status epilepticus has mortality rates of 35%~60%. About

40% of patients with the first episode of status epilepticus develop subsequent epilepsy, and there is a 25% ~ 30% risk of recurrent status epilepticus after the first episode. Mortality with status epilepticus may reach up to 30% in adults. Age over 60, female, treatment in smaller-sized hospitals, the presence of comorbidities (e.g., hypertension, diabetes mellitus, previous stroke), status epilepticus complications (e.g., respiratory failure, sepsis), and etiologies such as status epilepticus postcardiopulmonary resuscitation are associated with worse discharge outcomes. SE has long-term consequences, including neuronal injury and seizures with severe associated disabilities.

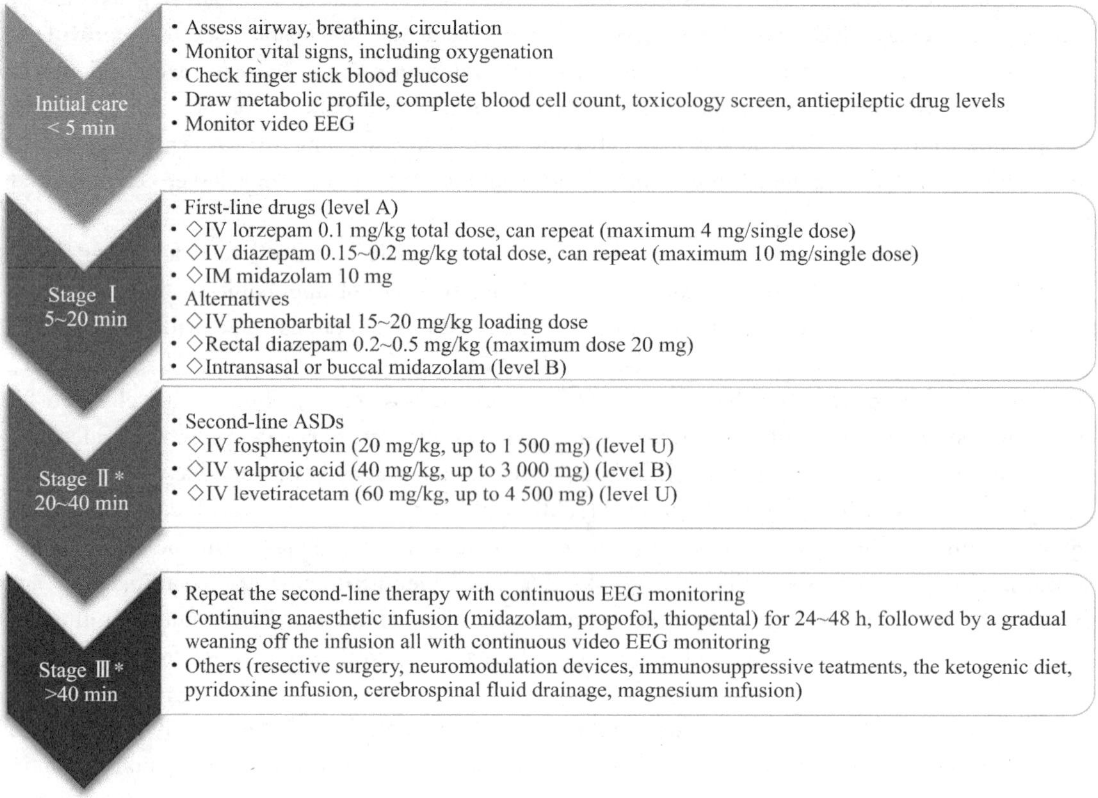

Fig. 13.3 Proposed hospital management of SE

* There is no clear evidence to guide therapy in this phase (level U).

References

[1] SCHEFFER I E, BERKOVIC S, CAPOVILLA G, et al. ILAE classification of the epilepsies: position paper of the ILAE commission for classification and terminology [J]. Epilepsia, 2017,58(4):512-521.

[2] PACK A M. Epilepsy overview and revised classification of seizures and epilepsies [J]. Continuum: Lifelong Learning in Neurology, 2019,25(2):306-321.

[3] FEYISSA A M, TATUM W O. Adult EEG[J]. Handbook of Clinical Neurology, 2019,160:103-124.

[4] GAVVALA J R, SCHUELE S U. New-onset seizure in adults and adolescents: a review[J]. JAMA, 2016,316(24):2657-2668.

[5] PERUCCA P, SCHEFFER I E, KILEY M. The management of epilepsy in children and adults[J]. Medical Journal of Australia, 2018,208(5):226-233.

[6] FRANCO V, PERUCCA E. Pharmacological and therapeutic properties of cannabidiol for Epilepsy[J]. Drugs, 2019,79(13):1435-1454.

[7] KIM H, KIM D W, LEE S T, et al. Antiepileptic drug selection according to seizure type in adult patients with epilepsy[J]. Journal of Clinical Neurology, 2020,16(4):547-555.

[8] CONSALES A, CASCIATO S, ASIOLI S, et al. The surgical treatment of epilepsy [J]. Neurological Sciences, 2021,42(6):2249-2260.

[9] WELLS J, SWAMINATHAN A, PASEKA J, et al. Efficacy and safety of a ketogenic diet in children and adolescents with refractory epilepsy-a review[J]. Nutrients, 2020,12(6): 1809.

[10] BETJEMANN J P, LOWENSTEIN D H. Status epilepticus in adults[J]. The Lancet Neurology, 2015,14(6):615-624.

[11] TRINKA E, LOCK H, HESDORFFER D, et al. A definition and classification of status epilepticus-report of the ILAE task force on classification of status epilepticus [J]. Epilepsia, 2015,56(10):1515-1523.

[12] GLAUSER T, SHINNAR S, GLOSS D, et al. Evidence-based guideline: treatment of convulsive status epilepticus in children and adults: report of the Guideline Committee of the American Epilepsy Society[J]. Epilepsy Currents, 2016,16(1):48-61.

[13] HARDEN C L. Pregnancy and epilepsy[J]. Continuum, 2014,20:60-79.

(Wang Xiaoshan, Jiang Ping)

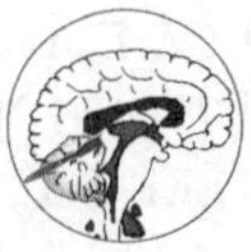

Chapter 14

Headache and Facial pain

Headache is the most frequent and the most common reason for seeking medical help. It is caused by a pain pathway to the cerebral cortex. Interestingly, headache is practically the only pain sensation produced by pain-sensitive cranial structures, which include skin, subcutaneous tissue, muscles, extracranial arteries, and periosteum of the skull; delicate structures of the eye, ear, nasal cavities, and paranasal sinuses; intracranial venous sinuses and their large tributaries, especially pericavernous structures; parts of the dura at the base of the brain and the arteries within the dura, particularly the proximal parts of the anterior and middle cerebral arteries and the intracranial segment of the internal carotid artery; the middle meningeal and superficial temporal arteries; the optic, oculomotor, trigeminal, glossopharyngeal, vagus, and the first three cervical nerves. Headache can be classified as primary and secondary. Significant underlying neurologic pathology cannot be found in the former, but the latter is due to some other intracranial process such as a mass lesion, raised intracranial pressure, inflammatory or infectious process. Detailed history can provide first-hand information for the diagnosis of headache. The mode of onset, the variation of the pain over time, and duration of the headache, with respect both to a single attack and to the profile of the headache over a period of years, are also useful data. In the diagnosis of headache, the primary or secondary headache should be distinguished firstly. Any diagnosis of primary headache should be based on the exclusion of secondary headache.

International headache society (IHS) makes an international classification of headache disorders (3nd edition), ICHD-3 (beta version) in 2013 as follows.

Part 1: primary headache

Migraine;

Tension-type headache;

Trigeminal autonomic cephalalgia;

Other primary headache disorders.

Part 2: secondary headache

Headache attributed to trauma or injury to the head and/or neck;

Headache attributed to cranial or cervical vascular disorder;

Headache attributed to non-vascular intracranial disorder;

Headache attributed to a substance or its withdrawal;

Headache attributed to infection;

Headache attributed to disorder of homoeostasis;

Headache or facial pain attributed to disorder of the cranium, neck, eyes, ears, nose, sinuses, teeth, mouth or other facial or cervical stracture;

Headache attributed to psychiatric disorder.

Part 3: painful cranial neuropathies, other facial pains and headaches
Painful cranial neuropathies and other facial pains;
Other headache disorders.

14.1 Migraine

Migraine is a common primary headache clinically with a prevalence of 5% ~ 10%, characterized by episotic, unilateral, moderate to severe, pulsatile headache. It generally lasts 4~72 hours and can be accompanied by nausea and vomiting. Headache can be aggravated by sound and light stimulation or daily activities, and can be relieved by quiet environment and rest. Food rich in tyramine is incriminated as a provocative factor in migraine. Alcohol, particularly red wine or port, regularly provokes an attack in some persons.

(1) Etiology and pathogenesis

Migraine has genetic predisposition. About 60% of migraine sufferers have a family history, and the risk of migraine in their relatives is 3~6 times higher than in the general population. Environmental factors also play a role in migraine attacks. Certain food and medicaments can induce migraine. Additional bright light, overwork, morpheus obstacle, tension are also the inducement factors of migraine. The underlying mechanisms of the premonitory, aura, headache, and postdrome phases of migraine become more well understood. Identification of this complex pain network which involves calcitonin gene-related peptide (CGRP), the trigeminal and upper cervical afferents, the trigeminal nucleus caudalis, the thalamus, hypothalamus, limbic, cortical structures and descending inhibitory nociceptive pathways, helps explain the affective, cognitive, and autonomic symptoms involved in migraine.

(2) Clinical feature

Migraine headache is unilateral in two-thirds of attacks and is commonly associated with nausea, vomiting, and sensitivity to light, sound, and smells. Two closely related clinical syndromes have been identified, the first called migraine with aura, as classic or neurologic migraine, and the second called migraine without aura, as common migraine. The ratio of classic migraine to common migraine is 1 : 5. Either type may be preceded by vague premonitory changes in mood and appetite. Migraine with aura is ushered in by a disturbance of nervous function, most often visual, followed in a few minutes to hours by hemicranial (or, in about one-third of cases, bilateral) headache, nausea, and sometimes vomiting, all of which last for hours or as long as a day or more. Migraine without aura is characterized by an unheralded onset over minutes or longer of increasing hemicranial headache or, less often, by generalized headache with or without nausea and vomiting, which then follows the same temporal pattern as the migraine with aura. Sensitivity to light, noise, and often smells attends both types, and intensification with movement of the head is common. If the pain is severe, the patient prefers to lie down in a quiet, darkened room and tries to sleep. The hemicranial and the throbbing (pulsating) aspects of migraine are its most characteristic features in comparison to other headache types. Each patient displays a proclivity for the pain to affect one side or the other of the cranium, but not exclusively so that some bouts are on the other side.

Classification of migraine is demonstrated in Fig. 14.1.

- Classification of migraine
  - Migraine without aura
  - Migraine with aura
    - Migraine with typical aura
      - Typical aura with headache
      - Typical aura without headache
    - Migraine with brainstem aura
    - Hemiplegic migraine
      - Familial hemiplegic migraine
        - Familial hemiplegic migraine type 1 (FHM1)
        - Familial hemiplegic migraine type 2 (FHM2)
        - Familial hemiplegic migraine type 3 (FHM3)
        - Familial hemiplegic migraine, other loci
      - Sporadic hemiplegic migraine
    - Retinal migraine
  - Chronic migraine
  - Complications of migraine
    - Status migrainosus
    - Persistent aura without infarction
    - Migrainous infarction
    - Migraine aura-triggered seizure
  - Probable migraine
    - Probable migraine without aura
    - Probable migraine with aura
  - Episodic syndromes that may be associated with migraine
    - Recurrent gastrointestinal disturbance
      - Cyclical vomiting syndrome
      - Abdominal migraine
    - Benign paroxysmal vertigo
    - Benign paroxysmal torticollis

Fig. 14.1 Classification of migraine

There are special subtypes of migraine.

a. Basilar migraine, preferably called "migraine with brainstem aura", is a less-common form of migraine syndrome, with prominent brainstem symptoms. There may be associated vertigo, staggering, incoordination of the limbs, dysarthria, and tingling in both hands and feet and sometimes around both sides of the mouth. Aura is clearly derived from the brain stem. Headache with the characteristics of migraine occurs at the same time or within 60 minutes of aura, often accompanied by nausea and vomiting.

b. Ophthalmoplegic and retinal migraine are recurrent unilateral headaches associated with weakness of extraocular muscles, including flickering, dark spots, or blindness. Ophthalmic examination is normal on interictal.

c. Familial hemiplegic migraine, known as hemiplegic migraine, is a condition mostly of infants and children (rarely adults), there are episodes of unilateral paralysis that may long outlast the headache. Several families have been described in which this condition is the result of a mutation in an ion channel.

(3) Diagnosis

A clinical diagnosis is usually made based on the type of migraine attack, family history and neurological examination. Brain CT, CTA, MRI, MRA can exclude cerebral vascular disease, intracranial aneurysm, space-occupying lesions and other intracranial organic diseases.

Diagnostic criteria for ICHD-3 migraine are in Tab. 14.1~Tab. 14.3.

Tab. 14.1 Diagnostic criteria of migraine without aura

A	At least five attacks fulfilling criteria B~D
B	Headache attacks lasting 4~72 hours (when untreated or unsuccessfully treated)
C	Headache has at least two of the following four characteristics: ① unilateral location; ② pulsating quality; ③ moderate or severe pain intensity; ④ aggravation by or causing avoidance of routine physical activity (e.g., walking or climbing stairs)
D	During headache at least one of the following: ① nausea and/or vomiting; ② photophobia and phonophobia
E	Not better accounted for by another ICHD-3 diagnosis

Tab. 14.2 Diagnostic criteria of migraine with aura

A	At least two attacks fulfilling criteria B and C
B	One or more of the following fully reversible aura symptoms: visual/sensory/speech and/or language/motor/brainstem/retinal
C	At least three of the following six characteristics: ① at least one aura symptom spreads gradually over 5 minutes; ② two or more aura symptoms occur in succession; ③ each individual aura symptom lasts 5~60 minutes; ④ at least one aura symptom is unilateral; ⑤ at least one aura symptom is positive; ⑥ the aura is accompanied, or followed within 60 minutes, by headache
D	Not better accounted for by another ICHD-3 diagnosis

Tab. 14.3 Diagnostic criteria of chronic migraine

A	Headache (migraine-like or tension-type-like) on 15 days/month for >3 months, and fulfilling criteria B and C
B	Occurring in a patient who has had at least five attacks fulfilling criteria B ~ D for migraine without aura and/or criteria B and C for migraine with aura
C	On 8 days/month for >3 months, fulfilling any of the following: ① criteria C and D for migraine without aura; ② criteria B and C for migraine with aura; ③ believed by the patient to be migraine at onset and relieved by a triptan or ergot derivative
D	Not better accounted for by another ICHD-3 diagnosis

(4) Differential diagnosis

a. Tension-type headache is usually bilateral, with occipitonuchal, temporal, or frontal predominance, or diffuse extension over the top of the cranium (Fig. 14.2).

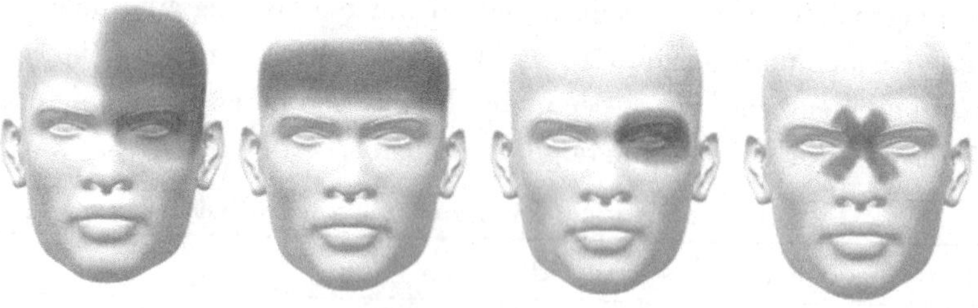

Fig. 14.2 Location of different headache

b. Cluster headache is a less common form of intense paraphernial pain, which lasts 15 minutes to 3 hours and occurs between once every other day and eight times a day. It is characterized by repeated intensive attacks, unilateral headache, ipsolateral conjunctiva congestion, tearing, runny nose, forehead and facial sweating, and Horner sign.

c. Inflammation of an extracranial artery causes pain localized to the site of the vessel. Lesions of the paranasal sinuses, teeth, eyes, and upper cervical vertebrae induce a less sharply localized pain but still one that is referred to a certain region, usually the forehead or maxilla or around the eyes.

d. Symptomatic headache can also be similar to migraine, accompanied by nausea, vomiting, but no typical migraine attack process. Most cases have focal nerve function loss or stimulation symptoms, craniocerebral imaging examination can show lesions.

(5) Treatment and prognosis

The purpose of migraine treatment is to relieve or terminate headache attack, relieve concomitant symptoms, and prevent headache recurrence. Treatment includes drug therapy and non-drug therapy. Drug treatment is divided into episodic treatment and preventive treatment. Mild to moderate migraine can be treated with nonsteroidal anti-inflammatory drugs (NSAIDs) alone. If it fails, migraine-specific medications can be used. Moderate to severe migraine can directly choose migraine-specific medications. Triptans are the first migraine-specific drug class developed and have proven efficacy in treatment of this neurological disease. They are contraindicated in patients with cardiovascular disease and possibly others, owning to their vasoconstrictive properties. "Ditans" and "Neurally acting anti-migraine agent", designed to selectively agonize the serotonin 5-HT 1F receptor subtype, provide anti-migraine effects without concomitant vasoconstriction. The drugs used now are listed in Tab. 14.4 and Tab. 14.5. Non-drug treatment is mainly to strengthen propaganda and education, to help patients establish scientific and correct concepts for prevention and treatment, to maintain a healthy lifestyle, to find and avoid all kinds of migraine triggers.

Most migraine sufferers have a good prognosis. Migraine symptoms can gradually ease with age, and some patients can no longer have migraine by the age of 60~70.

Tab. 14.4 Migraine-specific agents

	Agent	Recommended dose	Maximum daily dose
Ergots	Ergotamine	1~2 mg PO/SL/PR	6 mg PO/SL/PR
	Dihydroergotamine	1~2 mg IM/1~3 mg PO	4 mg IM/9 mg PO
Triptans	Sumatriptan	6 mg SC/25~100 mg PO	12 mg SC/300 mg PO
	Nalatriptan	2.5 mg PO	5 mg PO
	Rizatriptan	5~10 mg PO	30 mg PO
	Zolmitriptan	2.5~5 mg PO	10 mg PO
	Amotriptan	6.25~12.5 mg PO	25 mg PO
Ditans	Lasmiditan	100 mg	—
	Rimegepan	75 mg	—

Note: PO, per os; SL, sublingual; PR, per rectum; IM, intramuscular; SC, subcutaneous.

Tab. 14.5 Migraine preventive therapy

	Agent	Recommended dose
β-blockers	Propranolol	10~60 mg bid
	Metoprolol	100~200 mg/d
Calcium-channel antagonist	Flunarizine	5~10 mg qn
	Verapamil	160~320 mg/d
Antiepileptic drugs	Valproate	400~600 mg bid
	Topiramate	25~200 mg/d
	Gabapentin	900~1 800 mg/d
Antidepressant	Amitriptyline	25~75 mg/d
5-HT receptor antagonist	Pizotifen	0.5~3 mg/d

14.2 Tension-type Headache

Tension-type headache (TTH) is the most common primary headache disorder, with a worldwide lifetime prevalence of 46% and the male to female ratio is 4 : 5. The etiology of TTH is thought to be multifactorial, involving genetic and environmental factors. Clinical features of

TTH resemble common manifestations of muscle referred pain. Episodic TTH may evolve into the chronic form by different aspects and several triggers may be involved at the same time. Both peripheral and central sensitization mechanisms seem to be clearly involved in this process. Individuals with episodic TTH exhibit higher levels of peripheral excitability whereas chronic TTH clearly show central sensitization manifestations.

(1) Clinical feature

It is usually bilateral, with occipitonuchal, temporal, or frontal predominance, or diffuse extension over the top of the cranium. Patients typically describe headache pain as pressing, dull, and with the sensation of a tight band around the head. Physical examination detects tenderness of the muscle at the site of pain. Sometimes neck and shoulder muscle feels stiff and comfortable when pressed. The three subtypes of TTH are infrequent episodic, frequent episodic, and chronic.

① Infrequent episodic tension-type headache is typically bilateral, pressing or tightening in quality and of mild to moderate intensity, lasting minutes to days. The pain does not worsen with routine physical activity and is not associated with nausea, although photophobia or phonophobia may be present. Its frequency is at least 10 episodes of headache occurring on <1 day/month on average (<12 days/year).

② Frequent episodic tension-type headache is at least 10 episodes of headache occurring on 1~14 days/month on average for >3 months (≥ 12 and <180 days/year). Its nature is the same as infrequent episodic tension-type headache.

③ Chronic tension-type headache is a disorder evolving from frequent episodic tension-type headache, with daily or very frequent episodes of headache, typically bilateral, pressing or tightening in quality and of mild to moderate intensity, lasting hours to days, or unremitting. The pain does not worsen with routine physical activity, but may be associated with mild nausea, photophobia or phonophobia.

④ Probable tension-type headache missing one of the features required to fulfill all criteria for a type or subtype of tension-type headache coded above, and not fulfilling criteria for another headache disorder.

(2) Treatment

Simple analgesics, such as aspirin or acetaminophen or other NSAIDs, may be helpful, if only for brief periods. Persistent or frequent tension headaches respond best to cautious use of one of the several drugs that relieve anxiety or depression such as amitriptyline, especially when symptoms of these conditions are present. Some patients respond to ancillary measures such as massage, meditation, and biofeedback techniques. Some patients benefit from acupuncture, physical therapy, biofeedback, cognitive-behavioral therapy.

14.3 Cluster Headache

Cluster headache occurs predominantly in adult men (age range: 20 to 50; male-to-female ratio: approximately 5 : 1). The cause and mechanism of the cluster headache syndrome are unknown. Calcitonin gene-related peptide (CGRP) in brain venous blood of patients with cluster headache increased significantly, suggesting that trigeminal neurovascular complex is involved in the onset of cluster headache. Cluster headache has circadian rhythm and autonomic nerve symptoms in ipsilateral face, which may be related to hypothalamic nerve dysfunction.

(1) Clinical feature and diagnosis

Cluster headache is characterized by a consistent unilateral orbital localization. The pain is felt deep in and around the eye, is very intense and nonthrobbing as a rule, and often radiates into the forehead, temple, and checkless often to the ear, occiput, and neck. The pain is associated with ipsilateral conjunctival injection, lacrimation, nasal congestion, rhinorrhoea, forehead and facial sweating, miosis, ptosis and/or eyelid oedema, and/or with restlessness or agitation. The other characteristic feature is a nightly recurrence, 1~2 hours after the onset of sleep, or several times during the night; less often, it occurs during the day, unattended by aura or vomiting. The headache is called "alarm clock headache" because it recurs with remarkable regularity each night for periods extending over 6~12 weeks, followed thereafter by complete freedom for many months or even years. However, in approximately 10% of patients, the headache becomes chronic (without a remission period, or with remissions lasting <3 months, for at least 1 year), persisting over days, months, or even years. Cluster headache is usually so characteristic that it can not be confused with any other disease, although those unfamiliar with it may entertain a diagnosis of migraine, trigeminal neuralgia, carotid aneurysm, or temporal arteritis. Its diagnostic criteria are in Tab. 14.6.

Tab. 14.6 Diagnostic criteria of cluster headache

A	At least five attacks fulfilling criteria B~D
B	Severe or very severe unilateral orbital, supraorbital and/or temporal pain lasting 15~180 minutes (when untreated)
C	Either or both of the following: a. at least one of the following symptoms or signs, ipsilateral to the headache: conjunctival injection and/or lacrimation, nasal congestion and/or rhinorrhoea, eyelid oedema, forehead and facial sweating, miosis and/or ptosis; b. a sense of restlessness or agitation
D	Occurring with a frequency between once every other day and 8 times per day
E	Not better accounted for by another ICHD-3 diagnosis

(2) Treatment

Treatment of cluster headache entails a combination of fastacting abortive treatment, transitional treatment and preventive treatment. Inhalation of 100% or high flow oxygen via mask for 10~15 minutes at the onset of cluster headache may also abort the attack, but about 70% patients respond to this way. Intranasal lidocaine or sumatriptan can also be used to abort an acute attack. Ergotamine given once or twice during the day is helpful. Treatment in the acute phase does not shorten the duration or frequency of cluster attacks. Therefore, preventive treatment should be given immediately once cluster headache is diagnosed. Prophylactic drugs include verapamil, glucocorticoid and lithium. Verapamil can be started with 80 mg qid and increased the dose over days, and electrocardiogram (ECG) monitoring is recommended.

14.4 Intracranial Hypotension Headache

The cardinal feature is orthostatic headache. There are spontaneous and secondary types, which follow lumbar puncture occurs after straining, a nonhurtful fall, or for unknown reason.

Continuous leakage of CSF results from head trauma or surgery, ventricular shunt, spinal trauma or surgery. Dehydration, uremia, severe systemic infections, hypotension, and others can lead to reduced production of cerebrospinal fluid. As a result of the reduction of cerebrospinal fluid volume, pressure, brain tissue displacement and subsidence, intracranial pain sensitive structure is stretched thereby causing headache.

(1) Clinical feature and diagnosis

Patients often have headache or headache aggravation within 15 minutes of standing upright, headache relief or disappear after recumbent position. It is characterized by a steady occipitonuchal and frontal pain coming on within a few minutes after arising from a recumbent position and is relieved within one minute or two by lying down. It may be accompanied by posterior neck pain or stiffness, nausea, vomiting, fear of voice or photophobia, tinnitus, dizziness. A few cases have presented with stupor as a result of downward transtentorial displacement of the diencephalic region or an upper cervical myelopathy caused by downward deformation and displacement of the spinal cord. In these cases, the CSF pressure is low or not measurable; the fluid may contain a few mononuclear cells but is most often normal. A helpful diagnostic sign is diffuse pachymeningeal enhancement on MRI. The leak can be found by radionuclide cisternography or CT myelography. Most spontaneous CSF leaks occur at the cervical-thoracic junction or at the thoracic spine. So the diagnosis can be made by lumbar puncture measurement of decreased CSF pressure (60 mmH_2O or less) based on the typical clinical features of postural headache.

(2) Treatment and prognosis

Patients can be supine or in a position with head low and feet high. The ingestion of large volumes of fluids and the infusion of 1 000~2 000 mL of 5% glucose (or 3 500~4 000 mL of normal saline) are usually recommended. The administration of caffeine-ergotamine preparations or intravenous caffeine may also have a salutary though temporary effect on the headache. The most dependable treatment is a "blood patch" (spinal epidural injection of a few milliliters of the patient's own blood). Moreover, the volume of blood injected is usually about 20 mL. Blood can compress the dural sac and block leakage of cerebrospinal fluid. Secondary hypotensive headache can be treated for specific causes, such as fistula repair for cerebrospinal fluid leakage after surgery or trauma.

Some patients with spontaneous hypotensive headache experience remission within 2 weeks, some of which last for months or even years.

14.5 Trigeminal Neuralgia (Tic Douloureux)

Trigeminal neuralgia (TN) is a severe facial pain disease of unknown cause and unclear genetic background. TN is further subclassified into classical, secondary or idiopathic, depending on the underlying cause. The classical type, which accounts for 75% of cases, is diagnosed when there is trigeminal neurovascular compression with morphological changes ipsilateral to the side of the pain, demonstrated either on MR imaging with appropriate trigeminal sequences or during surgery. The current pathophysiological hypothesis for classical TN suggests that the pain mechanisms are precipitated by a proximal compression of the trigeminal sensory root near the brainstem (root entry zone, considered a vulnerable area to demyelination) by a blood vessel. The vascular compression may start a process of focal demyelination and remyelination, probably mediated by microvascular ischaemic damages. The secondary type, accounting for approximately 15% of cases, is attributable to an identifiable underlying neurological disease that is known to cause TN, such as cerebellopontine angle tumour, arteriovenous malformation and multiple sclerosis. The idiopathic type, accounting for approximately 10% of cases, is diagnosed when no apparent cause for TN can be found.

(1) Clinical feature

1) Clinical manifestation

TN is a common disorder of middle age and later life, consisting of paroxysms of intense, stabbing pain in the distribution of the mandibular and maxillary divisions of the fifth cranial nerve. The pain seldom lasts more than 2 minutes, but it may be so intense that the patient winces involuntarily. The paroxysms recur frequently, both day and night, for several weeks at a time. Another characteristic feature is the initiation of a jab or a series of jabs of pain by stimulation of certain areas of the face, lips, or gums, as in shaving or brushing the teeth, or by movement of these parts in chewing, talking, or yawning, or even by a breeze, the so-called trigger points. In addition to the paroxysmal pain, some patients complain of a more or less continuous discomfort, itching, or sensitivity of restricted areas of the face, features regarded as atypical even though not infrequent. Usually a spatial and temporal summation of impulses is necessary to trigger a paroxysm of pain, which is followed by a refractory period of up to 2 or 3 minutes.

2) Diagnostic investigation

MR of the brain is the gold-standard investigation to exclude secondary causes of TN. Detailed trigeminal MR brain scan sequences are pivotal to detecting the presence of a trigeminal neurovascular conflict, the type of vascular structure (artery or vein or both) and the degree of compression. If MR is contraindicated, a CT scan of the head, CT cerebral angiogram and trigeminal-evoked potentials and/or neurophysiological recordings of trigeminal reflexes should be used.

(2) Diagnosis

The diagnosis of TN must rest on the strict clinical criteria enumerated below (Tab. 14.7), and the condition must be distinguished from other forms of facial and cephalic neuralgia and pain arising from diseases of the jaw, teeth, or sinuses.

Tab. 14.7 ICHD-3 diagnostic criteria for TN

A	Recurrent paroxysms of unilateral facial pain in the distribution (s) of one or more divisions of the trigeminal nerve, with no radiation beyond, and fulfilling criteria B and C
B	Pain has all of the following characteristics: ① lasting from a fraction of 1 s to 2 minutes; ② severe intensity; ③ electric shock-like shooting, stabbing or sharp in quality
C	Precipitated by innocuous stimuli within the affected trigeminal distribution
D	Not better accounted for by another ICHD-3 diagnosis

(3) Treatment and prognosis

Antiepileptic drugs such as phenytoin (300~400 mg/d), valproic acid (800~1 200 mg/d), clonazepam (2~6 mg/d), gabapentin (300~900 mg/d or more), pregabalin (150~300 mg/d), and carbamazepine (600 ~ 1 200 mg/d), alone or in combination, suppress or shorten the duration and severity of the attacks. Baclofen may be useful in patients who cannot tolerate carbamazepine or gabapentin, but it is most effective as an adjunct to one of the anticonvulsant drugs. Most of the patients with intractable pain, however, come to surgery or an equivalent form of root destruction. There are four types of surgical intervention available: a. microvascular decompression; b. controlled lesioning of the trigeminal ganglion or root by mechanical, thermal or chemical means; c. separation of trigeminal nerve fascicles in the posterior fossa; d. non-invasive ablative (stereotactic radiosurgery which focuses radiation at the trigeminal root entry zone). TN is characterised by recurrences and remissions. Many people have periods of remission with no pain lasting months or years but in many, TN becomes more severe and less responsive to treatment over time, despite increasing pharmacological intervention. Most patients with TN are initially managed medically, and approximately 50% eventually have a surgical procedure.

References

[1] Headache Classfication Committee of the International Headache Society (IHS). The international classification of headache disorders, 3rd ed (beta version) [J]. Cephalalgia, 2013,33(9):629-808.

[2] ROPPER H A, SAMUELS A M. Adams and Victor's principles of neurology[M]. 9th ed. New York: McGraw-Hill Education/Medical, 2009.

[3] RECOBER A. Pathophysiology of migraine [J]. Continuum: Lifelong Learning in Neurology, 2021,27(3):586-596.

[4] OLLA D, SAWYER J, SOMMER N, et al. Migraine treatment[J]. Clinics in Plastic Surgery, 2020,47(2):295-303.

[5] SCRIPTER C. Headache: tension-type headache[J]. FP Essentials, 2018,473:17-20.

[6] BRANDT B R, DOESBORG P G G, HAAN J, et al. Pharmacotherapy for cluster headache[J]. CNS Drugs, 2020,34(2):171-184.

[7] LAMBRU G, ZAKRZEWSKA J, MATHARU M. Trigeminal neuralgia: a practical guide[J]. Practical Neurology, 2021,21(5):392-402.

(Zhu Wenli, Wu Wenqi)

SECTION III

Disciplines Linked to Neurology

Chapter 15
Neurorehabilitation

Neural rehabilitation is an important branch of clinical rehabilitation and an integral part of clinical treatment of nervous system diseases. The core guiding ideology of neurorehabilitation is functional recovery and reconstruction. The goal of neural rehabilitation is to adopt a variety of effective measures based on functional training to speed up the recovery of neural function, eliminate or reduce the functional disorders caused by nervous system lesions, make patients return to their family and society, and improve their quality of life.

15.1 Theoretical Basis of Neural Rehabilitation

(1) The plasticity theory of the central nervous system

The central nervous system is variable in order to regulate various adaptive responses, and this variability is also known as modifiability or plasticity. This plasticity is manifested in short-term functional changes and long-term structural changes.

(2) Schwann cells

Schwann cells secrete a variety of neurotrophic factors and extracellular matrix, which participate in the microenvironment of peripheral nerve regeneration and affect nerve regeneration.

15.2 Methods of Rehabilitation Evaluation for Stroke

a. The commonly used scoring scales for evaluating the severity of brain damage include the Glasgow coma scale (GCS) and the National Institute of Health Stroke Scale (NIHSS). The former can be used to determine the severity of brain damage, while the latter can be used to evaluate the degree of neurological impairment.

b. Brunnstrom motor function evaluation method. The motor function recovery of stroke hemiplegia is divided into 6 stages by Brunnstorm, and the motor function recovery is evaluated according to the changes of muscle tension and movement pattern of upper limb, hand and lower limb.

c. Three-level balance test is often used in clinic. Berg balance scale is the most commonly used scale in clinical rehabilitation and research of stroke.

d. The assessment of activities of daily living (ADL) is a common functional assessment in clinical rehabilitation of stroke. The main methods are Barthel index and function independent measure (FIM).

15.3 Rehabilitation Treatment of Stroke

(1) Acute rehabilitation treatment

During this period, the patients begin to recover from no active movement of the affected limb to muscle tension, and have weak flexor and extensor muscle movement together.

a. Passive movement of hemiplegic limbs. In this period, the stroke affects limbs of most patients. In order to maintain the range of motion of joints, prevent joint swelling and stiffness, and promote the early emergence of active activities of hemiplegic limbs, passive hemiplegic limbs are mainly used. The order of activity is from proximal joint to distal joint, generally 2 ~ 3 times a day, more than 5 minutes each time, until the active movement of hemiplegic limbs recovers. At the same time, the patient is told to turn his head to the hemiplegic side, through visual feedback and therapist speech stimulation, contributing to the patient's active participation.

b. Physical factor therapy. Commonly used local mechanical stimulation (such as hand slapping on the corresponding muscle surface), ice stimulation, functional electrical stimulation, EMG biofeedback and local air pressure therapy can make paralyzed limb muscles gradually improve tension through passive contraction and relaxation.

c. Traditional therapy. Commonly used massage and acupuncture treatment, through deep and shallow sensory stimulation, contribute to local muscle contraction and blood circulation, thus promoting the improvement of limb function on the affected side.

(2) Early rehabilitation treatment

From the joint movement of the weak flexor and extensor of the affected limb to the obvious spasm, the patient can actively move the affected limb, but the muscle activity is common exercise.

1) Bedside and bedside activities

When the hemiplegic upper limb can not complete the action independently, the method of bilateral simultaneous movement is adopted, but the degree of active participation of the hemiplegic upper limb increases. Bedside sitting and bedside station: on the basis of lying on the side, gradually change to bedside sitting (feet can not be suspended). When patients begin to practise this action, it should be completed with the help of the therapist. When standing at the bedside, the therapist should stand on the hemiplegic side of the patient and give some help to the hemiplegic knee to prevent knee weakness or knee overextension, requiring both lower limbs to bear weight at the same time in the process of sitting-station transfer to prevent the center of gravity from deviating to one side.

2) Sitting activity

Through the center of gravity (left, right, front, back) transfer to train the motor control ability of the sitting trunk, the therapist should give help and guidance on the hemiplegic side at the beginning of the training, gradually reduce support as appropriate, and transition to activities of daily life.

3) Standing activities

Through the center of gravity transfer, training the movement control ability of the lower limbs and trunk in the standing position, at the beginning, the therapist should give support to the legs and knees on the hemiplegic side, gradually reduce the support as appropriate, and pay attention to the weight bearing of both lower limbs at the beginning of the standing position.

4) Weight loss walking training

Weight loss walking training can be carried out on the premise that the hemiplegic lower limbs can not adapt to one leg support, the training can lighten the weight of the lower limbs by supporting part of the body weight, and make the affected lower limbs bear weight as soon as possible, provide symmetrical weight transfer for both lower limbs, repeat complete walking cycle training and increase the safety of training.

5) Walking in parallel bars

Walking in parallel bars can be carried out on the premise that the lower limbs of the hemiplegic side can adapt to the support of one leg. In order to avoid insufficient extension of pulp, knee hyperextension or knee weakness on the hemiplegic side, the therapist should give help and guidance on the hemiplegic side, if the ankle dorsiflexion of the affected side is insufficient, ankle-foot orthosis can be worn to prevent possible hemiplegic gait.

6) Physical factor therapy

The focus is to improve the function of elbow extension, wrist extension and finger extension of the upper limb on the hemiplegic side (such as triceps brachii and forearm extensor), and the flexors of the lower extremities on the hemiplegic side (such as biceps femoris, tibialis anterior muscle and long and short fibula muscle). To improve knee flexion and ankle dorsiflexion function, the commonly used methods include functional electrical stimulation, EMG biofeedback and low and medium frequency electrical stimulation.

7) Traditional rehabilitation therapy

The commonly used methods are acupuncture and massage. The hemiplegic upper limb extensor and lower limb flexor should be selected to improve their corresponding function.

8) Speech therapy

Stroke patients with dysarthria or aphasia should be given early speech function training to improve their communication ability and their overall functional level.

(3) Recovery of mid-term rehabilitation

The goal of rehabilitation therapy in this period is to strengthen coordination and the practical function of upper limbs and lower extremities. The focus of motor function training in stroke patients should be on the recovery of normal motor mode and motor control ability. It is very important to improve the rehabilitation training of various sensory functions for the recovery of motor function.

a. Therapeutic movements of the upper limbs and hands. In the therapeutic activities of hemiplegic upper limbs and hands, especially in the training of motor control ability, special attention should be paid to the recovery law of "from near to far, from thick to fine". The active control ability of the proximal joint directly affects the functional recovery of the distal joint of the limb (such as the improvement and recovery of hand function).

b. Therapeutic activities of the lower extremities. The function of lower limbs is not only weight-bearing, but also walking. People can better participate in daily life, family life and community life by walking. If the patient has severe brain damage and other functional disorders (such as cognitive dysfunction), which affect the recovery of limb motor function, a wheelchair can be used.

(4) Rehabilitation treatment in the later stage of recovery

Most of the muscle activities of the patients in this period are selective, patients can move independently, and are not affected by the common movement of the limbs, until the muscle spasm of the limbs disappears, the muscle activity is selective, the separation movement is stable, the coordination is good, but the speed is slow.

a. Ability training for activities of daily living. Strengthen self-care ability training in daily life, such as decoration, toilet use, bathing, going up and down stairs, and increase necessary housework and outdoor activity training.

b. Speech therapy. On the basis of the previous speech therapy, increase the content related to daily life in order to adapt to the activities of daily life in the future.

c. Cognitive function training. Carry on the related training combined with the daily life activities, see the relevant chapter for details.

d. Psychotherapy. Encouragement and psychological counseling are helpful to strengthen patients' confidence in rehabilitation treatment, so as to ensure the smooth progress of the whole rehabilitation treatment.

e. The application of brace and orthosis, such as hand brace, affected foot orthosis and walker, is helpful to improve the independent living ability of patients.

(5) Rehabilitation treatment of sequelae

Stroke sequela period refers to the brain damage caused by dysfunction after a variety of treatment, the damaged function will not be significantly improved in a long time.

The rehabilitation treatment in this period is three-level rehabilitation, and the recovery of residual and existing functions should be strengthened, that is, compensatory functional training, including the application of orthoses, walkers and wheelchairs, as well as environmental transformation and necessary vocational skills training to meet the needs of daily life. At the same time, pay attention to prevent the further aggravation of abnormal muscle tone and contracture, avoid the occurrence of disuse syndrome, osteoporosis and other complications, help patients get out of bed and carry out appropriate outdoor activities, pay attention to more communication with patients and necessary psychological counseling, stimulate their awareness of active participation, and play the role of family and society.

References

[1] KHAN F, AMATYA B, GALEA M P, et al. Neurorehabilitation: applied neuroplasticity[J]. Journal of Neurology, 2017,264(3):603-615.

[3] ANAYA M A, BRANSCHEIDT M. Neurorehabilitation after stroke[J]. Stroke, 2019,50(7):e180-e182.

[3] DONNAN G A. Neurorehabilitation[J]. International Journal of Stroke, 2016,11(4):385.

(Pu Lang, Zhang Lei)

Chapter 16
Neurological Intensive Care

The critical nervous system diseases mainly include disturbance of consciousness, mental disorder, increased intracranial pressure, epileptic state and so on. The above diseases mainly occur in cerebrovascular disease, central nervous system infection, spinal neuromuscular disease, poisoning and so on. As brain is an organ with special anatomical structure and physiological functions, severe brain injury is often accompanied by heart, lung, liver, kidney, gastrointestinal, metabolic and immune injury and other organ systems. With the progress of society and medicine, more and more critically ill patients with nervous system are placed in the neuro-intensive care unit (NCU), and are monitored and treated by medical staff with advanced instruments and professional expertise. As a result, the mortality rate decreases significantly. The degree of neurological disability is significantly reduced. This chapter focuses on the monitoring and treatment of several common critical nervous system diseases.

16.1 Brain Herniation

Brain herniation refers to the displacement of part of the brain tissue due to intracranial pressure differences that exceed certain anatomical boundaries. When intracranial pressure increases, the pressure in the lesion site and ventricle first increase, and then transfer to the surrounding sites and ventricles with lower pressure. Due to the barrier between falx and tentorium, the pressure is cushioned, but at the same time, parts of the brain are forced to move towards openings or crevices. When displaced brain tissue affects vital centers, it can lead to poor prognosis and even death. Therefore, cerebral hernia is the most serious consequence of increased intracranial pressure, which is clinically common in transtentorial herniation and transforamen magnum herniation.

(1) Pathogenesis

1) Transtentorial herniation

Increased intracranial pressure pushes displaced brain tissue down into the tentorial hiatus, which is called transtentorial hernia. The serious results of cerebellar tentorial hiatus hernia include not only the entrapment and necrosis of the herniated brain tissue, but also the extrusion, traction and damage of the adjacent structures caused by herniated material, such as the midbrain, oculomotor nerve, basilar artery and its branches, which block cerebrospinal fluid circulation pathway. There are two types of cerebellar tentorial hiatus hernia: lateral (uncinate hernia) and central (central hernia).

① Uncinate hernia

The uncinate hernia is formed by herniating the structures of hippocampus and uncinate gyrus in the medial temporal lobe into the tentorial hiatus. Uncinate hernia first involves ipsilateral midbrain cerebral peduncle and oculomotor nerve roots (the parasympathetic fibers regulated by the dorsal internal eye muscles are the first to be involved). If it continues to develop, the posterior cerebral artery will be pulled, and the brain damage range can be extended to thalamus, hypothalamus, temporal lobe and occipital lobe (Fig. 16.1).

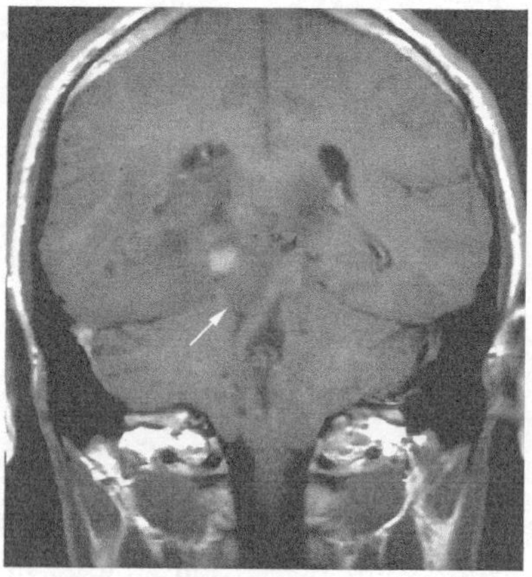

Fig. 16.1 Uncinate hernia (white arrow)

② Central hernia

Different from uncinate hernia, midline or deep brain structure cause bilateral compression and downward displacement where the supratentorial thalamus, third ventricle and basal ganglia are located. So it is also called midline hernia. The displaced tissue first presses the hypothalamus, thus the diencephalon is the first part involved. If it continues to develop, the upper middle brain is involved and the entire brain stem is involved from top to bottom (Fig. 16.2). Central hernia cannot be accompanied with uncinate hernia, but severe uncinate hernia often coexists with central hernia.

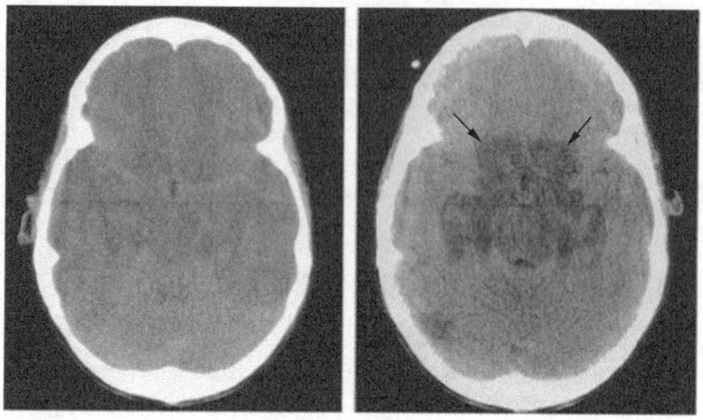

(a) (b)

Fig. 16.2 Axial non-contrast CT scan

2) Transforamen magna herniation

The small pressure difference can push the cerebellar tonsil to herniate downward into the spinal canal through the foramen magnum. Foramen magnum hernia is more common in space occupying lesions of posterior fossa and can be seen in diffuse intracranial lesions with severe cerebral edema (Fig. 16.3a). Supratentorial lesions may occur tentorial hernia firstly and foramen magnum hernia lately (Fig. 16.3b). Herniated cerebellar tonsils can be compressed, displaced, deformed, resulting in congestion, edema, bleeding, more importantly, the movement of cerebellar tonsils to the front can press the lower part of the medulla oblongata, thus the respiratory and circulation centers involved. Compression of cerebellar tonsils into the outlet of the fourth ventricle can lead to obstructive hydrocephalus, further increasing intracranial pressure. Of course, glossopharynx, vagus, accessory nerve and upper neck segment of spinal nerve root can be injured due to compression.

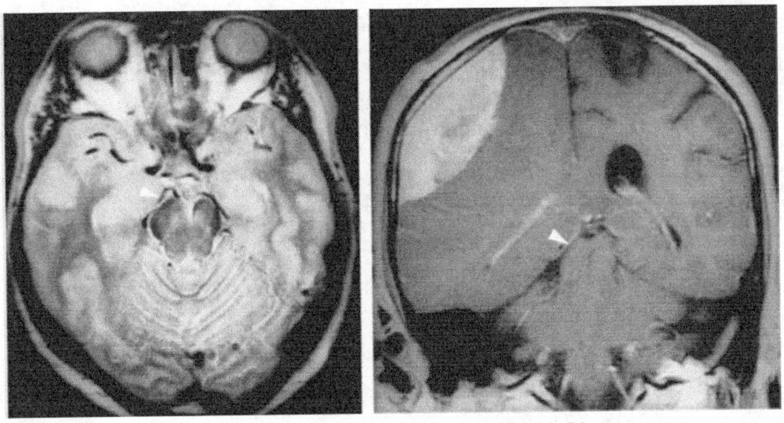

(a) (b)

Fig. 16.3 Transforamen magna herniation (arrow)

(2) Clinical manifestation

1) Uncinate hernia

Patient may present with headache (mild headache in early time, severe headache accompanied by vomiting in late time), disturbance of consciousness (early drowsiness, late lethargy or coma), oculomotor nerve paralysis (early intraocular muscle paralysis, pupil shrinkage, but most of which are transient too hard to be found, then the pupil dilates, the light response is slow or disappear and extraocular muscle paralysis occurs in late stage), pyramidal tract sign (contralateral pyramidal tract sign is positive or contralateral limb paralysis occurs in early stage, bilateral pyramidal tract sign or bilateral limb paralysis occur in late stage), decerebrate rigidity (contralateral limb upper limb become straightened, internally rotated in early stage. Spontaneous, intermittent or continuous limb stretching ankylosis occurs in late stage), and changes of vital signs (body temperature and blood pressure increase, heart rate and breathing decrease in early stage; vital center failures, temperature and blood pressure drop, irregular respiration occurs, heart rate increases and finally respiratory and cardiac arrest in the late stage).

2) Central hernia

The clinical manifestations are associated with the site involved, that is, the disease progresses from the initial diencephalon to the upper and lower brain stem in a top-down processing manner.

a. Early drowsiness, lethargy or shallow coma, normal or tidal breathing, existing bilateral pupil response to light; bilateral pyramidal tract sign, orbital pressing inducing upper limb defense action or cortical ankylosis (diencephalon involvement).

b. Moderate coma, central neurogenic hyperventilation, disappearance of bilateral pupil response to light, retardation or disappearance of cephalo-ocular response and vestibular response, diencephalic ankylosis (upper brain stem involvement).

c. Late deep coma, shallow fast or irregular breathing, flaccid paralysis of limbs (lower brain stem involvement).

3) Transforamen magna herniation

a. Neck stiffness or forced head position: early occipital and neck pain, late neck stiffness or forced head position (cervical nerve root is stimulated).

b. Posterior cerebral nerve palsy: early articulation, hoarseness, drinking cough and dysphagia, late aphonia, dysphagia (posterior cerebral nerve is pulled and damaged).

c. Changes in vital signs: The changes of vital signs are most obvious in acute foramen magnum hernia, which is manifested as rapid respiratory and circulatory failure, and sudden respiratory arrest is the most characteristic manifestation. Chronic foramen magnum hernia is characterized by shallow and slow breathing, irregular breathing and eventual apnea. Sometimes the circulatory function can be maintained for a short time under mechanical ventilation, which is manifested as respiratory and circulatory separation (the respiratory center located in the lower portion of the medulla oblong is more easily damaged than the cardiovascular center, or the heart has automatic rhythmic pacing).

(3) Diagnosis

Uncinate hernia, central hernia and foramen magnum hernia may occur independently, simultaneously or sequentially. The common features are compression and displacement of the brain stem. The diagnosis principles of uncinate hernia include supratentorial lesion, varying degrees of disturbance of consciousness and pupil changes on the side of hernia. The main diagnostic principles of central hernia include the supratentorial lesion and descending damage of diencephalon, upper brainstem and lower brainstem, which is manifested as disturbance of consciousness and breathing, and gradual occurrence and aggravation of brainstem reflex and limb movement disorders. The diagnosis principles of foramen magnum hernia include supratentorial lesion, rapid respiratory and circulatory failure and sudden respiratory arrest, which is the most characteristic manifestation.

(4) Treatment of cerebral hernia

Treatment is aimed at relieving the swelling and pressure inside the brain early. It may prevent further brain damage or death. To reduce swelling and pressure, treatment may involve surgery to remove a tumor, blood clot, or abscess, ventriculostomy, a surgery that places a drain through a hole in the skull to get rid of fluids, osmotic therapy or diuretics (such as mannitol or hypertonic saline) to pull fluid out of the brain tissue, corticosteroids to reduce inflammation, craniectomy, a surgery that removes a part of the skull to make more room. Endotracheal intubation or (and) mechanical ventilation are required if the patient is in hypopnea or his respiratory arrests.

16.2 Central Nervous Respiratory Pump Failure

Several anatomical structures of the central nervous system are associated with respiratory movement. The medulla oblongata is the origin of respiratory rhythm and controls inhalation and exhalation. The diencephalon, midbrain and pons are the respiratory regulation centers, which improve the respiratory rhythm. The cerebral cortex is the control center of voluntary breathing (conscious or unconscious), making breathing more controlled. Damage of any part of these structures can result in central nervous respiratory pump failure.

(1) Etiology and pathogenesis

The causes of central nervous respiratory pump failure can be divided into organic causes and nonorganic causes. Organic causes include craniocerebral trauma, cerebral hemorrhage, cerebral infarction, brain tumor and so on. Nonorganic causes include poisoning of drugs (such as narcotics, sedatives) and poisons (such as organophosphorus pesticides).

The mechanism of central nervous respiratory pump failure is that the central controlling respiratory muscle movement cannot produce nerve impulse normally to weaken respiratory movement. Its clinical features include reduced respiratory rate and tidal volume, which lead to respiratory acidosis and hypoxemia. In addition, central nervous respiratory pump failure can coexist with neurogenic pulmonary edema. Pathological studies find that almost all patients with severe brain injury and rapid death have pulmonary edema, namely neurogenic pulmonary edema, whose respiratory failure is characterized by the higher degree of hypoxemia compared with hypercapnia. The exact mechanism of neurogenic pulmonary edema is unclear and may be related to hyperreactive pulmonary vascular tone caused by autonomic nerve injury. Although neurogenic pulmonary edema is indistinguishable from other types of pulmonary edema, it is characterized by its rapid onset and resolution.

(2) Clinical manifestation

The respiratory frequency, rhythm and amplitude of central nervous pump failure vary differently, showing special respiratory types. In cerebral hemisphere lesions, the midbrain or diencephalon respiratory regulation center can not be controlled, resulting in respiratory fluctuations that amplitude varies from small to large, and then from large to small, and even chyne-stokes respiration occur after gradual disappearance (pause). When the midbrain tegmental is damaged, the pons reticular respiratory center can not be controlled, resulting in central neurogenic hyperrespiration. The respiratory center of the medulla oblongata is out of control, and prolonged inspiratory time alternates with apnea. When the lower part of the pons is damaged, the respiratory center of the medulla oblongata is out of control, resulting in clustered breathing of apnea after 4 ~ 5 breaths. When the medulla oblongata (the lowest center of respiration) is affected, ataxic breathing occurs, that is, the frequency and amplitude of breathing changes from time to time, followed by irregular apnea, mandibular breathing, and even apnea.

(3) Diagnosis

The diagnosis principles of central nervous system respiratory pump failure include clear diagnosis of central nervous system diseases; coexistence of decreased respiratory drive and uncontrollable respiratory rhythm, which are manifested as changes of respiratory frequency, rhythm and amplitude related to brain anatomical structure injury; $PaO_2 < 60$ mmHg and/or $PaCO_2 > 50$ mmHg.

(4) Treatment

The treatment principle of central nervous pump failure is to establish artificial airway and mechanical ventilation immediately to assist respiration, avoiding respiratory arrest or more serious acid-base imbalance and electrolyte disorder. The treatment principles of neurogenic pulmonary edema include: a. Actively treat the primary disease; b. Reduce intracranial pressure; c. Reduce pulmonary edema (methylprednisolone and other adrenocorticosteroid drugs); d. Reduce cardiac preload by diuretic; e. High flow oxygen or mechanical ventilation; f. Remove respiratory secretions and keep the airway unobstructed.

16.3 Peripheral Nerve Respiratory Pump Failure

Multiple anatomical sites of the peripheral nervous system are associated with respiratory movement, such as nerves, nerve-muscle joints, and muscles. Although spinal cord is classified as central nervous system according to the anatomical classification of nervous system, the innervation of respiratory muscle movement is only the connection between brain and respiratory muscle and the integration of respiratory reflex, and does not produce respiratory rhythm, thus they are described here together. Damage of any part of these structures can result in peripheral nerve respiratory pump failure.

(1) Etiology

1) Myelopathy

Spinal cord injury, such as ischemia, inflammation, and trauma, can reduce respiratory muscle contraction through damage of the anterior horn of the spinal cord. When acute spinal cord injury occurs above the fourth cervical plane, the respiratory muscles including the diaphragm are paralyzed, and respiratory failure is rapid and serious. Respiratory failure may occur when spinal cord injury occurs under the fourth cervical plane, although diaphragmatic movement is preserved.

2) Peripheral neuropathy

Guillain-Barré syndrome is the most representative disease that manifests decreased respiratory muscle contractility caused by motor nerve damage. With the progression of the disease, neuromuscular dystrophy can occur, which weakens and aggravates respiratory muscle contractility.

3) Neuromuscular junction disease

Myasthenia gravis, botulism and drug poisoning (such as muscle relaxants) can induce nerve impulse conduction disorder of neuromuscular junction and weaken respiratory muscle contractility.

4) Myopathy

Progressive muscular dystrophy, polymyositis or dermatomyositis may weaken respiratory muscle contractility due to damage of the motor endplate. Patients with chronic progress are often accompanied by respiratory muscle atrophy, which weakens and aggravates respiratory muscle contractility.

(2) Pathogenesis

The mechanism of peripheral nerve respiratory pump failure is that the nerve controlling the movement of respiratory muscles can not conduct nerve impulse normally, thus the contraction of respiratory muscles is weakened and ventilation is insufficient. The pulmonary parenchyma of patients with peripheral nerve respiratory pump failure is mostly normal, and the ventilatory dysfunction caused by weakened respiratory muscle contractility manifests high respiratory rate and low tidal volume. Mild patients can keep ventilatory volume stable by increasing respiratory rate, and severe patients can improve ventilatory volume quickly by mechanical ventilation treatment. However, if the patient fails to improve ventilation as early as possible, it can cause complications such as airway obstruction, mis-aspiration or asphyxia, bacterial pneumonia, atelectasis and other complications, inducing cough weakness and poor sputum excretion, and resulting in ventilation dysfunction, hypoxemia and metabolic acidosis.

(3) Clinical manifestation

Peripheral nervous respiratory pump failure manifests shallow, rapid and weak breathing. Patients with phrenic paralysis have dyspnea, shortness of breath, cyanosis, reverse breathing (paradoxical movement of outward chest and inward abdomen when inhaling), which can be relieved after head elevation or sitting up. Diaphragmatic paralysis of acute peripheral nervous system disease progresses rapidly and requires ventilator assistance. Phrenic paralysis of chronic peripheral nervous system disease progresses slowly, but it can only be maintained by mechanical ventilation in late stages.

(4) Diagnosis

The diagnostic principle of peripheral nerve respiratory pump failure include: the diagnosis of spinal cord and peripheral nervous system diseases is clear; weakened respiratory muscle contraction is prominent, that is, high respiratory rate and low tidal volume (shallow and rapid breathing); PaO_2<60 mmHg and $PaCO_2$>50 mmHg; lung capacity <55% and/or <1 500 mL; complications such as aspiration/asphyxia, bacterial pneumonia and atelectasis are common.

(5) Treatment

In addition to the treatment of the primary disease, the most significant measure is to establish an artificial airway as early as possible, if necessary, using mechanical ventilation to assist breathing. For mild acute patients, non-invasive ventilator can be used for assisted breathing, while for severe patients, endotracheal intubation (or tracheotomy) and invasive ventilator can be used to assist breathing.

References

[1] KOENING M. Cerebral herniation syndromes and intracranial hypertension[M]. New Jersey: Rutgers University Press, 2016.

[2] SARAH E, NYQUIST P A. Neurointensive care unit clinical practice and organization [M]. Berlin: Springer, 2020.

(Han Wei, Xu Yuhao)

Chapter 17
Neuropsychology

Neuropsychology studies psychological problems from the perspective of neuroscience. People need to understand how the human brain reflects things in the external environment, how to reflect social phenomena, how to produce psychological activities, and the relationship between psychological activities and physiological activities of the brain. Neuropsychology regards brain as the material noumenon of psychological activities to study the relationship between brain and psychology or brain and behavior.

17.1 Delirium

Delirium is a common syndrome found across many medical specialties and has many other names (i. e., encephalopathy, acute brain syndrome, acute brain failure, toxic psychosis, etc.). In 2018, the World Health Organization defined delirium as acute or subacute onset attention disorder and consciousness disorder. The symptoms often fluctuate within 1 day, accompanied by other cognitive disorders (such as memory, language, visuospatial function or sensory perception disorder), which can affect the sleep arousal cycle, and its cause is usually the intoxication or withdrawal of non psycho behavioral disorder substances.

The pathophysiological mechanism of delirium is complex and not fully understood. Because there are many causes and risk factors of delirium and various clinical manifestations, it is difficult to explain the occurrence and development of delirium with a single pathophysiological mechanism. The theory of neurotransmitter imbalance mechanism plays an important role in the pathogenesis of delirium and is the theoretical basis of drug treatment for delirium.

(1) Clinical manifestation

The basic feature of delirium is the disorder of acute or subacute attention and consciousness state, which can be manifested in the impairment of consciousness content (decreased attention and poor orientation) and consciousness level (impairment of awakening degree) significantly different from the basic level, as well as language disorder, perception and behavior disorder. It mostly presents a fluctuating course of disease, which generally lasts for several hours to several days, and worsens in the evening and at night. Delirium mainly has the following core manifestations.

a. Attention disorder: The ability to orient, focus, continue and change attention is reduced, the patient's attention is distracted, easy to be disturbed by irrelevant stimuli, and patients are unable to properly answer or change topics according to the inquiry content.

b. Disturbance of consciousness content: It shows that the orientation to the environment is weakened, sometimes the orientation to their own state is weakened, accompanied by decrease of consciousness activities such as the degree of awakening, indifference and drowsiness, or the excessive enhancement of consciousness states such as alertness, irritability, aggressiveness and refusal to cooperate with diagnosis and treatment activities.

c. Cognitive impairment: It can mainly include sensory and perceptual impairment (such as illusion or hallucination), memory and learning impairment, abstract thinking and understanding impairment, executive dysfunction (i.e. the ability to determine goals, formulate and revise plans, implement plans and carry out purposeful activities), and language impairment.

d. Biological rhythm and mood regulation disorder are characterized by disorder of sleep wake cycle, fear, irritability and anxiety.

(2) Classification

At present, delirium can be divided into five clinical subtypes:

a. Hyperactivity: Patients present highly alertness, irritability, hallucinations and delusions, and aggressive mental behavior abnormalities, which is the most easily found type.

b. Activity inhibition type: It can be characterized by increased sleep, indifferent expression, slow speech and movement, and the diagnosis is often missed because the symptoms are not easy to be detected.

c. Mixed delirium: The above two types of delirium appear alternately and fluctuate repeatedly.

d. Subsyndromal type: It shows partial delirium symptoms, which only meets the diagnostic criteria of partial delirium and is often ignored.

e. Persistent delirium: It is relatively few, mostly in patients with previous cognitive impairment, or delirium secondary to new intracranial lesions.

(3) Supplementary examination

It is recommended that medical staff use cam, 4AT, DRS and other scales for delirium assessment. The following tests should be performed routinely in patients with delirium: blood routine, liver and kidney function, blood glucose, blood electrolyte, arterial blood gas analysis, body fluid balance and C-reactive protein, urine routine, blood, urine and body fluid culture and chest film, ECG, etc. Specific examination according to medical history and physical examination clues to determine the etiology or trigger factors.

(4) Diagnosis

Diagnostic and statistical manual of mental disorders (DSM-V) criteria is currently recommended as the gold standard for delirium diagnosis, and delirium can be diagnosed if the five items are met, as shown in Tab. 17.1.

Tab. 17.1 Diagnostic and statistical manual of mental disorders (DSM-V)

	Content
A	Attention disorder (decreased ability to point, focus, maintain and divert attention) and consciousness (decreased orientation to the environment)
B	The disorder occurs in a short period of time (usually hours to days), which is characterized by changes in attention and consciousness compared with baseline, and fluctuations in severity over the course of 1 day
C	Accompanied by cognitive impairment (such as memory, orientation, language, visuospatial ability or perception)

Continued

	Content
D	The disorders of diagnostic criteria A and C can neither be better explained by other existing, confirmed or progressive neurocognitive disorders, nor do they occur in the context of a severe reduction in the level of arousal (such as coma)
E	Medical history, physical examination or laboratory evidence indicates that the disorder is a direct physiological result of other physical diseases, substance poisoning or withdrawal (i.e., due to abused drugs or drugs), or exposure to toxins, or multiple causes

(5) Treatment

Treatment of delirium trigger factors: it is the focus of delirium treatment. There are many trigger factors of delirium, among which infection and pain are the most common inducing factors. According to the corresponding diagnosis and treatment routine, the treatable trigger factors should be treated actively, the symptoms of delirium should be reduced and the prognosis should be improved.

17.2 Generalized Anxiety Disorder

Anxiety is a kind of unpleasant emotional experience in which one is nervous, worried or has a premonition that an adverse situation which is difficult to deal with will happen. Not all anxiety is pathological. In daily life, anxiety is everyone's defensive emotion, which inspires us to take positive actions and achieve better results. Pathological anxiety, also known as anxiety symptoms, refers to continuous tension and feeling that there is going to be a great disaster without sufficient realistic basis.

Anxiety disorder is the general name of a group of mental disorders with the above pathological anxiety symptoms as the main clinical phase. Common anxiety disorders include generalized anxiety disorder (GAD), phobic anxiety disorder (social phobia, square phobia and specific phobia), panic disorder (also known as acute anxiety disorder), etc. GAD is the most common anxiety disorder. It has no clear objective object, it is not limited to any specific external environment, and its symptoms are generalized, persistent and fluctuating. The course of disease is often chronic and recurrent, so it is also known as chronic anxiety. Patients often have a certain personality basis, and their onset is often related to life stress events, especially threatening events, such as interpersonal relationships, physical diseases and work stress.

(1) Epidemiology

Anxiety disorder is one of the most common mental disorders in people. In 2004, the World Health Organization (WHO) conducted the World Mental Health Survey (WMHS) and cross-cultural research in 28 countries and regions around the world. It has found that the lifelong prevalence rate of anxiety disorder is 13.6% ~ 28.8%, and the annual prevalence rate is 5.6% ~ 19.3%. The annual prevalence of GAD in the general population of the United States is about 3.1%, and the lifetime prevalence is 5.7%.

Anxiety disorder is very common in patients treated in general hospitals and grass-roots medical and health institutions. GAD exists in 7% ~ 8% of patients in primary medical and health institutions. 33% ~ 55% of the patients with non cardiogenic chest pain who repeatedly visited the emergency department suffered from panic disorder.

(2) Clinical manifestation

a. Mental anxiety: Excessive worry is the core symptom of mental anxiety. It is often expressed by worrying about some unpredictable danger or misfortune that may occur in the future.

b. Somatic anxiety: It includes sports anxiety and muscle tension. Motor restlessness can be manifested as rubbing hands and feet, unable to sit still, constantly walking back and forth, and many aimless small movements.

c. Autonomic nervous dysfunction: The manifestations include tachycardia, chest tightness, shortness of breath, dizziness and headache, skin flushing, sweating or pallor, dry mouth, feeling of swallowing obstruction, stomach discomfort, nausea, abdominal pain, abdominal distension, constipation or diarrhea, frequent urination, etc.

d. Other symptoms: GAD patients often experience fatigue, depression, compulsion, fear, panic attack, depersonalization and other symptoms.

(3) Diagnosis

The main clinical symptoms of patients with different GAD are quite different, but the following complaints are common: nervous tension, trembling, muscle tension, sweating, heavy head and light feet, palpitation, dizziness and upper abdominal discomfort. The course of disease is uncertain, but tends to fluctuate and become chronic.

The key points of diagnosis are as follows.

a. In an attack, the patient must have primary symptoms of anxiety for most of the time in a few weeks (usually several months). These symptoms usually include panic, motor tension and hyperactivity of autonomic nerve activity.

b. The prominent performance of children may be the frequent need for comfort and repeated complaints of physical discomfort.

c. There are other transient symptoms, especially depression, but the patient shall not fully meet the criteria of depression, phobic anxiety disorder, panic disorder and obsessive-compulsive disorder.

d. To determine the diagnosis of GAD, the duration of the disease should last more than 6 months.

(4) Differential diagnosis

a. Depression: The main symptoms of depression are depressive mood, lack of pleasure, decreased interest, lack of self-confidence, suicidal concept and behavior, while the main symptoms of anxiety disorder include fear anxiety, autonomic hyperfunction related symptoms, exercise anxiety, avoidance behavior and so on.

b. Schizophrenia: Sometimes schizophrenic patients also have obvious anxiety, but their anxiety is often secondary to psychotic symptoms, such as hallucinations, and delusions.

c. Dementia: The obvious impairment of cognitive function is the characteristic of dementia. The examination of cognitive function, especially memory function, and brain imaging is beneficial to the definite diagnosis.

d. Psychoactive substance withdrawal: Such patients often show prominent anxiety and may also have a chronic course of disease. Clearly asking all patients about the use history of psychoactive substances (especially tobacco and alcohol) and whether these substances will be suddenly interrupted in the near future is very important for diagnosis.

(5) Treatment

The basic treatment principles of GAD should cover comprehensive treatment, whole course treatment and individualized treatment. The specific goal is to alleviate or eliminate anxiety symptoms and accompanying symptoms, restore the social function of patients, improve the quality of life and prevent recurrence.

Medication principle: The drug treatment should pay attention to "dose titration administration" and "maintenance administration". The main drugs for treatment of GAD are benzodiazepines, 5-HT 1A receptor partial agonists, antidepressants with anti-anxiety effect and other drugs. The goal of psychotherapy is to eliminate current symptoms. Psychotherapy should limit the duration of treatment, prevent excessive occupation of medical resources and increase patients' attention to themselves. It is necessary to reevaluate and replace or combine drugs if the symptoms are neither improved after 6 weeks of treatment nor completely relieved by a whole course treatment of 12 weeks.

17.3 Depression

Depressive disorder is a kind of mood disorder caused by various reasons and characterized by significant and lasting depression. Clinically, it is mainly manifested in low mood, which is not commensurate with its situation. It can range from depression to grief, and even numbness. Some patients have obvious anxiety and motor agitation, and in serious cases, there can be psychotic symptoms such as hallucinations and delusions. There are great differences in the prevalence of depression reported in different countries and regions around the world. The lifetime prevalence of depression in most countries is 8%~12%.

Major depressive disorder (MDD) is the most common type of depressive disorder, which is characterized by single attack or repeated attack, and has a high risk of recurrence. There are significant emotional, cognitive and physical symptoms in the attack period, and the symptoms can be relieved in the interval.

(1) Clinical feature and diagnosis

Depressive symptoms mainly include emotional symptoms, physical symptoms and cognitive symptoms, while emotional symptoms are the core symptoms.

According to the 10th edition of the *International Classification of Diseases* (ICD-10), the symptomatic standard of depression includes 3 core symptoms and 7 other symptoms (Tab. 17.2). When there are at least 2 core symptoms and 2 other symptoms at the same time, it meets the symptomatic criteria of depression.

Tab. 17.2 Symptoms of depression

Core symptoms	Other symptoms
① low mood; ② Loss of interest and pleasure; ③ Fatigue, decreased vitality or loss	① Decreased attention; ② Lower self-evaluation and self-confidence; ③ Self guilt and sense of worthlessness; ④ Bleak and pessimistic attitude towards future; ⑤ Idea or behavior of self injury or suicide; ⑥ Sleep disorders; ⑦ Loss of appetite

(2) Treatment

The treatment goal of depression is to diagnose as early as possible, standardize treatment in time, control symptoms, improve the clinical cure rate, minimize the disability rate and suicide rate, and prevent recurrence. The treatment methods include drug therapy, psychotherapy and biophysical therapy.

a. Medication. Antidepressants can be divided into the following categories according to the mechanism of action or chemical structure: selective serotonin reuptake inhibitors (SSRIs), serotonin and norepinephrine reuptake inhibitors (SNRIs), noradrenergic and specific serotonin antidepressants (Nassa), tricyclic and tetracyclic antidepressants (TCAs), monoamine oxidase inhibitors (MAOIs), etc.

b. Psychotherapy. It is similar to that of antidepressants for mild to moderate depression, but it can not be used alone for severe depressive attacks, and it needs to be used in combination on the basis of drug treatment.

c. Biophysical therapy. Studies have confirmed that some physical therapy measures can improve depressive symptoms and treat depression, including modified electroconvulsive therapy (MECT), transcranial magnetic stimulation, vagus nerve stimulation, deep brain stimulation, etc.

17.4 Somatic Symptom Disorder

Somatic symptom disorder (SSD) is a kind of neurosis somatic disorder characterized by persistent worry or belief in the dominant concept of various somatic symptoms. Its core symptom is somatization. The clinical manifestations of SSD are complex and diverse, as its physical symptoms are closely related to psychological conflict. SSD can be seen in many clinical departments (digestive department, neurology department, cardiovascular department, pain department, gynecology department, etc.), because most patients believe that they have physical diseases and deny the social and psychological factors of diseases, it leads to difficulties in doctor-patient communication. It is estimated that the prevalence of somatic symptom disorder is about 1%~19%, and in general adults, the prevalence may be 5%~7%. There are more women than men, so it is estimated that the prevalence of somatic disorders is high in women.

(1) Clinical feature

Patients reported one or more exaggerated, ambiguous, and inconsistent symptoms within 6 months. Excessive thinking, feelings or behaviors is related to physical symptoms or health problems. After seeing multiple doctors, they usually turn to psychiatrists, but there is no improvement. It usually has high neuroticism and anxiety/depression comorbidity. Their lives are often chaotic, manifested in marital discord, employment problems, suicidal thoughts and other damaged social functions. SSD is usually a chronic disease, which usually aggravates fluctuations during stress.

(2) Diagnosis

One or more physical symptoms that cause pain or significant damage to an individual's daily life. Excessive thoughts, feelings or behaviors related to physical symptoms, or excessive concerns related to health, manifested in at least one of the following: a. thoughts that are not commensurate with the severity of individual symptoms and persistent; b. persistent high-level anxiety about symptoms; c. invest too much time and energy in these symptoms or health concerns. Although physical symptom may not persist, some symptoms are persistent (usually more than 6 months). The main manifestation is pain all the time. The current severity is marked by continuous course of disease (more than 6 months) characterized by severe symptoms, significant damage and disease period.

(3) Treatment

Establishing a true therapeutic relationship is the most important way to help patients with somatic symptoms.

a. Psychotherapy: The purpose of psychotherapy is to make patients gradually understand the essence of the disease, change their wrong ideas, eliminate or reduce the influence of psychological factors, and enable patients to correctly evaluate their physical and health status.

b. Medication: Antidepressants can improve depression, anxiety and physical symptoms. Relevant studies have shown that the combination of low-dose antipsychotics and other drugs shows better effect than single drug.

c. Transcranial magnetic stimulation: Repetitive transcranial magnetic stimulation (rTMS) has been gradually used in the treatment of mental diseases in recent years. It is a non-invasive, safe and physical therapy method that directly affects the function of cerebral cortex. Its main indications include depression, schizophrenia, dementia and cognitive impairment.

References

[1] INOUYE S K, WESTENDORP R G J, SACZYNSKI J S. Delirium in elderly people [J]. Lancet, 2014,3832(9920):911-922.

[2] BELLELLI G, MORANDI A, DI SANTO S G, et al. "Delirium day": a nation wide point prevalence study of delirium in older hospital patients using an easy standardized diagnostic tool[J]. BMC Medicine, 2016,14:106.

[3] STEIN M B, SAREEN J. Clinical practice. Generalized anxiety disorder[J]. New England Journal of Medicine, 2015,373(21):2059-2068.

[4] STERN T A, FRICCHION G L. 麻省总医院精神病学手册[M]. 许毅, 译. 北京: 人民卫生出版社, 2017:137-138.

[5] KESSLER R C, CHIU W T, DEMLER O, et al. Prevalence, severity, and comorbidity of 12-month DSM-Ⅳ disorders in the National Comorbidity Survey Replication[J]. Archives of General Psychiatry, 2005,62(6):617-627.

[6] HUANG Y, WANG Y, WANG H, et al. Prevalence of mental disorders in China: a cross sectional epidemiological study[J]. Lancet Psychiatry, 2019,6(3):211-224.

[7] NOYES R Jr, CLARKSON C, CROWE R R, et al. A family study of generalized anxiety disorder[J]. American Journal of Psychiatry, 1987,144(8):1019-1024.

[8] 唐宏宇, 方贻儒. 精神病学[M]. 北京: 人民卫生出版社, 2014:114-120.

[9] TAYLOR D, PATON C, KAPUR S. Maudsley 精神科处方指南[M]. 司天梅, 译. 北京: 人民卫生出版社, 2015.

[10] INDU P S, ANILKUMAR T V, PISHARODY R, et al. Prevalence of depression and past suicide attempt in primary care[J]. Asian Journal of Psychiatry, 2017,27:48-52.

(Cai Zhirong, Yang Yi)

Chapter 18
Neurointerventional Technique

In recent years, with the rapid development of neuroimaging, catheter technology, materials, computers and other sciences, intravascular interventional technology has become one of the important prevention and treatment methods of cerebrovascular diseases. Its basic principle is to deliver contrast agent or special materials into the vascular lesion area of the central nervous system to achieve diagnosis and (or) treatment effect through the natural passage of human blood vessels with the help of guiding instruments (such as catheter, guide wire) under X-ray fluoroscopy monitoring. Diagnosis and treatment objects can be intracranial, head, neck, spinal canal vascular lesions. The therapeutic subjects include cerebral aneurysm, arteriovenous malformation (AVM), dural arteriovenous fistula (DAVF), arterial stenosis or occlusion and so on. Related treatment techniques include endovascular embolization, angioplasty, stent implantation, mechanical thrombectomy and so on. Because the whole process of diagnosis and treatment occurs in the vascular lumen associated with the disease, it is called intravascular interventional treatment.

18.1 Interventional Diagnosis

Digital subtraction angiography (DSA) is considered as the "gold standard" for the diagnosis of cerebrovascular diseases due to its comprehensive, accurate and dynamic display of cerebrovascular structure and related lesions.

(1) Indication

a. Diagnosis and efficacy follow-up of cerebrovascular diseases, such as aneurysm, arteriovenous malformation, moyamoya disease, stenosis or occlusion of great arteries. b. Recognition of the blood supply of tumors, such as meningioma, hemangioblastoma, jugular bulbar tumor and so on. c. Identification of vascular lesions of neck, face, eye and skull, scalp and spinal cord.

(2) Contraindication

a. Patients who are allergic to contrast agents and anesthetic; b. patients with severe bleeding tendency or bleeding diseases; c. patients with uncontrolled severe hypertension; d. patients with severe liver, kidney, heart or lung dysfunction; e. patients with systemic infection that uncontrolled or local infection at the puncture site; f. patients with poor general condition, unstable vital signs, shock or moribund state.

(3) Operation method and precaution

Methods of operation: Angiography is generally performed under local anesthesia, most are punctured through femoral artery, arterial sheath is inserted, and then different angiography catheters are used to perform angiography in different vessels according to patient's examination purposes. For some patients, radial artery or direct carotid artery puncture angiography can also be selected.

18.2 Preoperative Evaluation

Preoperative evaluation is the premise to ensure the safety of cerebrovascular interventional surgery. Patients who really need and can tolerate surgery can be screened through evaluation of patients' basic condition and brain functional reserve. Through evaluation of the local condition of the lesion and the surgical approach, surgical equipment can be ready and surgical plan can be designed reasonably.

18.2.1 Basic Condition

The patient's basic condition largely determines whether the patient can tolerate surgical treatment and the necessity of surgery.

(1) General conditions

Old age, advanced malignant tumors or other malignant diseases, life expectancy less than 2 years, responsible vessels have caused severe changes in modified Rankin scale (mRS≥3), or imaging shows large cerebral infarction in the blood supply area of responsible vessels, great surgical risk are contraindications. Patients with diabetes mellitus under poor control of blood glucose, uncontrolled hyperthyroidism and obvious active inflammation in the body are not suitable for surgery.

(2) Cardiopulmonary function

Patients with grade Ⅲ or higher cardiac function and obvious lung function abnormalities have poor tolerance to general anesthesia and high surgical risk. Patients with basal heart rate ≤50 beats/minutes, positive atropine test or long interval of dynamic ECG monitoring should be operated under the protection of temporary cardiac pacemaker. Patients with severe coronary artery stenosis should avoid prolonged hypotension during and after operation to prevent acute coronary syndrome caused by low blood flow perfusion.

(3) Renal function

Preoperative, intraoperative and postoperative patients should be provided with sufficient intravenous fluid to strengthen hydration, and the renal function needs intensive supervision. Any drugs with renal toxicity should be avoided, such as diuretics, mannitol and dopamine. It is reasonable to choose suitable contrast agent and limit the amount of contrast agent as far as possible. For patients taking metformin, if estimated glomerular filtration rate (eGFR) ≥ 60 mL/(minutes · 1.73 m^2), metformin is not required to be discontinued before surgery, but stopped for 2~3 days after using contrast agent, resume drug treatment according to the renal function review. If eGFR is 30~59 mL/(minutes · 1.73 m^2), metformin should be stopped for 48 hours before surgery, and whether to resume application 48 hours after surgery should be determined according to reassessment of renal function. Metformin and iodine contrast agent should be avoided when eGFR<30 mL/(minutes · 1.73 m^2).

(4) Hemorrhage risk assessment

It is necessary to consider whether the patient can tolerate dual antiplatelet drug therapy after surgery, whether the patient has uncontrolled peptic ulcer, or unknown fecal occult blood, or other uncontrolled hemorrhagic diseases and so on. For those who take warfarin orally for a long time, warfarin is usually stopped about 5 days before surgery, and the INR should be controlled below 1.5. Low molecular weight heparin or regular heparin can be used in patients at high risk of thrombosis.

18.2.2 Evaluation of Diseased Blood Vessels

(1) Evaluation method

Carotid artery color ultrasound, TCD and contrast-enhanced ultrasound (CEUS) are applied for evaluations of shape, diameter, vascular intima, vascular stenosis, blood flow, microemboli shedding, plaque shape and stability, etc. MRA is a widely used vascular evaluation method in clinical. CTA can display very severe stenosis that cannot be manifested on MRA or even DSA due to hemodynamic reasons. The collateral compensation of intracranial artery stenosis or occlusion can be clearly demonstrated. In addition to providing the information about vascular morphology and collateral compensation, DSA can also provide information about the whole surgical path. It is considered as a "gold indicator" for examining blood vessels. HRMRI can provide information about atherosclerotic plaque morphology, plaque composition (such as the degree of lipidosis, intra-plaque hemorrhage), inflammation, and help to distinguish it from other non-atherosclerotic vascular diseases. Optical coherence tomography (OCT) and intravenous ultra-sound (IVUS) have also been applied in clinic in recent years.

(2) Measurement of stenosis degree

Due to the defects of various non-invasive examinations, the calculation of vascular stenosis rate before stenting must be conducted via DSA, and be photographed and measured at the angle of the most severe stenosis. The degree of stenosis is a significant basis for operation and material selection for diseased vessels.

a. Intracranial vascular lesions: Refer to the treatment with Warfarin-Aspirin Symptomatic Intracranial Disease (WASID) trial method (Fig. 18.1).

$$\text{Stenosis degree }(\%)=\left(1-\frac{\text{Diameter of the most severe stenosis}}{\text{Diameter of normal vessel proximal to the stenosis}}\right)\times 100\% \quad (18.1)$$

b. Extracranial vascular lesions: Refer to the criteria of the collaborative study group in North American Symptomatic Carotid Endarterectomy (NASCE) trial method (Fig. 18.2).

$$\text{Stenosis degree }(\%)=\left(1-\frac{\text{Diameter of the most severe stenosis}}{\text{Diameter of normal vessel distal to the stenosis}}\right)\times 100\% \quad (18.2)$$

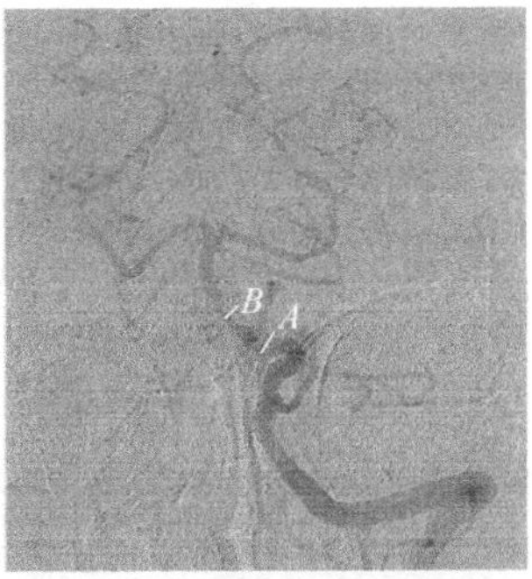

Intracranial artery stenosis degree (%)
$=(1-B/A)\times 100\%$

Fig. 18.1 Intracranial vascular lesions

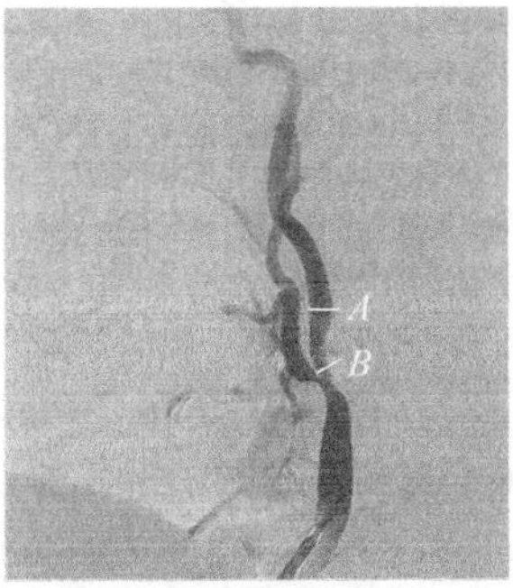

Extracranial artery stenosis degree (%)
$=(1-B/A)\times 100\%$

Fig. 18.2 Extracranial vascular lesions

(3) Evaluation of surgical path

Surgical path refers to the journey from the arterial puncture site to the expected landing point of guidewire tip. It is a significant basis for deciding whether surgical equipment (guidewire, catheter, stent, balloon, spring coil and so on) can be safely placed and can reduce the displacement of main vessels and the pulling and tearing of branch vessels. Evaluation about the shape and morphology of blood vessels as well as cerebrovascular reserve are essential. TCD, MRA, CTA and DSA can be used to directly observe collateral compensation. When DSA is not suitable or unconditional, the lateral branches of the pia meningeal can be evaluated by CTA and Willis circle can be evaluated by MRA. Tab. 18.1 shows direct evaluation methods of collateral assessment.

Tab. 18.1 Collateral circulation grading of cerebral arterial collateral based on DSA (ASITN/SIR method)

Collateral compensation level	DSA manifestations
Level 0	There is no collateral flow to the peripheral area of ischemia
Level 1	There is slow collateral flow to the peripheral area of ischemia, but some areas remain free of blood flow
Level 2	Rapid collateral flow to the peripheral area of ischemia is accompanied by continous perfusion defects, with only partial flow to the ischemic area
Level 3	Veins show slow but complete collateral flow to the ischemic area in the late stage
Level 4	The entire ischemic area is rapidly and completely perfused by collateral reverse perfusion

Note: Level 0~1 mean poor collateral circulation, level 2 means medium collateral circulation, and level 3~4 mean good collateral circulation.

18.3 Perioperative Medication

(1) Antiplatelet treatment

At present, the protocols adopted by clinical institutes are as follows: the combined application of aspirin 100~300 mg and clopidogrel 75 mg at least 3~5 days before elective surgery. If emergency intervention is required, oral load doses of antiplatelet drugs (aspirin 300 mg and clopidogrel 300 mg) should be used. Postoperative administration of aspirin 300 mg combined with clopidogrel 75 mg should be continued for at least 3 months, and then changed to aspirin or clopidogrel monotherapy for all life.

(2) Anticoagulant treatment

One-time intravenous infusion of heparin 2 000 U is recommended for angiographic surgery of ischemic cerebrovascular disease, and there is no consensus on whether whole-course infusion of heparin saline catheter is required. The initial heparin dose is 70 U/kg body weight, and 1/2 of the initial heparin dose is added every 1 hour after the operation time is extended. Anticoagulation is needed after venous sinus thrombosis.

(3) Blood pressure control

Blood pressure should be controlled closely to normal level before and during operation. In order to prevent the occurrence of hyperperfusion syndrome, postoperative blood pressure should be lower than preoperative basal blood pressure of 20 ~ 30 mmHg (but must be greater than 90/60 mmHg) for patients with severe stenosis or occlusive lesions. Postoperative control of blood pressure can use urapidil, and the use of nimodidi equal expansion of blood vessel drugs should be avoided.

(4) Statin treatment

For atherosclerotic vascular stenosis, routine preoperative and postoperative lifetime application of statin drugs, mostly high-intensity statin drugs are selected, such as atorvastatin calcium or rosuvastatin calcium, and the medication is adjusted according to the LDL standard (1.8 mmol/L) after treatment.

(5) Others

Routine intramuscular injection of phenobarbital sodium 0.1 ~ 0.2 mg is used for sedation before surgery. Intraoperative vasospasm, verapamil (5 mg diluted to 20 mL normal saline, 1 ~ 2 mL/minutes, 5 mg per vessel) or papaverine (diluted to 1 mg/mL, 1 ~ 5 mL each time, total <90 mg) can be intraductally injected. Note that papaverine has a short duration of action, which can lead to hypotension, intracranial hypertension, epilepsy and even vasospasm.

18.4 Equipment and Device

Angiography machine is the basic equipment for intravascular interventional operations. At present, digital subtraction angiography (DSA) system is widely used. DSA system mainly consists of five parts, including X-ray generation and imaging system, mechanical system, high-pressure syringes, image data storage system and computer system.

Interventional equipment comprises of vascular sheath, guide wire, catheter and accessory, which includes three-way valve, Y-type valve, infusion line, infusion tube, puncture needle, expander, pressure infusion bag and so on.

18.5 Interventional Treatment of Cerebrovascular Diseases

18.5.1 Interventional Treatment of Ischemic Cerebrovascular Disease

Ischemic cerebrovascular disease (ICVD) refers to the cerebrovascular diseases caused by blocked or narrowed external and intracranial artery, accounting for more than 80% of all cerebrovascular diseases. The key point of ICVD treatment is early diagnosis and intervention. In recent years, with the development of neurovascular imaging diagnosis and interventional therapy, interventional therapy has become one of the significant methods for prevention and treatment of ischemic cerebrovascular disease.

(1) Carotid artery stenosis

The lesions are mainly located in the bifurcation of common carotid artery and the initial segment of internal carotid artery. At present, there are many methods to calculate the degree of stenosis. According to the degree of carotid artery stenosis, carotid artery stenosis is divided into four grades: <50% stenosis is mild, 50% ~ 69% stenosis is moderate, 70% ~ 99% stenosis is severe, 99% ~ 100% stenosis is extremely severe or subtotal occlusion. According to the clinical manifestations, it can be divided into symptomatic and nonsymptomatic categories. Symptomatic patients may manifest TIA or cerebral infarction in the blood supply area of the internal carotid artery. Asymptomatic patients may be completely asymptomatic or may manifest atypical symptoms such as headache, light headedness, dizziness, memory loss and so on. The main examination methods include carotid ultrasound, MRA, CTA, DSA and so on.

In the early 1990s, carotid endarterectomy (CEA) was regarded as the "gold standard" for treatment of carotid artery stenosis. However, in recent years, with the rapid development of interventional technology and material science, carotid artery stenting (CAS) has gradually become an important alternative method for treatment of carotid artery stenosis. At present, the commonly used treatment methods include drug treatment, surgical treatment and interventional treatment. In general, surgical treatment refers to CEA while interventional therapy refers to CAS. They have some indications and contraindications respectively as follows.

1) Carotid endarterectomy (CEA)

① Indication

Absolute indication: Symptomatic carotid artery stenosis, non-invasive examination finds that carotid artery stenosis is larger than 70% or angiography finds stenosis is over 50%.

Relative indication: a. Asymptomatic carotid artery stenosis with stenosis ≥70% by non-invasive examination or ≥60% by angiography. b. Asymptomatic carotid artery stenosis with stenosis <70% by non-invasive examination, but angiography or other examination suggests that the stenosis is in an unstable state. c. Symptomatic carotid artery stenosis with stenosis reaching 50%~69% by non-invasive examination.

② Contraindication

a. Intracranial spontaneous hemorrhage within 12 months. b. Massive stroke or myocardial infarction occurs within 30 days. c. Progressive stroke within 3 months. d. Patients with relatively large intracranial aneurysms that cannot be treated in advance or simultaneously. e. Patients with chronic complete occlusion and without obvious cerebral ischemia symptoms. f. Patients with coagulation dysfunction and contraindications to heparin and antiplatelet drugs. g. Patients who cannot tolerate anesthesia. h. Patients with severe dysfunction of vital organs such as heart, lung, liver, and kidney.

2) Carotid artery stent (CAS) implantation

① Indication

a. Symptomatic patients: They have a non-disabling ischemic stroke or TIA in the responsible blood supply area of the diseased vessel within 6 months, and angiography confirms that stenosis of the diseased carotid artery is >50%, or noninvasive angiography confirms that stenosis of diseased carotid artery is >70%.

b. Asymptomatic patients: Although there are no neurological localization symptoms, angiography confirms that the stenosis of diseased internal carotid artery stenosis exceeds 60%, or noninvasive angiography confirms stenosis of diseased carotid artery is >70%.

② Contraindication

a. Patients with intracranial hemorrhage within 3 months. b. Patients with myocardial infarction or large cerebral infarction occurs within 3 weeks. c. Patients with intracranial aneurysm or vascular malformation and other lesions that cannot be treated in advance or simultaneously. d. Patients with gastrointestinal diseases accompanied by active bleeding. e. Patients with uncontrolled high blood pressure. f. Patients with contraindications to heparin and antiplatelet drugs. g. Patients who are allergic to contrast agents. h. Patients with severe dysfunction of vital organs such as heart, lung, liver, and kidney. i. Patients with placement difficulty in tortuous artery walking, catheter, balloon, stent and other instruments. j. Patients whose expected survival time is less than 2 years.

③ Complication

Common complications include cerebral embolism, cerebral hemorrhage, hyperperfusion syndrome, decreased blood pressure during the operation, myocardial infarction, arterial dissection, vasospasm, post-stent restenosis and so on.

(2) Intracranial artery stenosis

Lesions occur mostly in intracranial arteries with medium diameter and their main branches, including intracranial segment of internal carotid artery, middle cerebral artery, intracranial segment of vertebral artery, basilar artery and so on. The main examination methods include TCD, MRA, CTA, DSA and so on.

Treatment includes standard medication and interventional treatment. Interventional treatment includes balloon angioplasty or stenting for intracranial arterial stenosis (Fig. 18.3). There are some controversies about the indications of intracranial artery stenting on the international. It is generally believed that patients with symptomatic intracranial severe atherosclerotic stenosis (70% ~ 99%) can be performed if standard drug therapy is unfeasible. Intracranial balloon angioplasty is feasible for patients with difficulty or high risk of stenting. Its contraindications are basically as same as that of CAS. Common complications include subarachnoid hemorrhage, intracerebral hematoma, cerebral embolism, perforating artery occlusion, arterial dissection, stent thrombosis, vasospasm, post-stent restenosis and so on.

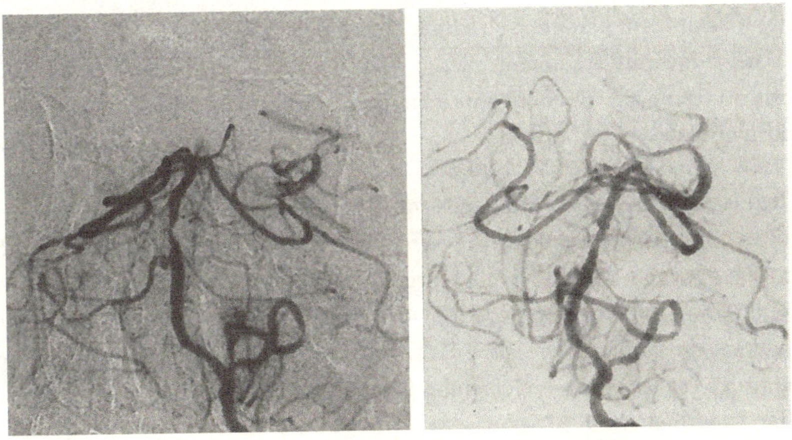

(a) (b)

Fig. 18.3 Intracranial arterial stent implantation

(3) Vertebral artery stenosis

Extracranial artery stenosis (ECAS) accounts for 25% ~ 40% cerebral artery stenoses, and the incidence of ECAS is only inferior to the extracranial stenosis of internal carotid artery. Stenosis prefers to occur at the initial segment of the vertebral artery. The stenosis degree is calculated by methods of vertebral artery stenting trial (VAST), as shown in Formula (18.2). The degree of stenosis is the same as that of carotid artery stenosis.

Drug treatment is preferred, including anti-platelet aggregation, lipid regulation, risk factors control and so on. Interventional treatment is suitable for the condition of symptomatic severe extracranial vertebral artery stenosis (70% ~ 99%) with ineffective medical therapy. The initial segment of vertebral artery contains a large number of elastic fibers and smooth muscle, and balloon angioplasty is tend to cause restenosis due to elastic retraction, so stent implantation is often selected. Complications of extracranial vertebral artery stenting are relatively rare comparing with carotid artery stenting, but the incidence of restenosis and stent rupture after stenting is higher due to local anatomical differences and the influence of vascular pulsation.

(4) Subclavian artery stenosis

About 11.6% of ischemic cerebrovascular diseases caused by atherosclerosis suffer subclavian artery stenosis. The stenosis is common on the left side. Compared with other atherosclerotic vascular diseases, this kind of patients are relatively young and common in male. Most patients are asymptomatic, and a few serious lesions may cause hemodynamic abnormalities, leading to Subclavian Steal Syndrome (SSS). It can manifest as follows. a. Posterior circulation ischemia: vertigo, syncope, diplopia, ataxia, dysphonia, dysphagia, limb sensory or motor abnormalities and so on. b. Upper limb ischemia: weakness after upper limb activity and improvement after rest, paresthesia, reduced or disappeared radial artery pulsation, ipsilateral blood pressure ≥20 mmHg lower than contralateral. The main examination methods include blood pressure difference measurement of both upper limb, cervical vascular ultrasound, CTA, DSA and so on. Interventional treatment mainly refers to subclavian artery stent implantation, which has gradually become the main treatment method for subclavian artery stenosis due to its simple technology and high safety (Fig. 18.4).

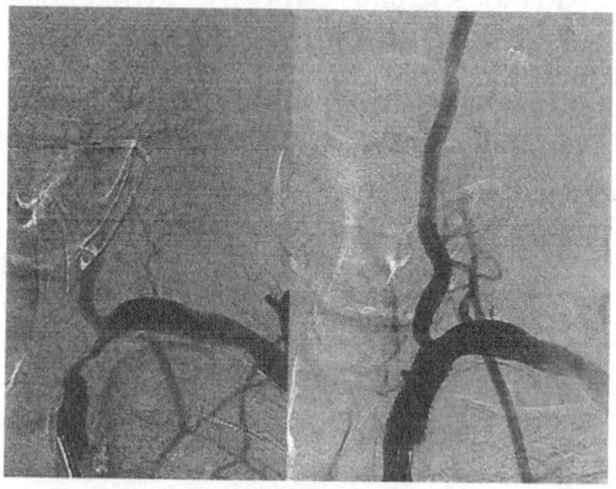

Fig. 18.4 Subclavian artery stent implantation

Q: What is subclavian steal syndrome (SSS)?

A: Subclavian steal syndrome, also called subclavian steal steno-occlusive disease, is a constellation of signs and symptoms that arise from retrograde blood flow in the vertebral artery or the internal thoracic artery, due to a proximal stenosis and/or occlusion of the subclavian artery. The arm may be supplied by blood flowing in a retrograde direction down the vertebral artery at the expense of vertebrobasilar circulation. It is more severe than typical vertebrobasilar insufficiency.

(5) Acute cerebral infarction

Acute cerebral infarction is one of the common severe cerebrovascular emergencies in clinic. In recent years, arterial thrombolysis and some new intravascular therapeutic devices (such as thrombus aspiration system and retractable thrombus stent) have been applied in clinical practice based on intravenous thrombolysis, which have significantly improved the recanalization rate of occluded vessels. The commonly used interventional treatment methods mainly include arterial thrombolysis, mechanical thrombectomy and so on.

1) Arterial thrombolysis

Under the supervision of DSA, thrombolytic drugs are directly injected into the occlusive location of the responsible vessel through microcatheter by intravascular intervention technology to achieve vascular recanalization. Compared with intravenous thrombolysis, this method can improve the concentration of thrombolytic drugs at the thrombus site, increase the contact surface between thrombolytic drugs and thrombus, and can control the administration and evaluate circulation in real time, reduce the dosage of thrombolytic drugs and improve the rate of vascular recanalization.

2) Mechanical thrombectomy

It refers to the use of special devices such as retrievable stents or thrombus aspiration systems to remove the thrombus under the supervision of DSA to achieve vascular recanalization. Some large randomized controlled studies have confirmed that mechanical thrombectomy with retrievable stents has a good effect on patients with acute aorta occlusion in recent years, and has now become the preferred interventional therapy for some acute cerebral infarction. For patients with acute ischemic stroke, large artery occlusion confirmed by non-invasive imaging examination, and poor intravenous thrombolytic effect, mechanical thrombectomy should be taken into account. At present, mechanical thrombectomy can be used within 6 hours after the onset of large artery occlusion of anterior circulation, and within 24 hours after the onset of large artery occlusion posterior circulation. However, with the rapid development of this field, the time window is gradually lengthening under the guidance of accurate imaging. But it has some contraindication as follows: a. Patients with active hemorrhage or known hemorrhagic tendency. b. CT or MRI shows large cerebral infarction (infarcts are larger than 1/3 of the middle cerebral artery supply area). c. Platelet count is lower than 100×10^9/L. d. Patients with severe heart, liver or kidney insufficiency or severe diabetes. e. Patients who experienced major surgery in the last two weeks. f. Patients with gastrointestinal or urinary bleeding in the last 3 weeks. g. Blood glucose <2.7 mmol/L or >22.2 mmol/L. h. Severe high blood pressure that cannot be controlled by drug. i. Expected survival <90 days. j. Pregnancy. Common complications include cerebral hemorrhage, cerebral embolism, ischemia-reperfusion injury, hyperperfusion syndrome, arterial dissection, secondary occlusion after recanalization and so on.

Mechanical thrombectomy

18.5.2 Interventional Treatment of Hemorrhagic Cerebrovascular Disease

Hemorrhagic cerebrovascular disease (HCVD) is a type of cerebrovascular disease that induces subarachnoid hemorrhage or parenchymal hemorrhage, including aneurysm, arteriovenous malformation, cavernous hemangioma, internal carotid cavernous sinus fistula, dural arteriovenous fistula, etc.

(1) Cerebral aneurysm

Cerebral aneurysm refers to the abnormal swelling on intracranial artery wall, which is the first cause of spontaneous subarachnoid hemorrhage (accounting for about 75% ~ 80%). Hypertension and cerebral arteriosclerosis are related to the occurrence and development of aneurysm. In addition, infection and trauma can also induce aneurysms. The prevalence of intracranial aneurysms worldwide is about 0.2% ~ 9%, most of which are sporadic, about 20% ~ 30% are multiple. They can appear at any age, the peak of incidence is at the age of 40 ~ 60, and there is a slight increase in females.

Intracranial aneurysms tend to occur in Willis circle and its main branches, especially at the bifurcation or hemodynamic changes. 80% ~ 90% of them are located in the anterior circulation and 10% ~ 20% of them are located in the posterior circulation. According to the different parent arteries, they can be divided into anterior communicating aneurysms, internal carotid artery-posterior communicating aneurysms, middle cerebral aneurysms, basal aneurysms and so on. According to the size, they can be divided into small aneurysms (< 5 mm), medium-sized aneurysms (5 ~ 10 mm), large aneurysms (11 ~ 25 mm) and giant aneurysms (>25 mm).

Unruptured aneurysms can be asymptomatic, while larger aneurysms can compress adjacent brain tissues or brain nerves and manifest corresponding focal symptoms, such as epilepsy, hemiplegia, aphasia, oculomotor nerve palsy, visual and visual filed impairment and so on. There can be prewarning symptoms before aneurysm rupture, such as pain of back head, dizziness, extraocular muscle paralysis, motor sensory disorders and so on. Once ruptured, aneurysms can cause subarachnoid hemorrhage, which manifests sudden and persistent severe headache, nausea, vomiting, photophobia, disturbance of consciousness, meningeal stimulation sign, hemiplegia and so on, and can induce death in severe cases. The main examination methods include CT, MRI, CTA, MRA, DSA and so on.

Interventional treatment includes various methods, among which, coil embolization is currently the preferred interventional treatment for intracranial aneurysm. Under the monitor of DSA, the coil is sent into the aneurysm cavity through microcatheter and released after indwelling. Mechanical occlusion of the coil and secondary intracavitary thrombosis can be performed through the coil. The aneurysm is separated from blood circulation of the parent artery to prevent aneurysm rupture. The common complications of intracranial aneurysm embolization include aneurysm rupture and hemorrhage, parent artery occlusion, vasospasm, coil displacement, aneurysm recurrence.

(2) Cerebrovascular malformation

Cerebrovascular malformation refers to the congenital non-neoplastic abnormal development of cerebrovascular, which includes arteriovenous malformation, cavernous hemangioma, telangiectasia and venous malformation. Arteriovenous malformation (AVM) is the most common type. AVM refers to the short capillaries between cerebral arteries and cerebral veins at the lesion site, which induces direct connection between artery and vein, forming a short circuit between artery and vein, and resulting in a series of cerebral hemodynamic disorders (Fig. 18.5). At present, the etiology is unclear, which may be related to the dysfunction of regulatory mechanism of embryonic angiogenesis. Its overall incidence is about 18/100 000 in adults, and it mostly occurs in people under the age of 40. The incidence of AVM is higher in males than in females. AVM can occur in any part of brain, and most of AVM are located in the tentorium of the cerebellum. Common clinical manifestations include intracranial hemorrhage, epilepsy, headache, focal neurological dysfunction and so on. DSA is the most reliable imaging examination.

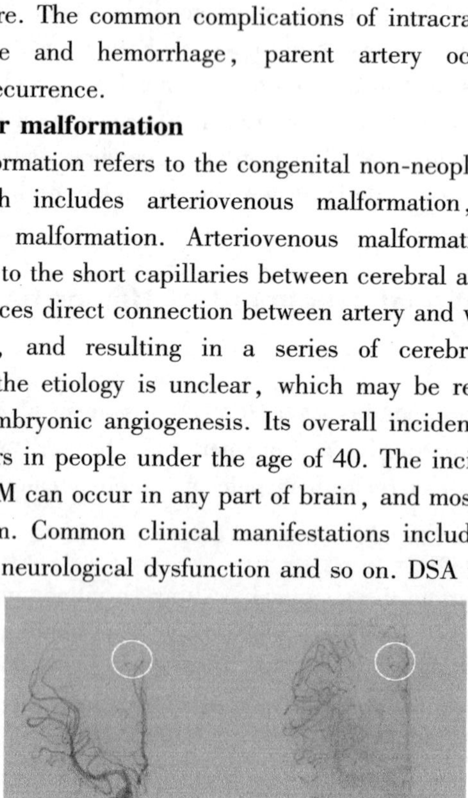

Fig. 18.5 Angiography of AVM

The selection of treatment methods should be considered in combination with the size, location and structure of the lesion, including microsurgical resection, interventional treatment, radiotherapy and combined therapy. At present, interventional embolization can be divided into pre-operative embolization, pre-radiation embolization, radical embolization and palliative embolization. Complications of AVM interventional embolization include cerebral hemorrhage, misocclusion of normal cerebral artery, translocation of embolized materials.

18.5.3 Interventional Treatment of Cerebral Venous Disease

Cerebral venous sinus thrombosis (CVST) is the most common type of cerebral venous disease and the mortality reaches up to 5% ~ 15%. For the formed blood clots, single anticoagulation is invalid. However, there is no definite medical evidence to support systemic intravenous thrombolytic treatment for CVST. Interventional treatment has therapeutic value, including transcatheter arterial embolus, contact venous embolus, transcatheter mechanical thrombectomy, balloon dilation, stent implantation. For complex and critically ill patients, multimodal treatments may be required.

(1) Thrombolytic therapy

Thrombolytic therapy includes catheterized contact venous thrombolysis and transcatheter arterial thrombolysis.

1) Catheterized contact venous thrombosis

It refers to sending the microcatheter into the intracranial venous sinus thrombosis through the jugular vein by catheterized intervention technique, and injecting a single dose of thrombolytic drugs through the microcatheter mass to convert plasminogen into plasmin and dissolve the fibrin in the thrombosis, achieving the purpose of thrombolytic. Patients without severe sinus stenosis, severe intracranial hemorrhage, with course < 1 week and with poor response to adequate anticoagulation treatment, could be treated with local thrombolysis of venous sinus carefully under close monitoring. The best type, dosage and administration method of thrombolytic drugs are still under exploration. Urokinase usage [$(0.5 \sim 1.5) \times 10^6$ U per day that are divided into 2 ~ 4 times, venous sinus pulse injection that can be 3 ~ 7 days] and rt-PA (a total dose of 23 ~ 300 mg, continuous infusion after a single injection) can be used. The specific course of medication depends on the patient's symptoms and imaging examinations to confirm that the venous sinus is basically unobstructed.

2) Transcatheter arterial embolus

The catheter is sent into intracranial artery through the carotid artery, and then thrombolytic drugs are injected through catheter. It is suitable for patients with cerebral deep vein thrombosis, cerebral cortex vein thrombosis. Arterial thrombolysis for intracranial venous thrombosis is based on partial venous opening, which is an effective complement to intravenous thrombolysis.

(2) Transcatheter mechanical thrombectomy

It refers to a method of vascular revascularization of venous sinus thrombosis by using auxiliary materials such as microguide wires, microcatheters, microballoons and recoverable stents through neural intervention technology. For patients with short course of disease, thrombolytic technology can also be combined. Acute and subacute CVST patients with persistent exacerbation of symptoms after the initiation of anticoagulant treatment, or with newly symptomatic hemorrhage after thrombolytic treatment, or consciousness impairment, or severe intracranial hemorrhage when admission, transcatheter mechanical thrombectomy can be used as an alternative treatment. However, its safety and effectiveness need to be confirmed by further studies with large samples.

(3) Balloon dilation and stenting

For patients with chronic venous sinus thrombosis, and with symptoms not relieved after more than 6 months of regular medical treatments, and with local venous sinus stenosis confirmed by imaging examinations, retrograde venography can be performed to measure the pressure at both ends of the stenosis. When the pressure difference between the two ends of the stenosis is greater than 10~12 mmHg, balloon dilation and stenting at the venous sinus of the stenosis site can be considered. However, their long-term efficacy and safety still need to be further evaluated.

References

[1] POWERS W J, DERDYN C P, BILLER J, et al. 2015 American heart association/American stroke association focused update of the 2013 guidelines for the early management of patients with acute ischemic stroke regarding endovascular treatment: a guideline for healthcare professionals from the american heart association/American stroke association[J]. Stroke, 2015,46(10):3020-3035.

[2] Chinese society of Neurology, Neurovascular Intervention Group of Chinese Society of Neurology, Writing Group of Guidelines for Interventional Therapy in Acute Ischemic Stroke. Guidelines for early endovascular diagnosis and treatment for acute ischemic stroke in China[J]. Chinese Journal of Neurology, 2015,48(5):356-361.

[3] Chinese society of Neurology, Neurovascular Intervention Group of Chinese Society of Neurology. Consensus on process and standard of early endovascular therapy in acute ischemic stroke[J]. Chinese Journal of Neurology, 2017,50(3):172-177.

[4] WRITING G, NAYLOR A R, RICCO J B, et al. 2017 ESC guidelines on the diagnosis and treatment of peripheral arterial diseases, in collaboration with the European society for vascular surgery (ESVS)[J]. European Journal of Vascular and Endovascular Surgery, 2018,55(4):457-464.

[5] THOMPSON B G, BROWN R D Jr, AMIN-HANJANI S, et al. Guidelines for the management of patients with unruptured intracranial aneurysms a guideline for healthcare professionals from the American heart association/American stroke association[J]. Stroke, 2015,46(8):2368-2400.

[6] CENZATO M, BOCCARDI E, BEGHI E, et al. European consensus conference on unruptured brain AVMs treatment (supported by EANS, ESMINT, EGKS, and SINCH)[J]. Acta Neurochirurgica, 2017,159(6):1059-1064.

[7] RUNGE V M. Critical questions regarding gadolinium deposition in the brain and body after injections of the gadolinium-based contrast agents, safety, and clinical recommendations in consideration of the EMA's Pharmacovigilance and risk assessment committee recommendation for suspension of the marketing authorizations for 4 linear agents[J]. Investigative Radiology, 2017,52(6):317-323.

[8] VENERMO M, WANG G, SEDRAKYAN A, et al. Carotid stenosis treatment: variation in international practice patterns, european journal of vascular and endovascular surgery[J]. European Journal of Vascular and Endovascular Surgery, 2017,53(4):511-519.

[9] NAYLOR A R, RICCO J B, DE Borst G J, et al. Management of atherosclerotic carotid and vertebral artery disease: 2017 clinical practice guidelines of the european society for vascular surgery (ESVS)[J]. European Journal of Vascular and Endovascular Surgery, 2018, 55(1):3-81.

[10] 中国卒中学会神经介入分会，中华医学会神经病学分会神经血管介入协作组. 脑静脉窦狭窄介入诊疗专家共识[J]. 中华内科杂志，2021,60(8):696-708.

(Zou Rong, Xu Jianhui, Yang Yi)

Appendixes

Ⅰ. Abbreviations

AC	Acetylcholine
ACA	Anterior Cerebral Artery
AChR	Acetylcholine Receptors
AD	Alzheimer's Disease
ADCA	Autosomal Dominant Cerebellar Ataxia
AE	Autoimmune Encephalitis
AF	Atrial Fibrillation
AHEM	Acute Hemorrhagic Encephalomyelitis
AHL	Acute Hemorrhagic Leukoencephalopathy
AIDP	Acute Inflammatory Demyelinating Polyradiculoneuropathy
ALS	Amyotrophic Lateral Sclerosis
AM	Acute Myelopathies
AMAN	Acute Motor Axonal Neuropathy
AMPAR	α-Amino-3-Hydroxy-5-Methyl-4-Isoxazole Propionate Receptor
AMSAN	Acute Motor-Sensory Axonal Neuropathy
ANHLE	Acute Necrotizing Hemorrhagic Leukoencephalitis
ApoE	Apolipoprotein E
APP	Amyloid Precusor Protein
AQP-4	Aquaporin-4
AQP4-IgG	Anti-Aquaporin-4 Antibody
ARF	Acute Rheumatic Fever
ART	Anti-Retroviral Therapy
ASDs	Anti-Seizure Drugs
A-T	Ataxia-Telangiectasia
ATM	Acute Transverse Myelitis
AVM	Arteriovenous Malformation
BA	Basilar Artery
BAEP	Brainstem Auditory Evoked Potentials

Continued

BMD	Becker Muscular Dystrophy
bvFTD	Behavioral Variant Frontotemporal Dementia
CAS	Carotid Artery Stenting
CASPR2	Contactin-Associated Protein-Like 2
CBD	Corticobasal Degeneration
CCA	Common Carotid Artery
CDC	Centre for Disease Control and Prevention
CEA	Carotid Endarterectomy
CEUS	Contrast-Enhanced Ultrasound
CGRP	Calcitonin Gene-Related Peptide
ChEI	Cholinesterase Inhibitor
CHMP2B	Chromatin Modifying Protein 2B
CIDP	Chronic Inflammatory Demyelinating Polyneuropathy
CIS	Clinically Isolated Syndrome
CJD	Creutzfeldt-Jakob Disease
CK	Creatine Kinase
CK-MB	Creatine Kinase-MB
CM	Cryptococcal Meningitis
CMD	Congenital Muscular Dystrophy
CMT	Charcot-Marie-Tooth Disease
CNS	Central Nervous System
CO	Carbon Monoxide
COHb	Carboxy-Hemoglobin
COMT	Catechol-*O*-Methyltransferase
CPEO	Chronic Progressive External Ophthalmoplegia
CSE	Convulsive Status Epilepticus
CSF	Cerebrospinal Fluid
CT	Computed Tomography
CTA	Computerized Tomography Angiography
CVD	Cerebrovascular Disease
CVS	Cerebrovascular Spasm
CVST	Cerebral Venous Sinus Thrombosis
CWSI	Cerebral Watershed Infarction
DAVF	Dural Arteriovenous Fistula
DBS	Deep Brain Stimulation
DCHS	Dysarthric-Clumsy Hand Syndrome
DEACMP	Delayed Encephalopathy due to Acute Carbon Monoxide Poisoning
DIS	Dissemination in Space

Continued

DIT	Dissemination in Time
DLB	Dementia with Lewy Bodies
DM	Distalmuscular Dystrophy
DMD	Duchenne Muscular Dystrophy
DRD	Dopa-Responsive Dystonia
DSA	Digital Subtraction Angiography
DTI	Diffusion Tensor Imaging
DVT	Deep Vein Thromhosis
DWI	Diffusion-Weighted Imaging
EA	Episodic Ataxia
EAE	Experimental Autoimmune Encephalomyelitis
EBV	Epstein-Barr Virus
ECA	External Carotid Artery
ECAS	Extracranial Artery Stenosis
EDMD	Emery-Dreifuss Muscular Dystrophy
EEG	Electroencephalogram
EIA	Enzyme Immunoassay
ELISA	Enzyme Linked Immunosorbent Assay
EMG	Electromyography
EP	Evoked Potential
EPO	Erythropoietin
ESR	Erythrocyte Sedimentation Rate
ETV	Endoscopic Third Ventriculo-Stomy
FARR	Friedreich Ataxia with Retained Reflexes
FFI	Fatal Familial Insomnia
FMRI	Functional Magnetic Resonance Imaging
FRDA	Friedreich Ataxia
FSHD	Facioscapulohumeral Muscular Dystrophy
FTA-ABS	Fluorescence Treponemal Antibody Absorption Test
FTD	Frontotemporal Dementia
GABABR	γ-Aminobutyricacid Acid B Receptor
GBS	Guillain-Barré Syndrome
GCIs	Glial Cytoplasmic Inclusions
GGEs	Genetic Generalized Epilepsies
GCS	Glasgow Coma Scale
HAART	Highly Active Antiroviral Therapy
HCVD	Hemorrhagic Cerebrovascular Disease
HD	Huntington's Disease

Continued

HIV	Human Immunodeficiency Virus
HLD	Hepatolenticular Degeneration
HRMRI	High Resolution Magnetic Resonance Imaging
HMSN	Hereditary Motor and Sensory Neuropathy
HSA	Hereditary Spastie Alaxia
HSV	Herpes Simplex Virus
ICA	Internal Carotid Artery
ICH	Intracerebral Hemorrhage
ICP	Intracranial Pressure
ICVD	Ischemic Cerebrovascular Disease
IDSA	Infectious Diseases Society of America
IGEs	Idiopathic Generalized Epilepsies
IHS	International Headache Society
INO	Internuclear Ophthalmoplegia
IVIG	Intravenous Immunoglobulin
KDT	Ketogenic Diet Therapy
KSS	Kearns-Sayre Syndrome
LA	Latex Agglutination
LAA	Large Artery Atherosclerosis
LC	Locus Coeruleus
LDH	Lactatedehydrogenase
LDL-C	Low Density Lipoprotein Cholesterol
LGD	Limb Girdle Dystrophy
LMN	Lower Motor Neurone
LOFA	Late-Onset Friedreich Ataxia
lvPPA	Logopenic Variant PPA
MAO-B	Monoamine Oxidase B
MAPT	Microtubule-Associated Protein Tau Gene
MCA	Middle Cerebral Artery
MNCV	Motor Nerve Conduction Velocity
MD	Myoclonus-Dystonia
MEG	Magnetoencephalography
MELASE	Mitochondrial Encelhalomyopath with Lactic Acidosis and Stroke-Like Episodes
MERRF	Myoclonus Epilepsy Ragged-Red Fibers
MFS	Miller Fisher Syndrome
MG	Myasthenia Gravis
MND	Motor Neuron Disease
MOG	Myelin Oligodendrocyte Glycoprotein

Continued

MPL	Methylprednisolone
MRA	Magnetic Resonance Angiography
MRC	Medical Research Council
MRI	Magnetic Resonance Imaging
MRS	Magnetic Resonance Spectroscopy
MRV	Magnetic Resonance Venography
MS	Multiple Sclerosis
MSA	Multiple-System Atrophy
mtDNA	Mitochondrial DNA
NASCET	North American Symptomatic Carotid Endarterectomy Trial
NCC	Neurocysticercosis
NCSE	Nonconvulsive Status Epilepticus
NCU	Neuro-Intensive Care Unit
NCV	Nerve Conduction Velocity
nDNA	Nucleus DNA
NDs	Neurodegenerative Diseases
NFT	Neurofibrillary Tangle
nfvPPA	Nonfluent/Agrammatic Variant PPA
NMDAR	N-Methyl-D-Aspartate Receptor
NMO	Neuromyelitis Optica
NMOSD	Neuromyelitis Optica Spectrum Disorder
NORSE	New-Onset Refractory Status Epilepticus
NREM	non-Rapid Eye Movement
NSAIDs	Nonsteroidal Anti-Inflammatory Drugs
OCB	Oligoclonal Bands
OH	Orthostatic Hypotension
OMD	Ocular Muscular Dystrophy
OPMD	Oculopharyngeal Muscular Dystrophy
PBP	Progressive Bulbar Palsy
PCR	Polymerase Chain Reaction
PD	Parkinson's Disease
PE	Pulmonary Embolism
PEG	Percutaneous Endoscopic Gastrostomy
PET	Position Emission Tomography
PGRN	Progranulin Gene
PLS	Primary Lateral Sclerosis
PM	Polymyositis
PMA	Progressive Muscular Atrophy

Continued

PMD	Progressive Muscular Dystrophy
PMH	Pure Motor Hemiparesis
PPA	Primary Progressive Aphasia
PPMS	Primary Progressive Multiple Sclerosis
PrPc	Cellular Prion Protein
PrPSc	Cellular Prion Protein Isoform
PSEN	Presenilin
PSP	Progressive Supranuclear Palsy
PSS	Pure Sensory Stroke
PSWCs	Periodic Sharp Wave Complexes
PWI	Perfusion Weighted Imaging
RBD	REM Sleep Behavior Disorder
RDP	Rapid-Onset Dystonia-Parkinsonism
REM	Rapid Eye Movement
RPR	Rapid Plasma Reagin
RRF	Raggedredfiber
RSE	Refractory Status Epilepticus
RT-QuIC	Real-Time Quaking-Induced Conversion
SAH	Subarachnoid Hemorrhage
SCA	Spinocerebellar Ataxia
SCD	Subacute Combined Degeneration
sCJD	Sporadic Creutzfeldt-Jakob Disease
SNCV	Sensory Nerve Conduction Velocity
SE	Status Epilepticus
SEP	Somatosensory Evoked Potential
SFEMG	Single Fiber Electromyography
SMS	Sensorimotor Stroke
SN	Substantia Nigra
SPECT	Single Photon Emission Computed Tomography
SQUID	Superconducting Quantum Interference Devices
SRSE	Super-Refractory Status Epilepticus
SSS	Subclavian Steal Syndrome
svPPA	Semantic Variant PPA
SWI	Sensitivity Weighted Imaging
TBM	Tuberculous Meningitis
TCD	Transcranial Doppler
TDP-43	Transactive Response DNA-Binding Protein-43
TEE	Transesophageal Echocardiography

Continued

TIA	Transient Ischemic Attack
TTE	Transthoracic Echocardiography
TLRs	Toll-Like Receptors
TN	Trigeminal Neuralgia
TPPA	*T. Pallidum* Particle Agglutination
TRUST	Toluidine Red Unheated Serum Test
TSE	Transmissible Spongiform Encephalopathies
TTH	Tension-Type Headache
UMN	Upper Motor Neurone
VA	Vertebral Artery
VAST	Vertebral Artery Stenting Trial
VCI	Vascular Cognitive Impairment
VCP	Valosin Containing Protein
VDRL	Venereal Disease Research Laboratory
VEP	Visual Evoked Potential
VLOFA	Very-Late-Onset Friedreich Ataxia
VNS	Vagus Nerve Stimulation
VPS	Ventriculo-Peritoneal Shunting
VRS	Virchow-Robin Spaces
WASID	Warfarin-Aspirin Symptomatic Intracranial Disease
WD	Wilson's Disease
WHO	World Health Organization

Ⅱ. NIH Stroke Scale (NIHSS)

NIH
STROKE
SCALE

Patient Identification. ____ ____-____ ____-____ ____

Hospital ______________(____ ____-________)

Date of Exam ____ ____/____ ____/____ ____

Person Administering Scale ______________

Administer stroke scale items in the order listed. Record performance in each category after each subscale exam. Do not go back and change scores. Follow directions provided for each exam technique. Scores should reflect what the patient does, not what the clinician thinks the patient can do. The clinician should record answers while administering the exam and work quickly. Except where indicated, the patient should not be coached (i.e., repeated requests to patient to make a special effort).

Instructions	Scale definition	Score
1a. Level of consciousness: The investigator must choose a response if a full evaluation is prevented by such obstacles as an endotracheal tube, language barrier, orotracheal trauma/bandages. The score is 3 only if the patient makes no movement (other than reflexive posturing) in response to noxious stimulation.	0 = Alert; keenly responsive 1 = Not alert; but arousable by minor stimulation to obey, answer, or respond 2 = Not alert; requires repeated stimulation to attend, or is obtunded and requires strong or painful stimulation to make movements (not stereotyped) 3 = Responds only with reflex motor or autonomic effects or totally unresponsive, flaccid, and areflexic	
1b. LOC questions: The patient is asked the month and his/her age. The answer must be correct—there is no partial credit for being close. Aphasic and stuporous patients who do not comprehend the questions will get a score of 2. Patients unable to speak because of endotracheal intubation, orotracheal trauma, severe dysarthria from any cause, language barrier, or any other problem not secondary to aphasia are given a score of 1. It is important that only the initial answer be graded and that the examiner can not "help" the patient with verbal or non-verbal cues.	0 = Answer both questions correctly 1 = Answer one question correctly 2 = Answer neither question correctly	
1c. LOC commands: The patient is asked to open and close the eyes and then to grip and release the non-paretic hand. Substitute another one step command if the hands cannot be used. Credit is given if an unequivocal attempt is made but not completed due to weakness. If the patient does not respond to command, the task should be demonstrated to him or her (pantomime), and the result scored (i.e., follows none, one or two commands). Patients with trauma, amputation, or other physical impediments should be given suitable one-step commands. Only the first attempt is scored.	0 = Perform both tasks correctly 1 = Perform one task correctly 2 = Perform neither task correctly	

Continued

Instructions	Scale definition	Score
2. Best gaze: Only horizontal eye movements will be tested. Voluntary or reflexive (oculocephalic) eye movements will be scored, but caloric testing is not done. If the patient has a conjugate deviation of the eyes that can be overcome by voluntary or reflexive activity, the score will be 1. If a patient has an isolated peripheral nerve paresis (CN Ⅲ, Ⅳ or Ⅵ), the score will be 1. Gaze is testable in all aphasic patients. Patients with ocular trauma, bandages, pre-existing blindness, or other disorder of visual acuity or fields should be tested with reflexive movements, and a choice made by the investigator. Establishing eye contact and then moving from side to side will occasionally clarify the presence of a partial gaze palsy	0 = Normal 1 = Partial gaze palsy; gaze is abnormal in one or both eyes, but forced deviation or total gaze paresis is not present 2 = Forced deviation, or total gaze paresis not overcome by the oculocephalic maneuver	
3. Visual: Visual fields (upper and lower quadrants) are tested by confrontation, using finger counting or visual threat, as appropriate. Patients may be encouraged, but if they look at the side of the moving fingers appropriately, this can be scored as normal. If there is unilateral blindness or enucleation, visual fields in the remaining eye are scored. Only if a clear-cut asymmetry, including quadrantanopia, is found can the score be 1. If the patient is blind from any cause, the score will be 3. Double simultaneous stimulation is performed at this point. If there is extinction, patient receives a score of 1, and the results are used to respond to item 11	0 = No visual loss 1 = Partial hemianopia 2 = Complete hemianopia 3 = Bilateral hemianopia (including cortical blindness)	
4. Facial palsy: Ask or use pantomime to encourage the patient to show teeth or raise eyebrows and close eyes. Score symmetry of grimace in response to noxious stimuli in the poorly responsive or non-comprehending patient. If facial trauma/bandages, orotracheal tube, tape or other physical barriers obscure the face, these should be removed to the extent possible	0 = Normal symmetrical movements 1 = Minor paralysis (flattened nasolabial fold, asymmetry on smiling) 2 = Partial paralysis (total or near-total paralysis of lower face) 3 = Complete paralysis of one or both sides (absence of facial movement in the upper and lower face)	____
5. Motor arm: The limb is placed in the appropriate position: extend the arms (palms down) 90° (if sitting) or 45° (if supine). Drift is scored if the arm falls within 10 seconds. The aphasic patient is encouraged to use urgency in the voice and pantomime, but not noxious stimulation. Limbs are tested in turn, beginning with the non-paretic arm. Only in the case of amputation or joint fusion at the shoulder, the examiner should record the score as untestable (UN), and clearly write the explanation for this choice	0 = No drift; limb holds 90° (or 45°) for full 10 seconds 1 = Drift; limb holds 90° (or 45°), but drifts down before full 10 seconds; without hitting bed or other support 2 = Some effort against gravity; limb cannot get to or maintain (if cued) 90° (or 45°), drifts down to bed, but some effort is made to against gravity 3 = No effort against gravity; limb falls 4 = No movement UN = Amputation or joint fusion, explain: ____ 5a. Left arm 5b. Right arm	

Continued

Instructions	Scale definition	Score
6. Motor leg: The limb is placed in the appropriate position: hold the leg at 30° (always tested supine). Drift is scored if the leg falls within 5 seconds. The aphasic patient is encouraged to use urgency in the voice and pantomime, but not noxious stimulation. Limbs are tested in turn, beginning with the non-paretic leg. Only in the case of amputation or joint fusion at the hip, the examiner should record the score as untestable (UN), and clearly write the explanation for this choice	0=No drift; leg holds 30° position for full 5 seconds 1=Drift; leg falls by the end of the 5-second period but does not hit bed 2=Some effort against gravity; leg falls to bed by 5 seconds, but some effort is made against gravity 3=No effort against gravity; leg falls to bed immediately 4=No movement UN=Amputation or joint fusion, explain: ____________________ 6a. Left leg 6b. Right leg	
7. Limb ataxia: This item is aimed at finding evidence of a unilateral cerebellar lesion. Test with eyes open. In case of visual defect, test must be done in intact visual field. The finger-nose-finger and heel-shin tests are performed on both sides, and ataxia is scored only if present out of proportion to weakness. Ataxia is absent in the patient who cannot understand or is paralyzed. Only in the case of amputation or joint fusion, the examiner should record the score as untestable (UN), and clearly write the explanation for this choice. In case of blindness, test by having the patient touch nose from extended arm position	0=Absent 1=Present in one limb 2=Present in two limbs UN=Amputation or joint fusion, explain: ____________________	
8. Sensory: Sensation or grimace to pinprick when tested, or withdrawal from noxious stimulus in the obtunded or aphasic patient. Only sensory loss attributed to stroke is scored as abnormal and the examiner should test as many body areas [arms (not hands), legs, trunk, face] as needed to accurately check for hemisensory loss. A score of 2 should only be given when a severe or total loss of sensation can be clearly demonstrated. Stuporous and aphasic patients will, therefore, probably be scored 1 or 0. The patient with brainstem stroke who has bilateral loss of sensation is scored 2. If the patient does not respond and is quadriplegic, score 2. Patients in a coma (item 1a=3) are automatically given a score of 2 on this item.	0=Normal; no sensory loss 1 = Mild-to-moderate sensory loss; patient feels pinprick is less sharp or is dull on the affected side; or there is a loss of superficial pain with pinprick, but patient is aware of being touched 2= Severe to total sensory loss; patient is not aware of being touched on the face, arm, and leg	

Continued

Instructions	Scale definition	Score
9. Best language: A great deal of information about comprehension will be obtained during the preceding sections of the examination. For this scale item, the patient is asked to describe what is happening in the attached picture, to name the items on the attached naming sheet and to read the sentences on the attached list. Comprehension is judged from responses here, as well as to all of the commands in the preceding general neurological exam. If visual loss interferes with the tests, the patient is asked to identify objects held in the hand, repeat, and produce speech. The intubated patient should be asked to write. The patient in a coma (item 1a=3) will automatically receive a score of 3 on this item. The examiner must choose a score for the patient with stupor or limited cooperation, but a score of 3 should be used only if the patient is mute and follows no one-step commands	0=No aphasia; normal 1 = Mild-to-moderate aphasia; some obvious loss of fluency or facility of comprehension, without significant limitation on ideas expressed or form of expression. Reduction of speech and/or comprehension, however, makes conversation about provided materials difficult or impossible. For example, in conversation about provided materials, examiner can identify picture or naming card content from patient's response 2 = Severe aphasia; all communication is through fragmentary expression; great need for inference, questioning, and guessing by the listener. Range of information that can be exchanged is limited; listener carries burden of communication. Examiner cannot identify materials provided from patient response 3 =Mute, global aphasia; no usable speech or auditory comprehension	
10. Dysarthria: If patient is thought to be normal, an adequate sample of speech must be obtained by asking patient to read or repeat words from the attached list. If the patient has severe aphasia, the clarity of articulation of spontaneous speech can be rated. Only if the patient is intubated or has other physical barriers to producing speech, the examiner should record the score as untestable (UN), and clearly write an explanation for this choice. Do not tell the patient why he or she is being tested	0=Normal 1 = Mild-to-moderate dysarthria; patient slurs at least some words and, at worst, can be understood with some difficulty 2=Severe dysarthria; patient's speech is so slurred as to be unintelligible in the absence of or out of proportion to any dysphasia, or is mute/anarthric UN = Intubated or other physical barrier, explain:________________	
11. Extinction and inattention (formerly neglect): Sufficient information to identify neglect may be obtained during the prior testing. If the patient has a severe visual loss preventing visual double simultaneous stimulation, and the cutaneous stimuli are normal, the score is normal. If the patient has aphasia but does appear to attend to both sides, the score is normal. The presence of visual spatial neglect or anosagnosia may also be taken as evidence of abnormality. Since the abnormality is scored only if present, the item is never untestable	0=No abnormality 1 = Visual, tactile, auditory, spatial, or personal inattention or extinction to bilateral simultaneous stimulation in one of the sensory modalities 2 = Profound hemi-inattention or extinction to more than one modality; patient does not recognize own hand or orients to only one side of space	

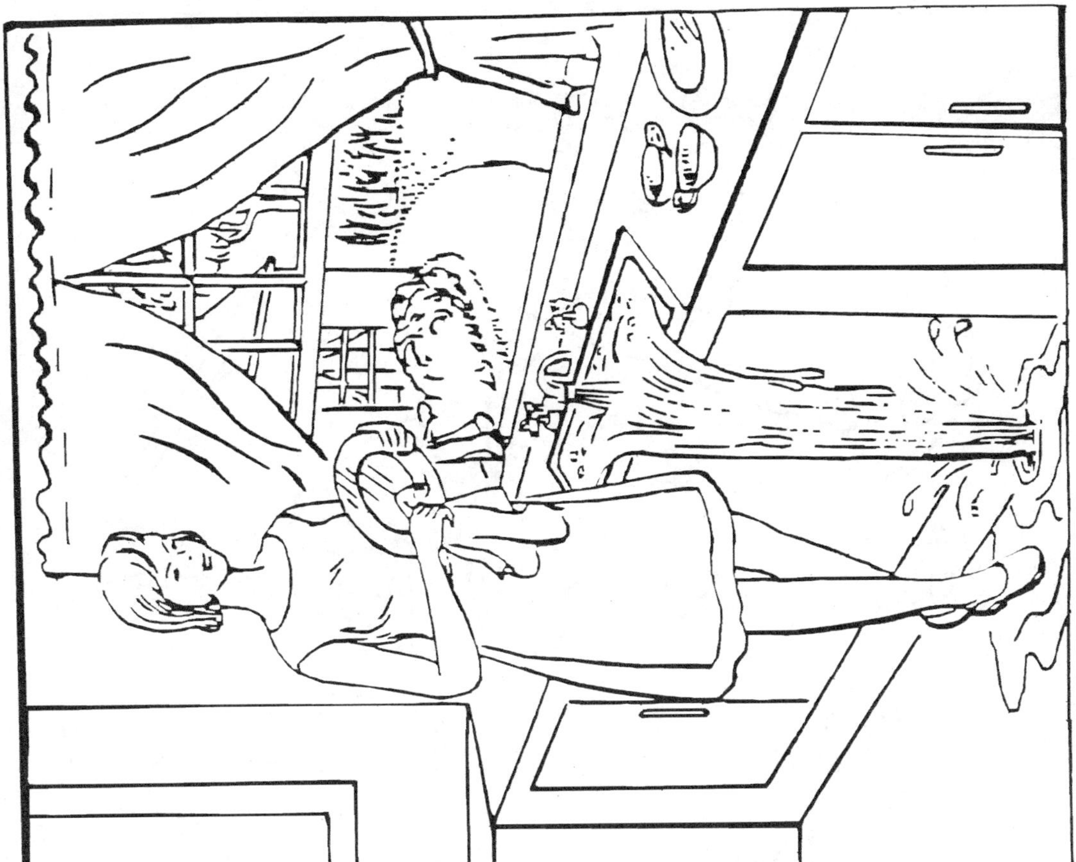
COOKIE
JAR

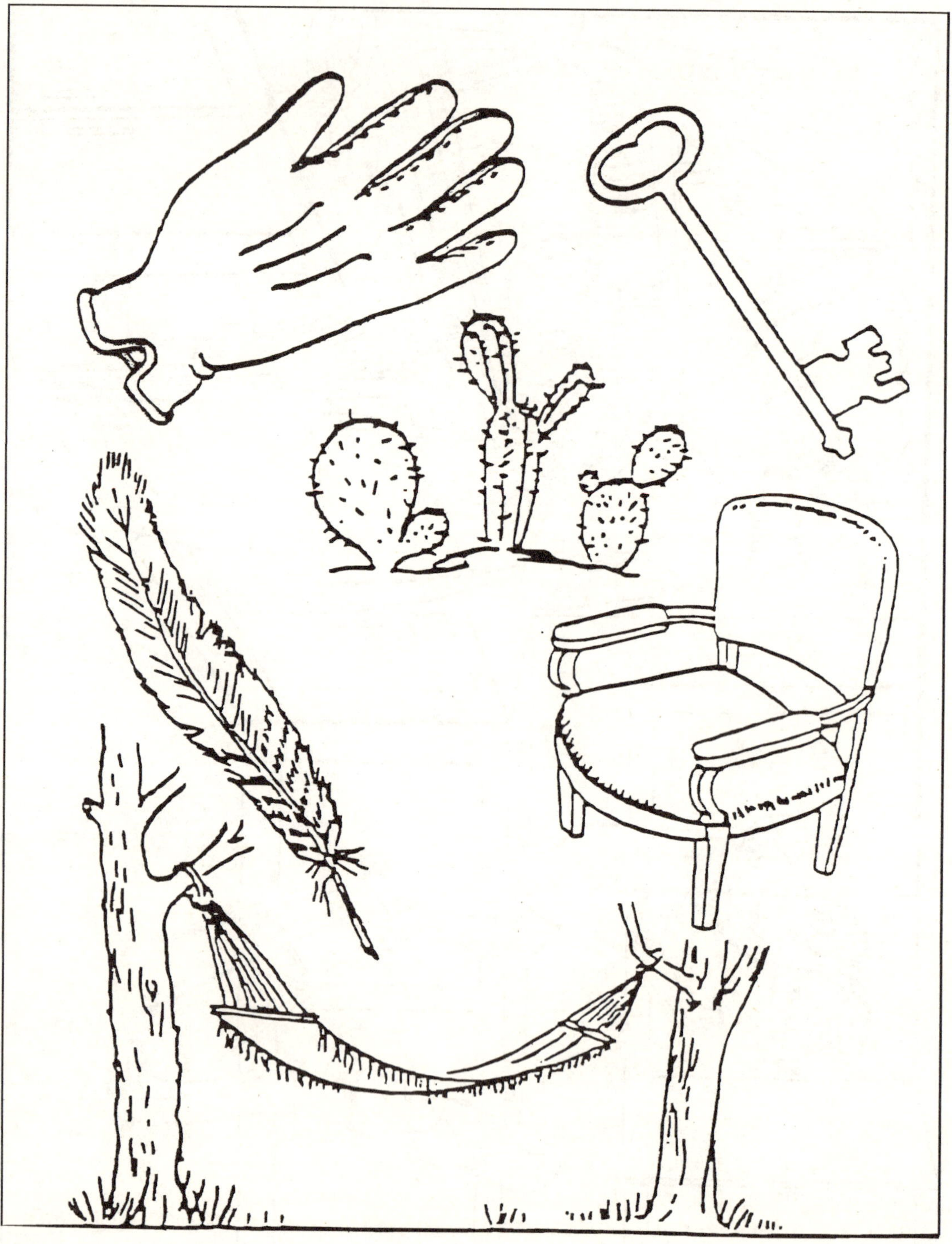

You know how.
Down to earth.
I got home from work.
Near the table in the dining room.
They heard him speak on the radio last night.

MAMA

TIP-TOP

FIFTY-FIFTY

THANKS

HUCKLEBERRY

BASEBALL PLAYER

Ⅲ. Mini-mental State Examination (MMSE)

Patient's Name: ______________________

Date: ______________________

<u>Instruction</u>: **Ask the questions in the order listed. Score one point for each correct response within each question or activity.**

Maximum Score	Patient's Score	Questions
5		"What is the year/season/date/day of the week/month?"
5		"Where are we now (State/County/Town(City)/Hospital/Floor)?"
3		The examiner names three unrelated objects clearly and slowly, then asks the patient to name all three of them. The patient's response is used for scoring. The examiner repeats them until patient learns all of them, if possible. Number of trials: ______
5		"I would like you to count backward from 100 by sevens." (93, 86, 79, 72, 65, …) Stop after five answers. Alternative: "Spell 'WORLD' backwards." (D-L-R-O-W)
3		"Earlier I told you the names of three things. Can you tell me what those were?"
2		Show the patient two simple objects, such as a wristwatch and a pencil, and ask the patient to name them.
1		"Repeat the phrase: 'No ifs, ands, or buts.'"
3		"Take the paper in your right hand, fold it in half, and put it on the floor." (The examiner gives the patient a piece of blank paper.)
1		"Please read this and do what it says." (Written instruction is "Close your eyes".)
1		"Make up and write a sentence about anything." (This sentence must contain a noun and a verb.)
1		"Please copy this picture." (The examiner gives the patient a blank piece of paper and asks him/her to draw the symbol below. All 10 angles must be present and two must intersect.) 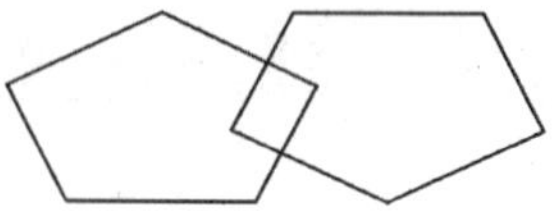
30		Total

(Adapted from Rovner and Folstein, 1987)

Ⅳ. Montreal Cognitive Assessment (MOCA)

NAME :
Education : Date of birth :
Sex : DATE :

Version 7.1 Original Version

		POINTS
VISUOSPATIAL / EXECUTIVE		

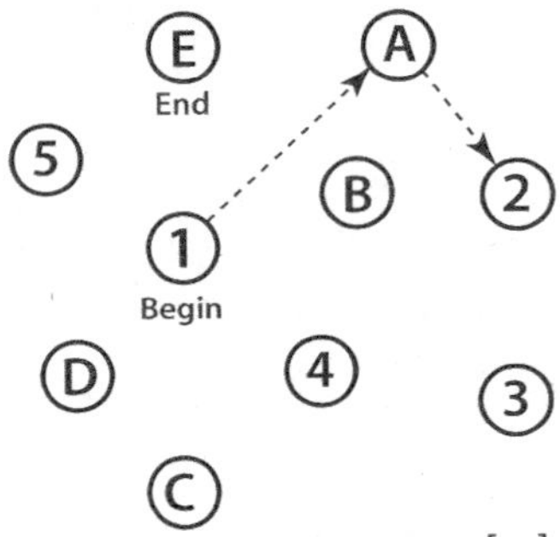

[ ]

Copy cube

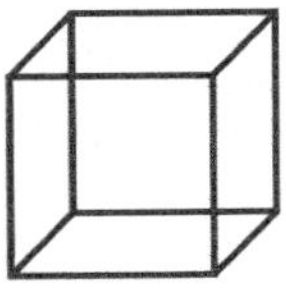

[ ]

Draw CLOCK (Ten past eleven)
(3 points)

[ ] Contour [ ] Numbers [ ] Hands

__/5

NAMING

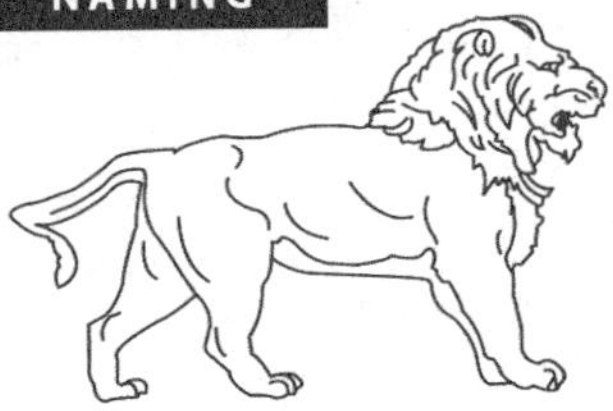

[ ]

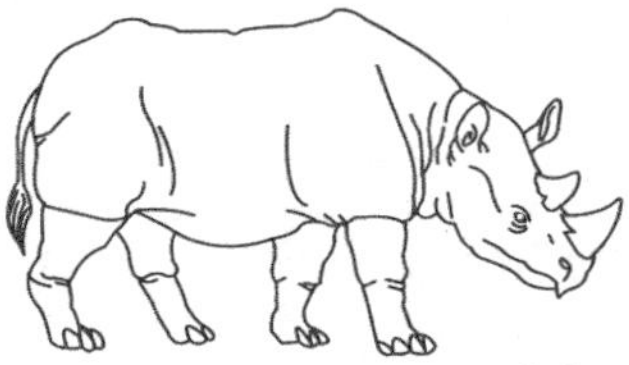

[ ]

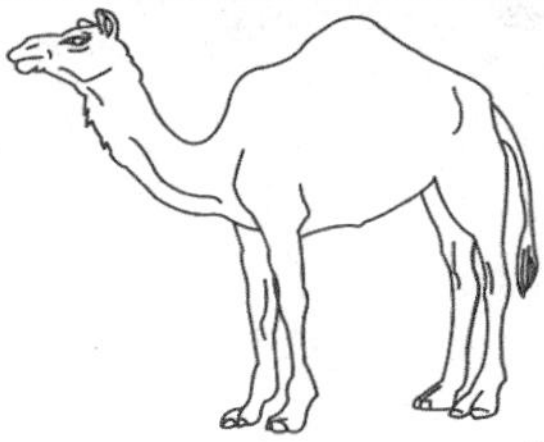

[ ]

__/3

MEMORY Read list of words, subject must repeat them. Do 2 trials, even if 1st trial is successful. Do a recall after 5 minutes.

	FACE	VELVET	CHURCH	DAISY	RED
1st trial					
2nd trial					

No points

ATTENTION Read list of digits (1 digit/ sec.).

Subject has to repeat them in the forward order	[ ] 2 1 8 5 4	
Subject has to repeat them in the backward order	[ ] 7 4 2	__/2

Read list of letters. The subject must tap with his hand at each letter A. No points if ≥ 2 errors

[ ] F B A C M N A A J K L B A F A K D E A A A J A M O F A A B __/1

Serial 7 subtraction starting at 100 [ ] 93 [ ] 86 [ ] 79 [ ] 72 [ ] 65

4 or 5 correct subtractions: **3 pts**, 2 or 3 correct: **2 pts**, 1 correct: **1 pt**, 0 correct: **0 pt** __/3

LANGUAGE Repeat : I only know that John is the one to help today. [ ]
The cat always hid under the couch when dogs were in the room. [ ] __/2

Fluency / Name maximum number of words in one minute that begin with the letter F [ ] ____ (N ≥ 11 words) __/1

ABSTRACTION Similarity between e.g. banana - orange = fruit [ ] train – bicycle [ ] watch - ruler __/2

DELAYED RECALL	Has to recall words **WITH NO CUE**	FACE [ ]	VELVET [ ]	CHURCH [ ]	DAISY [ ]	RED [ ]	Points for UNCUED recall only	__/5
Optional	Category cue							
	Multiple choice cue							

ORIENTATION [ ] Date [ ] Month [ ] Year [ ] Day [ ] Place [ ] City __/6

© Z.Nasreddine MD **www.mocatest.org** Normal ≥ 26 / 30 TOTAL __/30

Add 1 point if ≤ 12 yr edu

Administered by: ______________________________